MW00989809

ADHD MEDICATION

ADHD MEDICATION

Does It Work and Is It Safe?

Walt Karniski, MD

ROWMAN & LITTLEFIELD

Lanham • Boulder • New York • London

This book represents reference material only. It is not intended as a medical manual, and the data presented here are meant to assist the reader in making informed choices regarding wellness. This book is not a replacement for treatment(s) that the reader's personal physician may have suggested. If the reader believes he or she is experiencing a medical issue, professional medical help is recommended. Mention of particular products, companies, or authorities in this book does not entail endorsement by the publisher or author.

Published by Rowman & Littlefield
An imprint of The Rowman & Littlefield Publishing Group, Inc.
4501 Forbes Boulevard, Suite 200, Lanham, Maryland 20706
www.rowman.com

86-90 Paul Street, London EC2A 4NE, United Kingdom

British Library Cataloguing in Publication Information Available

Library of Congress Cataloging-in-Publication Data

Names: Karniski, Walt, 1950- author.
Title: ADHD medication : does it work and is it safe? / Walt Karniski.
Description: Lanham : Rowman & Littlefield, [2022] | Includes bibliographical
  references and index.
Identifiers: LCCN 2021047011 (print) | LCCN 2021047012 (ebook) | ISBN
  9781538155776 (cloth) | ISBN 9781538155783 (epub)
Subjects: LCSH: Attention-deficit-disordered children. | Attention-deficit-
  disordered children—Treatment. | Attention-deficit-disordered children—
  Counseling of.
Classification: LCC RJ506.H9 K38 2022 (print) | LCC RJ506.H9
  (ebook) | DDC 618.92/8589—dc23
LC record available at https://lccn.loc.gov/2021047011
LC ebook record available at https://lccn.loc.gov/2021047012

DEDICATION

This book is dedicated to three incredibly successful, intelligent, and nurturing women in my life.

Teresa is my wife of forty-three years. I knew that she would become my wife only a month after we met. She has been at my side for every moment that I have been confronted with a difficult decision, a major disappointment, or valued accomplishment. Her input to this book has been monumental, as a speech and language therapist, as the director of a preschool, and as a mother. She has read and weighed and smiled and frowned at every word of this book, many times over, to the point that I feel that I should list her as a fellow author. While writing this book, I would occasionally reach an impasse and start thrashing in my sleep at 3 a.m., and she was always there to talk me back to my dreams. Her wedding ring is engraved "You take my breath away." And I know that she will be with me, many years from now, when I take my last.

In addition to my wife, I am blessed by two magnificent and accomplished daughters, and I dedicate this book to them as well.

My oldest daughter, Alison, is a pediatrician in private practice. She started her career in business but left a highly lucrative position to become a physician. During her residency, I lost count of the number of times she would spontaneously comment, "I just love what I do." I cannot adequately express the pride that I feel, knowing the sacrifices that she has endured to follow a dream. And I have experienced great satisfaction through our experience of discussing both the science and emotional concerns associated with ADHD. On several occasions she has taught me a better way to approach a problem. Alison taught me that doing the right thing for the right reasons brings the greatest happiness.

My younger daughter, Caitlin, is an associate editor for a highly respected scientific journal. She writes the way a bird glides through the air. I believe that I have inherited my ability to write from her, but as an evolutionary biologist, she insists that that is not the way it works. As an editor for a prestigious scientific journal, Caitlin taught me how to present the science in this book in a scientifically accurate and empathetic way. She has walked with me as I have created this book, guiding me and calming me when the writing became difficult at times. But most important, I have learned from her how to live a life with passion and dignity and joy.

Finally, I dedicate this book to Jack Holland. We were friends at Rockhurst High School, and he and I often talked about our dreams to write a book. One day, we wrote out an agreement to dedicate our first book to each other, signed it, and then passed the agreement to the other. I kept that agreement in my wallet for fifteen years, until it was lost after purchasing a new wallet. So even though I have not seen Jack for more than fifty-three years, and even though I do not know where he lives (maybe Kansas City), a promise is a promise. Thank you, Jack.

Bill Read is my friend and a retired developmental pediatrician in Eau Claire, Wisconsin. Marty Cohen is my friend and one of the most recommended psychologists in Tampa, Florida. Michael Rapoff is my friend and a child psychologist and past president of the Society of Pediatric Psychology. I wish to thank each of them for their insight and help in producing this manuscript and for their friendship over the past forty-five years.

Three individuals had little to do with this manuscript, but without them it would not have been produced. Lois Delaney-Ogorek has been the director at Tampa Day School for the past twenty-four years, and Andrea Mowatt has been the school psychologist there for much of that time. They have been responsible for building Tampa Day School into a premier school for children who learn differently. However, before their affiliation at the school, they helped me set up a private practice. Much of what I know about children's education and learning has come from them. They are two of the most exquisitely competent and loving educators I have known. Thank you for your expertise, but even more important, thank you for your friendship.

Charles Oldham is not a physician, psychologist, or clinician. But he was my roommate in college and is my friend for life. Thank you, Charles, for a lifetime of memories and for "believing in miracles."

And thank you to the amazing staff at Rowman & Littlefield, especially Suzanne Staszak-Silva and Hannah Fisher. Without them this book would still just be a good idea.

Finally, I would like to thank the five thousand young boys and girls, men and women who have been my patients. These individuals were brought to me by parents and grandparents who did not know what to expect. They have taught me about the pain that ADHD brings to every facet of their lives. Together, we learned to recognize the unique benefits of ADHD medications and how to manage the irritating side effects. They taught me that every patient is different, that every child reacts to medication a little bit differently. They taught me that every child needs a customized approach, tailored to their specific needs and lifestyle. Without their insight, my knowledge of ADHD medication would be isolated to chemical formulas and reports from research studies. Thank you to them and to their families. This book has 5,001 authors, and I wish I could put each of their names on the cover. I could not have written it without them.

CONTENTS

1   What Is ADHD and How Has It Evolved?   1

2   What Is ADHD and How Does It Feel?   17

3   From Silk to Ritalin: A History of the Medical Treatment of Attention Deficit Hyperactivity Disorder   49

4   Is ADHD Really Real?   61

5   Could ADHD Medication Help My Child?   81

6   Why Are There So Many Different Medications for the Treatment of ADHD?   103

7   Which Medication Is Right for My Child?   125

8   Stimulant Medication Side Effects   139

9   Comorbidity: ADHD Does Not Dance Alone   177

10   Twenty Brand-Name Methylphenidate Medications to Treat ADHD   193

11   Sixteen Brand-Name Amphetamine Medications to Treat ADHD   227

12   Ten Non-Stimulant Medications to Treat ADHD   251

Afterword	267
Medication List	269
Notes	283
Index	309
About the Author	321

Chapter 1

WHAT IS ADHD AND HOW HAS IT EVOLVED?

STANDING IN LINE

Liz (Danny's mother): *As I stood in line at the pharmacy, all I could think of was,* What am I doing here? *Somehow, I felt like I had failed as a mother. When Danny was two, he seemed like the happiest, most inquisitive, and brightest child ever created. I used to think of all the great things that he would do when he grew up. And now that he is seven, I am standing in line at a pharmacy with a prescription in my hand, waiting to bring home a medication like a witch with a poison apple, a medication that is supposed to calm him down, a medication that will turn him into some kind of a bleary-eyed zombie, just because I can't control him, because I can't discipline him, because I can't be a good mother.*

Now wait a minute. That's not true. I am a good mother. I did all the things that my mother told me (at least all of the good things), and I read the books and magazine articles, and I listened to my sister-in-law; and when Chris comes home from work, I do everything I can to make sure that Danny is calmed down, and the house is picked up, and we can be a family. But three minutes before Chris walked in the door last night, Danny tried to pull the tail off the cat, so the cat was screaming, and the baby started crying, and Danny got mad and started throwing Legos at the cat, and the door opened, and into this chaos walked Chris. His smile rapidly melted into a scowl, and he looked at me, and he said, "Liz, what is going on here? Why can't you control him? Why can't you discipline him? Why can't you . . ."

And that's how I ended up seeing Dr. Lawrence this morning. I was lucky that he had a cancellation, and I got right in. Dr. Lawrence was great, and was trying to explain about ADHD and how it affects learning and how medication can help. I had a lot of questions, but during that time, Danny knocked over that little red box with the needles in it and put his foot in the wastebasket and broke the flashlight that Dr. Lawrence uses to look into kids' ears, and suddenly I couldn't remember a thing I wanted to say. Dr. Lawrence asked me some questions about Danny's birth, and then he asked me how he was doing in school, and then he asked me about my marriage, as if that had anything to do with the price of tea in China. But the fifteen minutes seemed like forever, because we were interrupted by Danny every thirty seconds, and then Dr. Lawrence took out his prescription pad. I had heard about Ritalin, but I never thought I would be holding a prescription for it in my hands. And then Danny opened the door and was down the hall, and by the time I dragged him back to the exam room, Dr. Lawrence was gone, and the nurse led me up to the desk, and they asked for my insurance card, and I was out the door.

So that's how I ended up here, waiting to drug my child.

But what am I doing here?

The first time your doctor suggested that your child might benefit from medication for an attention problem, you probably thought about a lot of things. You thought, *What did I do wrong? I should be a good parent. Why can't I?* You thought, *I need to get stricter with him and pay more attention to him. He needs to work harder, and there is no need for medication.* You thought, *You can't solve a complex problem like this with a pill. It's not that simple.* Oh, but if only you could.

Medication just doesn't seem like the right solution. And you wait a few weeks, and you talk to friends and neighbors. And things get worse at school, and things get worse at home. And you think, *Something's wrong*, and then you think, *Nothing's wrong*, and finally you think, *Something has to be done.*

And then you find yourself with a prescription in your hand at the pharmacy, and suddenly it seems like something's not right here, and you feel guilty and almost turn to look to make sure no one is watching. But no one is. You go ahead and fill the prescription and start the medication and things get better, maybe a little, maybe a lot, but something still is not right. And you think, *But I've got so many questions, such as Why does this medication work like this? and How long should he be on this medication? and Is he on the right dose? and Is he even on the right medication?* And on and on and on.

Your doctor answers many of your questions, but not the ones that pop into your head as you lie in bed at night. You find yourself getting a few answers from a magazine article. But that doesn't seem right, and you talk to more friends and neighbors and relatives, and you realize that the answers start to contradict each other. *Why is it so hard to get answers? I just want to do what's right for my child, but I don't know what is right.*

This book is written for parents who want more than a simple solution to a complex problem. This book is written for parents who have questions but do not feel that they are getting all the answers.

This book is *not* meant to replace your doctor. ADHD is one of the most common problems that pediatricians, pediatric neurologists, and pediatric psychiatrists manage. But in the beginning, it is best to see your pediatrician because she can work with your child in the context of other medical problems your child might have. Pediatricians are extremely knowledgeable, not only about ADHD, but about how to interact with teachers, about how to recognize learning disabilities and developmental problems, and about what to do about these problems. Some pediatricians even specialize in these areas and are very knowledgeable about both medication and non-medication treatments.

I would like to accomplish two things with this book. *First*, I will explain in depth about the medications used to treat ADHD. How do they work? Why are there so many different medications to treat ADHD? How long will my child need to be on medication? What are the side effects of medication? What are the long-term consequences of being on these medications?

Second, this book will attempt to deal with very practical questions. When appetite suppression occurs from medication, can I supplement my child's diet? If so, what supplements should I use? What should I do if my child refuses to take medication? What if he can't swallow a pill?

I wrote this book for parents of children with ADHD, to help you navigate the often-confusing waters of medication treatment of ADHD. This book is not meant to replace your physician, and it is definitely not written to encourage you to change aspects of your child's medical treatment without your physician's knowledge or agreement. But it *is* meant to help you understand what medication can do for your child, what it *cannot* do, and how to use medication for its benefits in a safe way. You are encouraged to discuss the information in this book with your doctor and with your spouse and with your child.

This book may help you stand in line at the pharmacy with knowledge and understanding . . . and without guilt.

WHO AM I?

I am a developmental pediatrician and have been a faculty member in the Department of Pediatrics at the University of South Florida in Tampa, Florida. In addition, I have also operated a private practice for 14 years. I specialize in problems that affect behavior, attention, and learning. Most of the children I saw in my university practice had ADHD, autism, or learning disabilities. Occasionally I would see a child with Down syndrome or cerebral palsy or rare disorders of metabolism.

I completed a four-year medical school program then a three-year residency in pediatrics and a two-year fellowship in developmental pediatrics at Children's Memorial Hospital in Boston. I began practicing in 1981. Over those forty years, I estimate that I have seen more than five thousand children (and occasionally an adult) with ADHD.

A developmental pediatrician is a cross between a pediatric neurologist and a pediatric psychiatrist. Developmental pediatricians start with the premise that every behavior of a child has both a neurological and a psychological basis. It is the developmental pediatrician's job to make a diagnosis and design a treatment strategy that addresses both a child's neurology and his feelings and emotions.

The recommended treatments might include counseling, tutoring, speech and language therapy, occupational therapy, and many other treatments. Many books have been written about these therapies. Sometimes the recommended treatment will include medication, and this is very often true when the diagnosis is ADHD. Unfortunately, very little information is available to parents about medication. This book is meant to fill that void. Although I am not writing about these non-medication treatments, that is not to deny their extreme importance.

I learned a great deal about developmental pediatrics during my training. I have also learned about new developments by reading medical journals, attending medical conferences, and talking to colleagues. My academic training taught me about diseases, disorders, conditions, and medications. But most of what I have learned about ADHD comes from my patients. My patients taught me about the embarrassment of a teacher asking a child in front of the whole class if he had taken his ADHD medication this morning. They taught me about the humiliation of having to repeat a grade. They taught me about being the last child picked to play softball. They taught me about the tears shed when a girl was not invited to her friend's birthday party.

This book has 5,001 authors, and I would love to put each of their names on its cover. I could not have written this book without them.

ADHD SEEMS LIKE A RECENTLY "INVENTED" DIAGNOSIS. WHERE DID IT COME FROM?

Sir Alexander Crichton, born in 1763, was a Scottish physician, an amateur geologist, and the physician in ordinary, or personal physician of Tsar Alexander of Russia. However, he is best known for his publication of the book *An Inquiry into the Nature and Origin of Mental Derangement* in 1798. It's not a title we would relish today, but in this work, he is credited with one of the earliest descriptions of ADHD:

> The incapacity of attending with a necessary degree of constancy to any one object, almost always arises from an unnatural or morbid sensibility of the nerves, by which means this faculty is incessantly withdrawn from one impression to another. It may be either born with a person, or it may be the effect of accidental diseases.
>
> When born with a person, it becomes evident at a very early period of life, and has a very bad effect, inasmuch as it renders him incapable of attending with constancy to any one object of education. But it seldom is in so great a degree as totally to impede all instruction; and what is very fortunate, it is generally diminished with age.[1]

Forty-five years later, a German physician, Heinrich Hoffman, would create amusing drawings to calm upset children so that he could complete his physical examination. In 1844 he created a storybook as a Christmas present for his three-year-old son, Carl Philip, with colorful drawings of Fidgety Phil. A year later, the book was published in multiple languages and was still being published and widely read in 1917 after the four hundredth edition of the book.

During World War II, American psychiatrists were asked to establish a system for the assessment and selection of soldiers. Partially in response to that experience, in 1952, the American Psychiatric Association published the first edition of the *Diagnostic and Statistical Manual (DSM) of Mental Disorders*. This was one of the first attempts to standardize the classification and diagnostic criteria of mental and behavioral disorders. This publication identified 106 different mental disorders, but the collection of symptoms that we know as ADHD was not included at all. Since the first publication of the *DSM* in 1952, it has been revised approximately every 7–15 years.

When the *Diagnostic and Statistical Manual* was revised in 1968, for the first time it included official recognition of the syndrome of behaviors that we now refer to as ADHD. This second edition of the *DSM* stated that the **hyperkinetic reaction of childhood** is a "disorder characterized by overactivity, restlessness, distractibility, and short attention span, especially in young children; the behavior usually diminishes by adolescence."

Clearly, as the title would suggest, the emphasis at that time was on the most obvious and disruptive of the symptoms (hyperactivity and impulsivity). However, as recognition of this disorder spread, many clinicians identified children who had trouble attending but were not hyperactive or impulsive. Over time, clinicians realized that even though hyperactivity was the most immediately disruptive symptom, the difficulty maintaining sustained attention was an even more disabling behavior, because it interfered with the process of learning.

In response to these observations, the third edition of the *DSM* (published in 1980) changed the name to Attention Deficit Disorder (ADD), which could occur in one of two subtypes, **ADD with hyperactivity** and **ADD without hyperactivity**.

Then in 1987 another revision of the DSM (*DSM-III-R*) changed the name to Attention Deficit *Hyperactivity* Disorder, dropping the subtype of ADD without hyperactivity.

Before the end of the millennium, an explosion of research began to suggest that more than a single type of ADHD was present in children. As a result, the 1994 revision (*DSM-IV*) introduced three subtypes of ADHD:

- ADHD—Primarily Hyperactive/Impulsive Type
- ADHD—Primarily Inattentive Type
- ADHD—Combined Type

This new classification system finally recognized the subtype of ADHD with the symptoms of inattention, but without the symptoms of hyperactivity and impulsivity and has been widely adopted as the current nomenclature, even after two further revisions of the *Diagnostic and Statistical Manual* (*DSM-IV-TR* [2000] and *DSM-5*[2] [2013]).

Many parents ask what the difference is between ADD and ADHD. Although the diagnostic criteria contain subtle differences, they are virtually the same disorder, with different names. Most physicians in the field now see ADD and ADHD as synonymous.

The reason that this history is so important is that most clinicians and scientists studying ADHD use the *DSM* diagnostic criteria to make a diagnosis. Although the diagnostic criteria have been hotly debated, having everyone use the same definition of ADHD, especially when conducting research, is a clear advantage. The diagnostic criteria are based upon current research; and as the research improves and progresses, presumably the diagnostic criteria will become more accurate. We can only anticipate a further name change at some future time.

SO HOW IS ADHD DIAGNOSED?

The diagnosis of ADHD is made mostly on a determination that a collection of behaviors exists in a child. Those behaviors might be identified by a physician observing the child in the office. Often, a psychologist will conduct a number of tests to assess cognitive intelligence, academic performance, attention, and many other behaviors. Rarely, a psychologist will actually watch the child in the classroom and on the playground. Most often, these behaviors are identified by questionnaires, filled out by the parents and teachers. The *DSM-5* lists nine inattentive behaviors (Table 1.1) and nine hyperactive or impulsive behaviors (Table 1.2). According to the current diagnostic criteria outlined in the *Diagnostic and Statistical Manual*[3] (*DSM-5*), the three subtypes can be diagnosed as follows:

arily Hyperactive/Impulsive Type: Must have six nine Hyperactive and Impulsive Symptoms (five than seventeen) without meeting the criteria for ...ention.

- ADHD—Primarily Inattentive Type: Must have six or more of the nine Inattentive Symptoms (five in persons older than seventeen) without meeting the criteria for Hyperactivity/ Impulsivity.
- ADHD—Combined Type: Must have six or more of symptoms of both Inattention and Hyperactivity/Impulsivity (five in persons older than seventeen).

But how are the inattentive and hyperactive/impulsive behaviors identified? Most physicians use a questionnaire that lists these behaviors, as well as many other behaviors that might be present in other problem areas (such as anxiety, anger, depression, etc.).

Table 1.1 American Psychiatric Association. (2013). Diagnostic and statistical manual of mental disorders (5th ed.). https://doi.org/10.1176/appi.books. 9780890425596.

Attention Deficit Hyperactivity Disorder
Inattention Symptoms

To make the diagnosis in children, 6 of the following 9 behaviors must be present, must be persistent and must significantly interfere with a person's ability to perform in multiple settings (school, work, social relations, etc.). Only 5 behaviors must be present in persons older than 17.

1. Doesn't pay close attention to details or makes careless mistakes in school or job tasks.
2. Has problems staying focused on tasks or activities, such as during lectures, conversations or long reading.
3. Does not seem to listen when spoken to (i.e., seems to be elsewhere).
4. Does not follow through on instructions and doesn't complete schoolwork, chores or job duties (may start tasks but quickly loses focus).
5. Has problems organizing tasks and work (for instance, does not manage time well; has messy, disorganized work; misses deadlines).
6. Avoids or dislikes tasks that require sustained mental effort, such as preparing reports and completing forms.
7. Often loses things needed for tasks or daily life, such as school papers, books, keys, wallet, cell phone, and eyeglasses.
8. Is easily distracted.
9. Forgets daily tasks, such as doing chores and running errands. Older teens and adults may forget to return phone calls, pay bills, and keep appointments.

Table 1.2 American Psychiatric Association. (2013). Diagnostic and statistical manual of mental disorders (5th ed.). https://doi.org/10.1176/appi.books.9780890425596

Attention Deficit Hyperactivity Disorder
Hyperactive and Impulsive Symptoms

To make the diagnosis in children, 6 of the following 9 behaviors must be present, must be persistent and must significantly interfere with a person's ability to perform in multiple settings (school, work, social relations, etc.). Only 5 behaviors must be present in persons older than 17.

1. Fidgets with or taps hands or feet, or squirms in seat.
2. Not able to stay seated (in classroom, workplace).
3. Runs about or climbs where it is inappropriate.
4. Unable to play or do leisure activities quietly.
5. Always "on the go," as if driven by a motor.
6. Talks too much.
7. Blurts out an answer before a question has been finished (for instance may finish people's sentences, can't wait to speak in conversations).
8. Has difficulty waiting his or her turn, such as while waiting in line.
9. Interrupts or intrudes on others (for instance, cuts into conversations, games or activities, or starts using other people's things without permission). Older teens and adults may take over what others are doing.

If you look closely at these behaviors, you might be struck by something. *Every single one of these behaviors occurs at **some time** in **everyone**.* We all forget things occasionally. Sometime we don't listen very well either. And we all lose things from time to time.

These behaviors are all normal behaviors, some of the time, in some places, by all people. And in some circumstances, these behaviors are actually beneficial (as we will see in a few pages). How can we say that these behaviors are symptoms of a medical problem?

To address this question, additional criteria confirm a diagnosis of ADHD. In addition to having at least six of the nine behaviors in one or both categories, **all** of the following additional criteria must be met as well:

- **These behaviors must be persistent and pervasive.** This means that these behaviors must occur frequently and in multiple settings (e.g., school, home, soccer, tutoring).
- **These behaviors must be sustained over time and not of recent onset.** In most children with ADHD, parents will relate that their child has had difficulty with attention or hyperactivity

or both since early on, such as preschool or kindergarten, or when the work and expectations got harder in third or fourth grade.

- **These behaviors must not be caused by some other medical condition**, such as a hearing problem or even a learning disability.
- Finally, *and most important,* **these behaviors must be severe and persistent enough that they are interfering with a child's ability to function at the tasks expected of him.** If these behaviors are affecting his learning in school, if they are affecting his social relations because he doesn't listen to the other kids, even if they are affecting his ability to listen to the baseball coach and, therefore, he is sitting on the bench frequently, then these behaviors are a problem.

DIAGNOSTIC CRITERIA: BLESSING OR CURSE?

We accept these criteria with a significant degree of confidence and credence for two reasons:

1. These behaviors have been documented by multiple research studies to co-occur together in children. This means that when one behavior is seen, the other behaviors will likely be present as well. When behaviors co-occur, it often means that the likelihood is greater than average that they have the same origin. A child who is more likely to be distracted (Criteria #8) is also likely to not pay close attention to detail (Criteria #1).
2. Even though one can debate whether these are the best behaviors to use to make a diagnosis of ADHD, they do provide a framework for the interpretation of research studies. When everyone is using the same definition, then the research studies can be more reliably compared and contrasted.

However, using such a diagnostic approach has drawbacks. The most prominent of these drawbacks is that these criteria are very subjective. This means that they are open to the judgment and past experiences and opinions of the individual who is tasked with evaluating these behaviors. And when a diagnosis relies totally on subjective criteria, physicians run the risk that they will be less consistent with the diagnosis. So, one child might be seen by a pediatrician, then by a psychologist, and then by a psychiatrist—and receive three different diagnoses. If that happened to your child, how much confidence would you have in the diagnosis?

The goal of the *Diagnostic and Statistical Manual* (*DSM*) was laudable: Replace the mysticism of psychoanalysis with the science of medical disorders of the brain. But the diagnosis is still based on subjective criteria. And when a diagnosis is seen as subjective, many people will suspect that the diagnosis is not a valid entity. They will claim that ADHD is invented by physicians and pharmaceutical companies so that they can sell more medication. They will claim that teachers complain about a child's inattention and refer to a doctor for medication treatment because they lack the simple ability to control children's behavior in the classroom. They will claim that parents want to pop a pill rather than appropriately discipline their child.

Because we cannot point to a specific laboratory test that is abnormal, we have difficulty refuting their arguments.

So, the *DSM* is the best we've got. Or is it? A medical diagnosis seems to have degenerated into a listing of symptoms with a seemingly arbitrary criteria of diagnosis. Why nine symptoms of inattention? Why not eight or twelve? In the next 30–40 pages, we will discover that ADHD has such a characteristic profile that it can be reliably diagnosed in most children and refute the claims above.

Although we do not know all the details, we do know that ADHD is a medical condition, and the basis of this medical condition will be discussed in detail in a few pages below. In 1998 the American Medical Association convened a group of the best researchers in the ADHD field. They published a consensus statement that summarized the diagnosis and treatment recommendations for the clinical assessment of ADHD in children and adults. Their summary statement concluded: "Overall, ADHD is one of the best researched disorders in medicine and the overall data on its validity are far more compelling than for many medical conditions."[4]

DAY OF JUDGMENT

Liz: *So last night, Danny had a lot of problems settling down and getting into bed. I let him watch a little TV, but he wanted more. I finally got him into the bathtub by promising him a popsicle after his bath, but during his bath he splashed so much water that I needed four towels just to wipe up the floor. I usually try to do counting games with Danny's toys in the bathtub, but tonight he was just too scattered. But finally, I got him into his pajamas. He ate his popsicle, we brushed his teeth, and he got into bed. He was not mad or angry or even irritable. He just still had too much energy. After reading three books, checking the closet and under the bed for monsters, and cuddling with him after I turned out the light, he finally fell asleep.*

I walked down the stairs to the kitchen, opened a bottle of wine and sat down on the couch in the family room. The TV was still on, but I turned it off and basked in the silence for a moment, knowing what was to come.

A few minutes later, Chris walked in and sat down next to me. We didn't say anything for a while, but then he asked, "So how did Danny's visit to Dr. Lawrence go? Is he growing?"

"Oh God, Chris. I don't know. I don't know."

"What do you mean?"

"Well, you know that Danny can be a little active, to say the least. He was at the top of his game today. He was all over Dr. Lawrence's office, even broke that special flashlight on the wall that the doctor uses to look in his ears. Dr. Lawrence asked me a bunch of questions, but it was really hard to answer him when Danny was being so wild. He gave me a couple of questionnaires to fill out, but the bottom line is that he thinks Danny has ADHD and that he may need medication to help him concentrate and that . . ."

"Wait a minute, Liz. What do you mean, ADHD? Medication? No way. End of story. We just need to start disciplining him better."

"Chris, I definitely don't want him on medication either, but something has to be done. He starts second grade next month, and they say that the work gets much harder, and they start sending home more homework. I can't get Danny to sit still for more than a minute, so I don't see how he is going to do twenty minutes of homework. You know how much trouble he had last year and . . ."

"Liz, you know that even though Mrs. Miller may have been a good teacher in her time, she is older now and can't handle the kids anymore."

"Then why don't the other kids in his class have the same problem? None of the other mothers say that their kids are having any trouble, and I always feel like they don't want their kids playing with Danny."

Chris stood up. *"I don't want him on medication. We need to start disciplining him more. End of story!"*

"OK, OK. I won't fill the prescription just now, but we have to fill out these questionnaires first anyway. They only have about fifty questions and should only take ten minutes. One for us to fill out and one for Mrs. Miller."

"Good. Now I'm going to watch the game."

*"First **we** will fill out the questionnaire. Together. And then you can watch the game. Here, I have it right here. Give me your pen. First question, 'Does he have trouble sitting still? Never, Some of the time, Often, or Always?'"*

"Well, some of the time, I guess."

"Chris, he is always moving. Won't sit at the dinner table for more than three minutes. He begs to watch a TV show, and then when we let him watch it, he runs to his room to get a toy."

"Yeah, OK, let's compromise and say, 'Often.'"

"Next question, 'Has trouble focusing?' Well, Mrs. Miller said that was a problem all day long."

"Trouble focusing? What does that mean? He can play a video game for an hour without moving. That's not focusing?"

"Yeah, but he has trouble focusing on something that doesn't interest him, and that is just about everything that happens at school."

"Liz, you know that I was a lot like Danny when I was a kid. And I turned out OK." Luckily Chris didn't see me roll my eyes.

This went on for the next forty-eight questions, but we completed the questionnaire. I told Chris that I would ask Mrs. Miller to fill out the other questionnaire and then take them both to Dr. Lawrence. And I agreed not to fill the prescription. Not yet. So, we had a plan.

Chris went over to turn on the TV. I took another sip of wine.

Every physician uses the medical history to delineate what symptoms are bothering a patient. Fever, chest pain, a rash, or a cough. And he or she then asks questions about those symptoms. How high was the fever? How long have you had the chest pain? When did it start? But with most medical conditions, the physician might say, "OK, your chest pain is mild, it is on the right, and it started about the same time as your fever and cough. I doubt that it is your heart, but we are going to get an EKG to be sure. And we are going to run some blood tests as well."

However, with ADHD, no specific medical test, X-ray, blood test, or other objective medical test can make the diagnosis of ADHD or definitively rule it out. So, we are left with symptoms. If the behaviors most commonly present in ADHD are present in your child, then that increases the likelihood of ADHD. If these behaviors are affecting your child's grades, or if other children avoid playing with your child because of those behaviors, then the likelihood of ADHD is increased again. If most of these behaviors are absent, then it decreases the likelihood of ADHD or even rules it out.

But we are still left with behaviors. And for children with ADHD, most of those behaviors are observed by others, rather than reported by the child. Children may feel bad about their dropping grades or about getting in trouble in school, but the younger the child, the less likely they will complain about their activity level, or their ability to focus, or their distractibility.

Both parents and physicians alike have a problem with this symptom-driven approach. The use of a questionnaire to determine the presence of symptoms is very subjective. Usually, a parent or both parents will fill out the questionnaire, and they have to make a judgment. And each parent's *interpretation* of those behaviors may differ, as they did between Liz and Chris. Further, the absence of a specific medical test that would allow a physician to point to a spot on the X-ray and say, "Here is your problem" makes people very uncomfortable. But the diagnosis of many medical conditions is dependent on the history, and specific medical tests are not available to assist the physician or to increase the confidence of the parents. For example, the symptoms of migraine headaches are subjective, without any changes on the physical exam and without any corroborating medical tests. As a matter of fact, when tests are run, it is usually to rule out something else rather than to make the diagnosis. And for conditions such as these, it is easy to doubt the credibility of the diagnosis.

The DSM criteria work, but they are not easy. I suspect that while you are reading these words, it is hard to hold all those symptoms in mind at the same time. So, in order to demonstrate what ADHD is and in order to show what the effects of ADHD are on the teacher, the mother, the father, *and especially* on the child, I am going to ask you to forget about everything you have just read about ADHD up to this point, including the previous fourteen pages. Let me paint a very different picture.

A number of years ago, I met Danny for the first time. His mother sat in front of my desk, with Danny to her right. He was not at all interested in our conversation, but he was in a good mood and smiled occasionally. While his mother was talking, he was fidgeting, looking out the window, moving around in his seat, and occasionally interrupting. When I asked her what was her biggest concern, she responded, "Well, he is highly intelligent, but he has a tough time staying focused and quiet in school. As a result, he has a difficult time learning. He is very scattered."

So, I began asking my usual questions. When did this start, how is he doing in school, how are his grades, how does he get along with other kids? She tried to answer each question, but she was clearly getting frustrated. I could hear a quiver in her voice, and I thought she was going to start crying. But then she stopped talking, reached into the bag sitting on the chair next to her, and pulled out a brightly colored, very ragged spiral notebook and handed it to me.

"Danny's teacher uses this calendar notebook to communicate with her students' parents. Each day the teacher will write a short note about how Danny did that day. I then can write a response or a question, and this notebook goes back and forth each day, from home to the school and back again."

I told her that I could not read the whole notebook at this time, but I would like to glance through the notebook now, and I would review it in more depth later. I then opened the notebook and began reading. By the time I got to the third page, I began to feel tears in *my* eyes. I already knew what was in the rest of the notebook, and I knew that I could not read any further without breaking into tears. I was so used to treating children with behavior and learning problems like a detective, objectively analyzing the facts, that I had forgotten what it *felt* like, to the child and his or her parents. Suddenly, reading this notebook, I could tell exactly how Danny and his mother must feel.

So, if someone asks me, "What is ADHD?," I can answer by showing them the two tables above and talk about finding six of nine behaviors in each category. Or I could show them Danny's notebook. Danny and his mother and teacher are real people who carried on a conversation through Danny's first-grade year by writing almost daily comments in a notebook that went home with Danny and back to the teacher in the morning. This notebook has about forty-five pages in it, one for each week of the year, and I can't reproduce all of those pages here. However, I have received permission from Danny's mother to reproduce some of these pages and to transcribe these notes in the next chapter.

The teacher's and mother's comments from the notebook are reproduced verbatim in the highlighted boxes. These "conversations" are real. The only editing I have done is to change the name of the child and to choose which "conversations" are included.

In addition, I have written short segments that represent what Danny and his mother might have been thinking at the moment. The sections are introduced with "Liz" or "Danny" in bold and the text in italics. An example is shown below.

> **Liz:** *Danny and I had just finished doing his homework when the phone rang. It was Danny's teacher, Mrs. Miller.*

Although these passages are fictional, they are not fictitious. They are inspired by forty years of listening to parents talk about a lifetime of frustration and joy that their children have experienced.

Forget the tables and the "six or more" symptoms and all of the definitions of ADHD.

What follows is truly ADHD in its rawest form.

Chapter 2

WHAT IS ADHD AND HOW DOES IT FEEL?

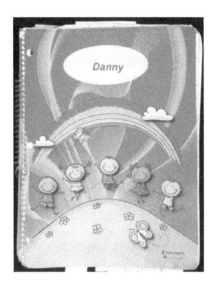

Danny: *Hi. My name is Danny. This summer, I am just a kid. But tomorrow I will be a first grader! I can't wait. Last year, in kindergarten, we did a lot of playing, and I got in a lot of trouble. But this year, I'm gonna be the smartest kid in the class. Last year, my brain wasn't very focused, and the teacher would want us to sing a song, and I wanted to play with my friends. But this year, I'm gonna pay attention to the teacher and just be smart and learn a lot. So, I'm going to bed now to get a good sleep so I will have a great day in first grade tomorrow. Talk to you later.*

Liz: *My son, Danny, seems so excited about starting school tomorrow. I know he had a rough year last year in kindergarten, but he seems like a different kid now, much more mature. And we were really lucky that Mrs. Miller will be his teacher this year because all of the parents of the older kids say that she is amazing and one of the best teachers in the school. She is so patient with the eighteen kids in her class. Danny was difficult in kindergarten last year, I know. But I think he has the hang of things now. This is going to be a good year.*

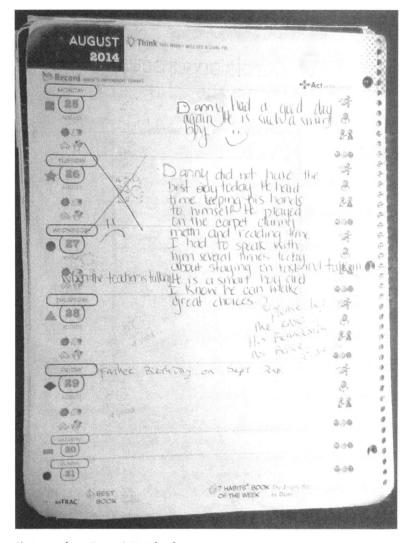

First page from Danny's Notebook.

August 26 (second week of school)
Teacher: Danny had a good day again. He is such a smart boy.

August 27
Teacher: Danny did not have the best day today. He had a hard time keeping his hands to himself. He played on the carpet during math and reading time. I had to speak with him several times today about staying on task and talking when the teacher is talking. He is a smart boy and I know he can make smart choices
Mother: Please let me know if his behavior is not better.

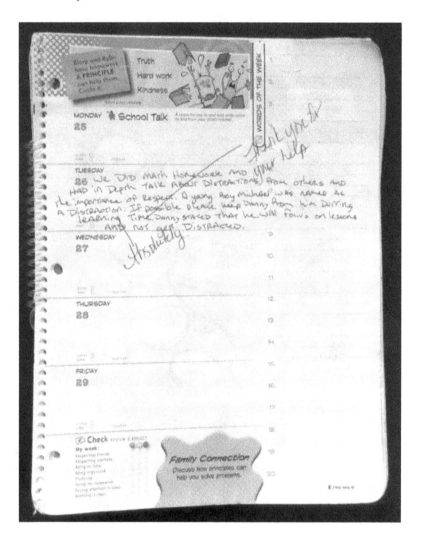

MONDAY 25

TUESDAY
26 We did math homework and had in depth talk about distractions from others and the importance of respect. A young boy Michael was named as a distraction. If possible please keep Danny from him during learning time. Danny stated that he will follow on lessons and not get distracted.

Thank you for your help

WEDNESDAY
27

Absolutely

THURSDAY
28

FRIDAY
29

Mother: We did math homework and had an in-depth talk about distractions from others and the importance of respect. A young boy Michael was named as a distraction. If possible, please keep Danny from him during learning time. Danny stated that he will focus on lessons and not get distracted.

Teacher: Absolutely. Thank you for your help.

September 3 (this page of the notebook not shown)

Teacher: Danny was very talkative today. He had a hard time staying on task.

Mother: We had a talk about staying focused & respectful by staying quiet during work time. Danny will try harder tomorrow.

September 4

Teacher: Danny had a better day; we are working on being an active listener. I moved him a little closer to me in hopes to help him stay engaged on the lesson.

> **Danny:** *So that's what it's like to be a first grader. It's cool, because I feel like one of the big kids now, in regular school, not kindergarten or preschool. But it's not cool because you have to work harder, and there are so many new rules. The teacher kept saying I needed to sit and stay on task. I don't even know what a task is! I'm not sure what she meant, because I was staying on my seat. But then Mom and I had a talk, and she explained that staying on task means to listen and pay attention. And that's what I was trying to do. But Michael kept laughing at me, and I don't know why, because I wasn't being funny. It's just hard to listen when someone is laughing at you.*

> **Liz:** *I am so proud of my big boy. It's been two weeks now since school started, and he has had a number of good days. And yes, he has had a few days like last year in kindergarten, but I am sure that this is just the newness of the new classroom and the new teacher and the new rules and the new demands. I just hope that this Michael kid doesn't interfere with Danny's ability to show how smart he is. Chris says that Danny is just "all boy," and maybe he is right.*
>
> *I talked to Danny about paying attention and staying on task, but he kept laughing about something and said that he would sit on his task from now on. Not sure if I was getting through to him or not.*

Hyperactivity and impulsivity are usually obvious and hard to miss. These behaviors occur in all children, occasionally. Danny's mother knows that things are not right, that Danny is starting the new school year the way he ended kindergarten, but she does not yet see this behavior as a problem. It is natural for a parent to search for the cause of these difficulties in the school, or the teacher, or the other kids in the classroom.

Parents will often brush off comments about a child's hyperactivity and impulsivity by saying, "He is all boy," or "Boys will be boys," but it is not really clear what this means. It certainly does not mean that any level of activity and aggressiveness is acceptable in any boy. There seems to be some unwritten law that boys are supposed to be active and aggressive and girls are quiet and reserved and passive. Nothing is wrong with a boy being active and nothing is wrong with a boy being aggressive, so long as he respects the rights of others. But if his activity or aggressiveness interferes with his ability to form cooperative friendships, then that is not just "*all boy*"; that is a concern.

The "all boy" reference to a male child with ADHD is common and represents the most "typical" presentation of ADHD. However, girls have ADHD as well. When a girl is hyperactive and impulsive, she seems to stand out even more.

When I started my training in the 1980s, research suggested that ADHD occurred in a ratio of 10 boys to 1 girl. Twenty years ago, the research indicated the ratio was 5 to 1. Currently, most studies suggest that the ratio is 3 to 1, and I strongly believe that the real ratio is closer to 1 to 1. Why has the ratio changed so much over the past forty years? Girls seem more likely to have the inattentive form of ADHD, without hyperactivity and impulsivity. As a result, girls are less disruptive in the classroom and less likely to be considered a problem. Many teachers describe a girl with the inattentive form of ADHD as "spacey." The inattentive behaviors in girls are just as likely to affect learning and, eventually, self-esteem as in boys, but girls with ADHD are more likely to be diagnosed later than boys, or not at all, partially because they often lack hyperactivity. The decreasing ratio over the past forty years seems to be caused by better recognition of the inattentive form of ADHD and, therefore, earlier recognition of these difficulties in girls.[1]

September 8

Teacher: I spoke with Danny a few times today about using gentle hands and keeping our hands to ourselves. I know that he is not trying to hurt a friend, but we talked about how it might make others feel when we touch them.

September 12
Mother: Thank you for talking with him on Monday. I'm glad his week got better.

September 15
Teacher: I spoke with Danny twice today about keeping his hands to himself and being an active listener.
Mother: We talked to Danny today about this, too. He said he would work very hard to keep his hands to himself and not touch anyone.

September 17
Mother: Yay! Another Great Day!
Mother: Super!

> **Danny:** *So, the teacher was teaching us sight words today, and we had to use them in a sentence. One of the words was "let," and I said, "We better hurry because we don't want to be let for school." Michael started laughing and pointing at me, so I pushed him, and Mrs. Miller got mad and said not to hit. But I didn't hit. I pushed. It's not the same thing.*

> **Liz:** *Danny got in trouble today for hitting, but I talked to him, and he insisted that he did not hit Michael. So, I believe Mrs. Miller, but I also believe Danny. Not sure what to think now.*

Danny's aggression is becoming a more frequent concern. If aggressive behaviors occur occasionally, if they occur without warning, if they occur with remorse, then these behaviors may be part of impulsivity. Impulsive behaviors occur without forethought, without malicious intent, without anger. Impulsive behaviors seem accidental.

On the other hand, aggression can be evidence that a child has not learned how to control his emotions. If aggressive behaviors occur in anger and with emotion, if they seem to be planned out, malicious, and without remorse, then these behaviors are much less likely to indicate the impulsivity of ADHD.

It is important to make the distinction between these two types of aggression. Impulsive aggression suggests ADHD. Emotional aggression may indicate a problem with mood control, such as oppositional defiant disorder, or a mood disorder (see Chapter 9 for much more detail).

In Danny's case, his aggressiveness seems more impulsive. This is an important but sometimes difficult distinction to make.

October 9

Teacher: Danny was not a great listener today. He had a hard time following directions. For example, when we went outside to go on a shape hunt Danny played in the sand box. He has a hard time staying focused at times. He is *very* bright but needs redirecting several times throughout the day.

Mother: I am very sorry. We had a long talk about his focus in school.

> **Danny:** *After dinner tonight, I wanted to play and watch TV, but Mom said no TV tonight and that we needed to talk. I'm so mad because my favorite program was on, and she wouldn't let me watch it. So, we talked, or actually Mom talked, and I pretended to listen. She kept saying that at school I need to pay attention when the teacher tells us what to do. But I am paying attention, or at least to those things that are interesting.*

> **Liz:** *I don't get it! Mrs. Miller had so many concerns today about Danny's difficulty following directions and needing redirection. But then she says he is very bright. If he is so bright (and I believe he is), then why can't he figure out that he needs to focus and attend? I apologized to Mrs. Miller about Danny's behavior. I guess we have been so absorbed in working with Danny about his sight words and letter and number skills that we have forgotten to teach him to focus and attend.*

Two months into the school year, and mother's tone has begun to change. Rather than see these behaviors as day-to-day anomalies, she is starting to see a pattern. She knows that Danny is intelligent, and on the one hand feels that paying attention is as natural as turning your head to the sound of a noise. However, she knows that something is not right. And because she does not feel that Danny is purposely trying to irritate the teacher, she feels that there is no one to blame but herself. So, she apologizes.

October 13

Mother: Hoping for a better week . . . We practiced sight words to prepare for this week's assessment.
Teacher: He did great. He knew all of them.
Mother: Go Danny!

October 16

Teacher: Danny was not a good listener today. I had to repeat directions multiple times because he was not listening. He selected a seat at my desk because he said "his brain won't let him think." He is extremely bright, but he has challenges staying on task. I am going to consult with the guidance counselor to see how we can help him stay focused in the classroom. If he truly is having difficulty, I don't want to reprimand him for something he feels he can't control. What are your thoughts?
Mother: Thank you for your concern for Danny. I e-mailed you to request a conference. He knows he had a bad day, and he told me that he was sorry (before I asked or prompted). I'd like to have a conference with the guidance counselor present at your earliest availability.

> **Danny:** *Mrs. Miller said I wasn't paying attention again today, but I was. I was paying attention to Michael's shirt. He had on a Bruins' jersey, and the Bruins are my favorite team. But I guess Mrs. Miller meant that I wasn't paying attention to her, so I moved closer to her desk so I wouldn't see Michael's jersey anymore. And at first it helped, and I could pay attention better. But then I couldn't stop thinking about Michael's Bruins' jersey, and I kept turning around to look at it. I wanted to pay attention, but I just couldn't. I don't think my brain works like everyone else's.*

Again, another change in tone, but this time the change comes from Danny. Even though it may be hard for his mother and teacher to see, Danny is trying to comply with what he knows that his teacher and his mother expect of him. When distractions overwhelm his ability to ignore them, he does not accept the blame as readily as his mother did when she apologized for him. He blames his brain. Then when his mother talks to him, he apologizes before she even prompts him. Danny is sorry, but he recognizes that something physical must be behind his inability to focus and pay attention.

Is ADHD a deficit of will? Does the ADHD child behave this way because he just doesn't care about school and learning? No. Danny is beginning to recognize that his ability to focus and attend must come from him, and when he cannot deliver, he blames his brain.

The next day, Danny's frustration reached its peak. For the fifth time, his teacher reminded him to pay attention. Danny didn't like being singled out in class, and he yelled at this teacher, "Shut up!" The next day, he wrote the following letter and gave it to his teacher (see next page):

I'm sorry Mrs Miller that I had told you to "shut up". I really didn't mean it. ~~~~~~ The reason that I talk is because every thing I think in my ~~head~~ hurts out of my mouth it's a bad habit. I'm not really *that* bad of a kid when I try very hard I can be the best kid in your class. Tommorw I will behave and try not to talk as much.

Sincerly Danny

Letter written by Danny to his teacher.

Im sorry Mrs Miller that I had told you to "shut up." I really didn't mean it. The reason that I talk so much is because every thing I think in my head blurts out of my mouth it's a bad habit. I'm not really that bad of a kid when I try very hard I can be the best kid in your class. Tomorrow I will behave and try not to talk as much.

Danny offers an explanation for his inappropriate behavior when he says, "everything I think in my head blurts out of my mouth. It's a bad habit." Danny is beginning to recognize that he is having difficulty in the classroom and that these difficulties are not completely under his control.

November 10–13

Mother: Danny said that he had a GREAT day and had FUN doing riddles with Mrs. Hammond.
Teacher: She said he did excellent. He is a genius.
Mother: WooHoo! Let's keep him humble though. LOL!

> **Danny:** *My teacher said I did soooooo good today and that I'm very smart. Well, I could have told her that! And I could have told my mom and everybody else the same thing! They just need to let me learn my own way.*

> **Liz:** *I think that Danny just needed a few months to get acclimated to the new expectations of first grade. He had a great week, with no concerns about his focusing or paying attention. I understand the concerns of his teacher, and I have talked to Danny about his behavior, and he has listened. Maybe Chris is right. I think that all those problems have melted away, and Danny is back to the "genius" that I always knew he was.*

Many aspects of ADHD are frustrating. Variability of these behaviors is at the top of the list. Some days are much better than others. Some days can be so good that they make you question whether it is really your child who has the problem.

But the next page shows that it didn't take long for Danny to return to his previous pattern of distractibility, impulsivity, and difficulty focusing and paying attention. If a child has ADHD, the one thing we can be sure of is that the behaviors will always return.

December 4

Teacher: Danny had a hard time staying focused today. He spent his day playing with his scissors instead of completing his work. He was not able to complete his science work. The students were given 20 minutes to complete it. He had a difficult time in Art today.

Father: We had a serious talk about not playing anymore. You will find the completed work attached. I have in his green folder his homework for Nov. and the first week of Dec. Please let me know if he is misbehaving in school. Thank you for everything.

Teacher: Thank you so much. I don't want his grades to suffer when I know he can do the work. I appreciate your help.

Danny: *Everybody tells me how smart I am. So, if I'm so smart, why did I get a C on my spelling homework? I got all the words right (except the two that I accidentally forgot to do). But then when it was time to turn in our homework yesterday, I was talking to Jacob, and I didn't hear Mrs. Miller tell us to turn it in. So, I turned it in today instead and got a C. Not fair!*

Liz: *After dinner, Danny went out to play in the backyard. I was at the sink, rinsing dishes for the dishwasher and watching Danny through the window. Chris was clearing the table.*

"You know, Danny should probably be doing this," Chris said.

"I know, I know, but he has so much energy and has so much trouble falling asleep that I think it is a good idea to let him run off some of that energy before he starts his homework. Oh, that reminds me, we got another note from Mrs. Miller today. She is concerned that because Danny has so much trouble focusing and paying attention that he is having trouble completing his work. Those incomplete assignments are beginning to affect his grades."

"But Mrs. Miller has told you so many times how smart he is. How is it going to affect his grades?"

"Yes, he is smart. He gets a hundred on every test, but when he forgets to hand in a homework assignment, he gets a zero. He has more homework than tests, so his grades can suffer big-time from just a few missed assignments. Actually, he has a spelling test tomorrow. Will you go over his words while I finish up in here?

"Sure." He opens the back door and calls out, "Danny, come here."

Danny: "OK, just a minute."

Dad: "Right now."

Danny: "I'm coming."

Dad (starting to get mad): "Danny, where are you?"

Danny (suddenly appearing): "Oh yeah, I forgot. What?"

Dad: "Don't you have a spelling test tomorrow?"

Danny: "I guess."

Dad: "Have you studied?"

Danny: "Yeah, I know it all."

Dad: "OK, Danny, how do you spell forest?"

Danny: "Oh, Dad, guess what story Mrs. Johnson read to us today? Robin Hood. *You know, it happened in Sherwood Forest, and they robbed the money from all these rich people . . ."*

Dad: "Danny, just spell the word forest."

Danny: "OK, forest, f-o, uh s; no, r. Is it spelled like four?"

Dad (forced, but patiently): "No, forest."

Danny: "Oh, yeah, f-o-s; no, r-s-t."

Dad: "Danny, fore . . ."

Danny: "Isn't there a forest down by that lake we went to Saturday?"

Dad (getting angry): "Danny, forest. Spell forest."

Danny: "F-o-r-e-s-t. Simple."

Dad: "OK, good. Now spell tower. And get your feet off the table. And sit up, Danny. You can't think all slouched over like that."

Danny: "Yeah, I can. See, I'm thinking."

Dad: "Danny, spell the word."

Danny: Oh, yeah . . . f-o-r . . ."

Dad: "Danny, you already spelled forest; the word is tower."

Danny: "Oh, yeah, tower, t-o, like the Eiffel Tower; that's in New York, right?"

Dad: "No, it's in France. Danny, spell Eiffel Tower; no, tower—spell tower."

Danny: "Ha, you said Eiffel Tower, too. It's . . ."

Dad (yelling): "Danny! Spell tower."

Danny: "OK, OK, t-o-w-e-r."

Dad: "Finally! Now spell . . ."

Danny: "Is the Eiffel Tower a water tower, or like a TV tower? TV towers have to be real big, don't they? Do they have TV in France? And what kind of shows do they have in France? Do they have Power Rangers? Hey, do ya think I could be a Power Ranger for next Halloween?"

January 8

Teacher: Not a great day. Danny was rolling and playing on the carpet. He was not able to complete his assignment in a timely manner because he was not listening to the instructions.

Mother: So disappointing. It's hard to get back to the swing of things after a long break, but we had a talk and Danny had consequences for his behavior. He promised to try harder tomorrow. He really wants to please and be a "good boy." Being 7 is tough sometimes. LOL!

Teacher: Thanks for speaking to him.

Danny: I don't know what Mrs. Miller and Mom are up to. Some days they tell me that I am so smart and such a good boy, but then there is today. Mrs. Miller was mad at me. And Mom was mad at me because Mrs. Miller was mad at me. And then Mom talked to me and said that I had to have consequences for my behaviors. That is Mom's way of saying that I am going to be grounded or punished. I really want to be a good first grader, and I will try harder. But maybe I'm just not as smart as Mom and Mrs. Miller think I am.

Liz: We had a really wonderful winter break. Danny was so excited about getting his presents that I had to put them up on the shelf so he couldn't get to them or he would have opened all of them right away. But he was in such a good mood the whole time, and I am sure that it was because he was not in school.

So, I thought after the break, he would do well once he returned to school. No such luck. The first couple of days, he was OK, but then came Thursday; not a good day.

He is in bed now. We had a talk about his behavior (again), and I had to tell him that he could not watch TV tonight before bed. I thought he would explode at this news, but he didn't get angry or mad. He just sat there quietly for about thirty seconds, then looked up at me with a tear rolling down his face. "OK, Mom. I will try harder tomorrow." He then stood up, walked back to his room, got his pajamas on, and got in bed.

I held it together until I got into bed. Chris asked me how things were with Danny, and I just broke down. Good day one day, bad day the next. Smiles and excitement one day, tears and sadness the next. Optimistic one day, dreading tomorrow the next. This roller-coaster ride is miserable.

January 12

Note from reading specialist about Danny's participation in the Accelerated Reader's Enrichment Program: "Congratulation! Your child has been selected to participate in the accelerated reader's enrichment program . . ."

January 15

Teacher: Danny had a difficult time listening and following directions today. I spoke with him multiple times about rolling on the carpet. He was not able to complete his assignment because he was playing with his crayons instead of listening to the directions. It was not the best day for Danny.

The contrast here between Danny's behavior and his academic performance is again striking. Danny can be selected for a special reading program, because he is advanced in his academic **abilities**, but his academic **performance** is another story. Research has shown that the intellectual potential (IQ) and academic potential (achievement) vary in the same way that they do in the general population. That is, ADHD can be seen in gifted children, in children with average abilities, in children with learning disabilities, and in children with more severe developmental problems. Children who are gifted with ADHD are more likely to be diagnosed later because they can use their intelligence to compensate for their ADHD, at least for a while. Most children with ADHD appear to have average cognitive abilities but lower than average academic performance, not because they lack the ability to perform academically, but because their ADHD interferes with their ability to do the work.

It is possible that ADHD may give a child some academic advantage. Because children with ADHD are usually impulsive, they are more comfortable with risk. As a result, they may be more likely to try a new task that is difficult and achieve more. On the other hand, they are more likely to lose interest in these activities and may not complete an assignment that they should have no difficulty completing.

January 27

Mother: Off to a good start!

January 28

Teacher: Not a good day! Talking back to the teacher when asked to do something. This afternoon I asked the students to put their things away, so they could listen. Danny continued to color. When I asked him to put his things away, he responded, "Why, I am still coloring?" Please speak with Danny about following directions the first time. He spent a few minutes in timeout. Afterwards, we talked about following directions.

Mother: Today's note is so disappointing. I am so sorry that he's giving you such a hard time. Danny is very sorry too and wants to apologize to you first thing tomorrow. Talking back is not tolerated. Not OK!

Teacher: Thank you for speaking with him. He apologized and was very sincere.

Mother: Danny told me he lost the privilege of going to the 100 party. We support that fully. He lost privileges and told me that he knows he "deserves to be consequenced."

Teacher: No, he did not lose that opportunity. He spent a few minutes in timeout. He lost the privilege to hear Silly Socks today. He will still celebrate the 100th day of school.

January 29

Teacher: Danny had a difficult time staying on task/focusing in order to complete his assignments. It is starting to impact him academically. I have spoken with Mrs. K (guidance counselor) for suggestions . . .

January 31

Mother: If he can read 100 books before school ends, we'll take him to Chuck E Cheese.

Teacher: LOL. Awesome. He told me he was extremely enthusiastic about it.

> **Liz:** *I am sitting in the family room, crying for the last half hour, trying not to let Chris hear me in the next room. Danny started out the year on such a positive note, and now that we are halfway through the year, things have only been getting worse. Danny's teacher has been amazingly*

*positive and willing to work with him, and Danny has recovered quickly
from his increasingly frequent disappointments. However, I am beginning
to believe that she is losing her patience. After all, Danny is not the only
kid in her class, and she has to be concerned about the behavior and learning of all of the other eighteen kids in the class as well. And most important, all of these problems are beginning to hit Danny hard, too. He talks
back, gets corrected, then feels guilty, then wants to apologize, and then
he talks back again. I know he is frustrated, because his usual carefree
attitude has begun to be replaced with a quiet angst that is worrying me.*

The frustration and exasperation of both Danny's teacher and mother
are glaring. Danny's difficulties are growing, and his mother's apolo-
gies have become more strident. Danny must be equally frustrated as he
wants to apologize as well (whether or not that has been encouraged by
his mother). In the past, while the teacher has been identifying a "bad
day" for Danny, she has been careful to point out what "an awesome
kid" he is.

> August 26: "He is such a smart boy!"
> October 9: "He is *very* bright, but needs redirecting several times
> throughout the day."
> October 16: "He is extremely bright, but he has challenges staying
> on task . . . I don't want to reprimand him for something he feels
> he can't control."
> November 10: "He is a genius."
> May 5: "I am blessed to have this time with Danny. Awesome
> kid!"

But it is becoming even more difficult for the teacher to draw from that
store of optimism in light of Danny's increasing difficulties.

It is important to draw your attention to the many positive comments this teacher made. It is very common in the early years of ADHD
to blame the school or the teacher. And in some cases, this blame is
justified. In some cases, the teacher may not have the experience needed
to address ADHD behavior in the classroom. In some cases, too many
children are in the classroom, or other children have behavior or learning difficulties, or the teacher is preoccupied with problems of her own.
But in Danny's case, it is clear that his teacher is exceptional. She not
only recognizes Danny's difficulties attending and focusing, but she

recognizes his superior academic and cognitive potential. And despite the fact that Danny's teacher is exceptional, and despite the fact that he is very bright, and despite the fact that Danny's mother tries to handle these concerns with patience and compassion and love, Danny still has difficulty learning.

February 17

Teacher: Danny was not a good listener today. He had a hard time staying focused during writing. He had to complete his assignments during recess time. During reading time, he was instructed to color only the pictures that begin with "U." He did not complete the assignment, even though he had 15 minutes to complete it. He currently has a "B" in reading, but he is capable of an "A." (Extremely smart.) Please speak with Danny about the importance of following directions. I don't want his grade to be affected by his poor listening choice.

Mother: Yesterday was a bad day for Danny. He has finished the assignment you sent home and he had consequences. We completely agree that he should not have "Bs" due to his inability to focus/follow directions. Please send home all incomplete assignments so we can complete them at home.

February 24

Teacher: Extremely talkative today. He had a hard time listening and following directions the first time.

Mother: We're working on this tonight! The first appointment we could get for an ADHD evaluation is on 7/31, but we're on a waiting list for something sooner.

Teacher: Sounds good. Thank you for your help. If you need paperwork completed over the summer, feel free to call me.

> **Liz:** *Chris had a meeting at corporate headquarters and had been out of town for a week. He got back from the airport about a half hour after Danny had fallen asleep. I was on the couch reading but almost asleep myself. I gave Chris a hug and told him I had missed him. He smiled and gave me a much longer hug than usual. His meeting had gone well, and his presentation was*

well received. He asked about my work, and then finally asked, "And how is Danny doing in school?"

"Same old stuff. Doing great one day, major problems the next. We had a follow-up appointment with Dr. Lawrence. He had received the questionnaires that we filled out and had one from Mrs. Miller as well."

"Yeah?"

"Yeah. So, Dr. Lawrence said that he had reviewed the questionnaires and feels that Danny needs to see a specialist."

His voice rising, "What kind of specialist?"

"Well, he recommended that we see someone at the university who is a specialist in ADHD and learning problems."

"Liz, I just got home and was in a good mood and all, and you have to hit me with this? Now?"

"If not now, when?"

"Well, I don't know. But you said he is supposed to see a specialist in ADHD and learning problems. First, Danny is smart and doesn't have a problem learning."

"Then why are his grades dropping?"

"And second, if you go see someone who is a specialist in ADHD, he is going to diagnose ADHD. That's what they do. And wasn't he supposed to see that guidance counselor lady at school?"

"He did. She spent a couple of hours in Danny's classroom, just watching him, and then she took him to her office for some testing. She said that she cannot diagnose ADHD, but that the testing was very consistent with that, and that he needs to see a doctor because he really might benefit from treatments for ADHD."

"Well, there you go again. Let's just drug him up. I told you that we need to discipline him more."

"Chris, I have. I get a note from Mrs. Miller almost every day. I have punished and grounded him and consequenced him, and each time Danny seems to feel so guilty. A couple of days ago, he apologized to me for being a bad kid. I will not do this anymore! I don't think it is his fault. I think he is smart and trying as hard as he can, and he wants to do well in school, but he thinks there is something wrong with his brain. I don't know about that, but I do know that he feels worse about this than I do or than Mrs. Miller does. So, I called the specialist that Dr. Lawrence recommended and got an appointment for this summer."

Chris did not respond but sat in silence for a few minutes. He then stood up, grabbed his suitcase, and walked back to the bedroom. He came out a few minutes later, walked to the kitchen, and opened a beer.

The silence was killing me more than the arguing. I couldn't move, and finally he said something. "Well, I'm going to bed. I had a really hard week, and I need to sleep on this. We can talk later." And he walked back to the bedroom. I came back about twenty minutes later. Chris was already in bed.

"Well, good night, Chris. I did really miss you while you were gone."

"Yeah. Me, too. Good night."

No more hugs tonight.

April 27

Teacher: Danny had a difficult time staying on task and following directions on Thursday and Friday (for the substitute). The substitute said that she had to speak with him several times about following directions. She sent him to Mrs. B's room (Kindergarten teacher next door) for the remainder of the day. On Friday, he was not allowed to participate in recess as a result of his behavior. We talked about showing adults respect and listening/following directions when asked. I was very sad to hear this. I spoke to the Kindergarten teacher and she said she witnessed Danny disrespect the substitutes. They said he was disrespectful and not listening. Very sad.

May 5

Mother: Happy Teacher Day! Thank you for all you do for Danny— all your kindness and patience. We are so incredibly blessed to have you in his life this year. We appreciate you more than you know. I hope you have a wonderful day!

Teacher: Thank you. You are too sweet. I am blessed to have this time with Danny. Awesome kid!

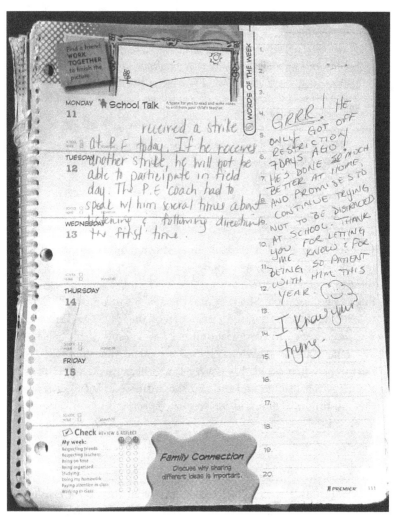

Page from Danny's Notebook, depicting teacher's and mother's frustration.

May 11

Teacher: Danny received a strike at PE today. If he receives another strike, he will not be able to participate in field day. The PE coach had to speak with him several times about listening and following directions the first time.

Mother: GRRR! He only got off restrictions 7 days ago. He's done so much better at home and promises to continue trying not to be distracted at school. Thank you for letting me know and for being so patient with him this year.

Teacher: I know you're trying.

May 12

Teacher: Danny received a warning by the TA for yelling in the caf-
eteria today. After lunch he continued to yell and play in the classroom. He is a smart boy and I know he can make better choices.
Mother: Very Disappointed. Danny will *NOT* be going on tomorrow's Field Trip.

May 14
Mother: I'm so very thankful he had a good day. He was REALLY
proud that you said he had a "MARVELOUS" day.

May 25

Mother: I've been meaning to email you. You are an amazing
teacher, THANK YOU!
Teacher: Thank you. It has been an absolute joy to have Danny in my
class this year. Not only is he "*brilliant*" but he is extremely funny
and witty. You should be extremely proud to have raised such an
amazing kid. Keep me posted over the years.
    No matter the results of the test, please know that he is a *brilliant*
child. I have taught for 7 years and I haven't encountered a child
who processes information and problem solves like Danny. His
scores were very impressive. He is a rock star!!!
Mother: Thank you for this.

I met Danny and his mother in my office at the University, shortly after
the beginning of the summer. Danny responded to questions appropriately
with an excellent vocabulary, occasional humor, and he occasionally commented on his mother's statements. During the evaluation, Danny's mother
stated that she felt that his difficulty focusing and attending "is all my fault."
She said that she would like to learn how to teach him to focus better. She
also felt that she is "too lenient." Danny's mother stated that she has laid out
consequences for Danny, which seems to help him control his behavior at
home but does not seem to carry over to his schoolwork.
    The history, questionnaire results from parents and teachers, and
psychoeducational testing were all highly indicative of Attention Deficit

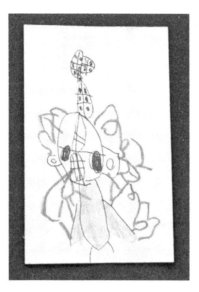

Danny's self-portrait.

Hyperactivity Disorder, Primarily Inattentive Type, without comorbid behaviors. The notebook made my job much easier, as it revealed an almost classic presentation for this disorder (it is unfortunate that such a notebook does not accompany every child who needs a full evaluation).

Danny started the new school year. Fortunately, Mrs. Miller, his first teacher from last year, was moved up to second grade and she requested that Danny attend her classroom. Danny and his mother loved Mrs. Miller and she appreciated the continuity. After two weeks medication was again started (this two-week delay gave Mrs. Miller the opportunity to observe Danny's ability to attend and learn both off medication and then again on medication). His teacher was not told when he started again on medication so that her responses could be more objective (see the teacher's and mother's notes on the following page). His mother and teacher reported a dramatic and immediate improvement. The first day on medication they were able to discern a significant difference in his ability to focus within 2–3 hours after taking medication.

Even on medication, Danny's parents' behavioral questionnaire did indicate some continuing mild problems with attention and especially hyperactivity, although markedly reduced from prior to starting medication. He had an excellent report card at midyear, with all As and one B and virtually no behavioral issues.

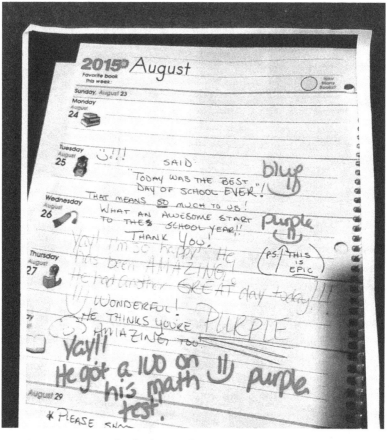

Page from Danny's Notebook after starting on ADHD medication.

August 25

Mother: Danny said today was the best day of school EVER! That means *so* much to us! What an awesome start to the school year!! Thank You!

Teacher: Yay! I'm so happy. He has been AMAZING. He had another GREAT day today!!!

Mother: Wonderful! He thinks you're AMAZING too.

Teacher: Yay!! He got a 100 on his math test.

Notice that Danny received three purple days in a row. Many teachers use a color system to let the kids know how they performed each day. (Red often being the worst, Orange, Yellow, Green, Blue, and Purple being the best.)

Danny did have some side effects from his medication. He "crashed" during the mid-afternoons, and by this his mother reported that he became extremely irritable (as the morning dose of medication was wearing off). A very small dose of short-acting medication was added in the afternoon, and the irritability resolved. These benefits were sustained over the next 2–3 years, with occasional "tweaks" in the timing and dosage of medication. (Side effects such as this are common but are usually easily managed, and they will be discussed in detail later in this book.)

CELEBRATION

Liz: *Chris took me out to dinner for my birthday at the end of October. He surprised me by taking me to Pavanti's, one of the best (and most expensive) restaurants in the city. The waiter sat us in a booth in the corner. The lights were low; two candles were on our table.*

We spent some time reviewing the extensive menu (thirteen kinds of caviar?) and then ordered appetizers and salads.

Danny was at my sister's home, so I didn't have to worry about him. He loved spending time with his younger cousin, Matthew. I am sure they were running and playing most of the evening.

"Well, Chris, you outdid yourself this time. What a beautiful place. What's the occasion?"

"Your birthday, of course."

"No, I mean, I've been wanting to come here for years, so why now?"

"Well, you deserve it. I know that this has been a rough year, with Danny's problems at school, and you taking him to see Dr. Lawrence and all. I just thought we needed a night away."

"Yes, it has been quite a year. But I am sure that we have turned a corner. Danny seems to be doing so well now. And he seems much happier, too. That makes it all worthwhile."

"Yeah, and I have to admit, he is doing much better and is much happier, although I am still very uncomfortable with his being on medication and all. And I still wonder if it was something we did, or didn't do."

"I know. Me, too. I still think, I could've disciplined him more."

"I know I said that a lot, that you could've disciplined him more. But when I see how he has responded to the medication, I doubt that medication could have reversed a lack of discipline. And the big thing for me is his

self-control. Not only is he better able to control his behavior and attention, but he seems aware that he's the one who's doing the controlling, not us. And that's huge. I thought that the medication was going to calm him down by sedating him, turning him into a zombie, but that's not what happened. He is quieter, but he seems so much more in control."

"Well, I had to fight you tooth and nail to get you to agree to start him on medication."

"True. But I am still a little nervous about what the medication is doing."

"You know, once I told the ADHD specialist at the university that we had agreed about the medication, he explained what it does, and then talked about the possible side effects. You might want to go with us the next time."

"Yeah, I think I will." We clinked glasses in agreement, and then they brought out the filet mignon.

For a few months, Danny continued to do well, both at school and at home. His grades were all A's, and his mood and self-esteem seemed to improve dramatically as well. However, one day, his mother received an e-mail from Danny's teacher. She said "he had a pretty rough day, not doing any work, trouble following directions and constantly talking. His new jacket was quite the distraction also." I did ask her if there was any chance that he did not receive medication that day, and Danny's mother responded that his father started to give him his medication, but he dropped it and couldn't find it, so Danny did not receive medication that day.

Because of his father's concern about side effects of the medication, and despite the fact that he saw significant improvement in Danny, Danny's medication was discontinued for the whole of third grade. His mother described this experiment as "a disaster." His grades suffered greatly. Dad finally compromised by agreeing to let him go back on medication, so long as he could be switched to another medication (Concerta or Vyvanse).

> **Danny:** *So, school is over for now. Can't wait for summer to start. FINALLY!! Last night, Mom made me go to the awards ceremony. So BORING. People talking . . . I don't know what they were saying. They gave out awards for lotsa different things. Last year I got one of the best reader awards. This year they said I was the most improved in science. Right, like that's any good. It's just an award they made up so that everyone could get some award.*

I had so many good days last year that I didn't know what to do. But this year, it's just gotten worse and worse. I don't know why. I am trying just as hard this year as last year. Maybe it's the medication that I was taking last year and not this year. I don't think so, because I think it is me who decides to be good or bad. It is me who decides whether to make good decisions or bad decisions. But I wanted to make good decisions this year; it just seems like everything turned out bad. Maybe it is the medicine, but I don't think so, but maybe. I think maybe I should tell Mom we should try it again. Maybe.

Chapter 3

FROM SILK TO RITALIN

A History of the Medical Treatment of
Attention Deficit Hyperactivity Disorder

Chinese medicine has used the ephedra plant for more than five thousand years as a treatment for colds, allergies, and hay fever,[1] and many consider it to be the oldest medicine known to man.[2] Without this plant, the current medication treatments for ADHD might not exist.

In 1887 Lazar Edeleano, a Romanian chemist, was attempting to develop an artificial fireproof silk. He felt that some of the new methods for producing artificial dyes might be helpful in his work with silk. Working with the ephedra plant, he was unsuccessful in producing artificial silk, but in the process, he accidentally synthesized the amphetamine base. To him, this was a useless by-product of his work. He did not recognize any of its psychoactive properties and did not pursue any further work with the molecule.

Nagayoshi Nagai was an organic chemist and the first doctor of pharmacy in Japan. He isolated ephedrine from the ephedra plant in 1885. A few years later, he synthesized pseudoephedrine. Today, pseudoephedrine is one of the most frequent medications sold over the counter for the treatment of colds, allergies, and sinus congestion.

But what does this have to do with ADHD? This is where the story becomes more surprising and fascinating than any of the chemists could have imagined.

Eight years after isolating ephedrine, Nagayoshi Nagai synthesized a new compound in 1893 from ephedra that he called phenylisopropylamine. We now call it methamphetamine.[3]

Nagai did not know it at the time, but he had just discovered a chemical substance that a hundred years later would become the basis for a multibillion-dollar industry to treat a medical condition that hadn't yet been recognized (ADHD). How did that happen?

After the synthesis of methamphetamine, not much happened right away. Then, in the 1920s, Gordon Alles was a twenty-five-year-old graduate student at the California Institute of Technology. He was initially interested in the synthesis of insulin, but his career took a very different turn two years after receiving his PhD when he synthesized the same molecule that Edeleano had discovered in 1887. However, Alles was the first to recognize the stimulant effects of amphetamine on the central nervous system. He patented his discovery and in 1934 sold his patent to the pharmaceutical company Smith, Klein & French (SKF). He later died from diabetes, caused by a lack of insulin, the same substance that started his career. SKF marketed Alles's amphetamine as an inhaler for allergies and congestion under the brand name Benzedrine and sold it over the counter, without a prescription.

FROM TEARS TO CALM: THE FIRST USE OF MEDICATION TO TREAT ADHD[4]

Emma Bradley was a beautiful seven-year-old in Pomfret, Connecticut, in 1886 who played with dolls and enjoyed school. But that year she developed a severe form of encephalitis. She survived but was left with chronic epilepsy, severe cognitive delays, and cerebral palsy. Her wealthy parents, George and Helen, embarked on a worldwide search for a cure for her condition, but met only frustration. Psychiatry and neurology were still developing fields of medicine. They were getting good at classifying symptoms into diseases but made little headway with cures or treatments for the newly described conditions, especially for children. They treated her at their sprawling home in Connecticut for twenty years, but Emma showed no improvement. George and Helen made arrangements that upon their death, their Providence, Rhode Island, estate would be converted into a home for children with severe neurological problems. In 1931, it became the Emma Pendleton Bradley Home. It is considered the first neuropsychiatric hospital in the country for children. Young children and teenagers were committed to the hospital because of a wide variety of neurological and psychiatric conditions.

The year after the hospital was founded, Charles Bradley, George's grandnephew, completed his psychiatric training and joined the hospital as its medical director. Most of the children in the hospital had severe behavioral problems, and to better understand what could be producing their intolerable behavior, he would often perform a spinal tap. This required restraining the child, then inserting a needle at the base of the spine into the fluid surrounding the spinal cord. Air was injected, which would then work its way up to the brain. This allowed for better visualization of the brain on X-ray. Unfortunately, this procedure left the child in tears with a tortuous headache that could remain for days. Bradley tried a number of treatments for the headaches, but they persisted, and the children remained in tears. In 1937, Dr. Bradley became aware of a new medication called Benzedrine, sold as an inhaler for the treatment of colds and congestion. Because it treated "head colds," he thought it might be helpful for the headaches. To his dismay, it had no effect on the headaches. But to his shock and surprise, many of the children showed an unexpected but dramatic improvement in their behavior.

> "There was a spectacular improvement in school performance in half of the children. A large proportion of the patients became emotionally subdued without, however, losing interest in their surroundings."[5] They "appeared subdued because they began to spend their leisure time playing quietly or reading, whereas formerly they had wandered aimlessly about antagonizing and annoying others."[6]
>
> The children who had become subdued exerted "more conscious control over their activities and the expression of their emotions" and conducted "themselves with increased consideration and regard for the feelings" of others.[7]

In addition to the change in behavior, the nursing staff noted something completely unexpected. They told Dr. Bradley that some of these children were now following directions, a skill that they did not seem capable of before. The children themselves were aware of the benefits and called the medication their "arithmetic pills."[8] Bradley noted that the improvements were seen on the first day after starting on Benzedrine and ceased the day after medication was discontinued. After only one week on medication, he noted,

> The most striking change in behavior occurred in the school activities of many of these patients. There appeared a definite "drive" to accomplish as much as possible. Fifteen of the 30 children responded to Benzedrine by becoming distinctly subdued in their emotional responses. Clinically in all cases, this was an improvement from the social viewpoint.[9]

Dr. Bradley quickly realized that Benzedrine had the potential for helping hundreds of thousands of children with neuropsychiatric difficulties, although he understood that Benzedrine did not *cure* the underlying neurologic problem. He advocated for a combination of medication, educational, and behavioral interventions.

> This approach in no sense replaces that of modifying a child's surroundings and so removing the sources of conflict . . . Neither can it offer the same assurance of mental health as do forms of psychotherapy which enable a child to work out his emotional problems.

Bradley[10] devoted the remainder of his career to further clarifying amphetamine's profound effects on children with neurologic difficulties and continued to publish papers into the 1960s and 1970s.

PHARMACEUTICAL COMPANIES GET INTERESTED[11]

Unfortunately, the psychiatric community was reveling in its application of Freud's psychotherapy and essentially ignored Dr. Bradley's finding for the next twenty years. But Bradley had inadvertently discovered a treatment for a disease that was not yet even named, and his work in the 1930s and 1940s has had a profound impact on the field of psychiatry, even to this day.

Smith, Klein, French Pharmaceuticals stopped producing the Benzedrine inhaler and sold it in pill form in the 1940s, which the company called Dexedrine. Dexedrine is the brand name, and dextroamphetamine is the generic. You are probably not aware that the Dexedrine used in the 1940s was identical to the Dexedrine that is still used today for the treatment of ADHD. And guess what? We will soon learn that almost half of the medications now used to treat ADHD contain the exact same ingredient as in Bradley's 1940 Dexedrine.

FROM OBETROL TO ADDERALL

The stockholders of Obetrol Pharmaceuticals were smiling all the way to the bank in 1960. They had been selling a drug called Obetrol since the early 1950s as a treatment for obesity, even though it had not been approved by the Food and Drug Administration. The FDA in those days did not have the teeth to enforce the requirement that all drugs prescribed in the United States be approved as safe and effective, but pharmaceutical companies could see the writing on the wall. The thalidomide deformities of newborn babies in the 1950s had frightened the public, and pressure was increasing for the federal government to guarantee the safety and effectiveness of all drugs prescribed in the United States. Eventually, this pressure resulted in the Kefauver-Harris amendment to the Federal Food, Drug, and Cosmetic Act in 1962 that required pharmaceutical companies to prove that their medications were safe and effective. Obetrol was ahead of the curve and was approved by the FDA for the treatment of obesity in 1960. At that time, many drugs were sold for treatment of obesity, but Obetrol, with its almost immediate reduction in appetite, was poised to become the most popular . . . and profitable.

Obetrol supressed appetite. And patients lost weight . . . in the beginning. However, the weight loss was only a few pounds and could not be substantiated by research studies. And not surprisingly, once patients stopped taking Obetrol, most put the weight right back on.

Original Obetrol was a mixture of amphetamine and methamphetamine. So, what is the difference between amphetamine and methamphetamine? Turns out, quite a lot. Amphetamine was the active ingredient in Benzedrine and most of the other medications marketed as diet pills. It would later become the critical ingredient in Dexedrine, Adderall, and Vyvanse, three of the most commonly prescribed medications for the treatment of ADHD. However, a decision was made to include methamphetamine in addition to amphetamine in Obetrol. Why?

Methamphetamine has many of the same properties of amphetamine. It decreases appetite as well, if not better than amphetamine. Like amphetamine, it keeps you awake and alert. So why use methamphetamine instead of amphetamine, which had been used for the past fifty years. Well, maybe it has something to do with one other property of methamphetamine. When you take methamphetamine, it gives you a very uplifting feeling. People who took methamphetamine seemed driven, in an almost frenetic way. And this gave way to a new nickname. Today we call methamphetamine *speed*.

So not only would Obetrol supposedly shave off inches around your waist, but it would make you feel great as well.

Obetrol quickly gained a reputation as a recreational drug. It was well known that Obetrol was Andy Warhol's drug of choice.[12] But as a result of this reputation, Obetrol was forced off the market.

That should have been the end of Obetrol. But then Rexar Pharmaceuticals, the company that produced Obetrol, did something unexpected. Rexar changed the formulation of the medication by doing two things. First, the company replaced methamphetamine with amphetamine, dramatically reducing the abuse potential of this medication. Although amphetamine can be abused, it does not produce the "high" that you would get from methamphetamine, and it is far less likely to be abused than methamphetamine. Further, it has clearly been demonstrated by multiple research studies that children who use stimulant medication (methylphenidate or amphetamine) to treat their ADHD are *less* likely to abuse drugs as adolescents and adults.[13]

In my forty years of clinical experience, I did have a few occurrences of diversion, where a patient would give his prescribed medication to a friend or roommate in college. I never had a situation where I suspected that an adolescent patient was abusing amphetamine. As a matter of fact, I had much more difficulty getting adolescents to *take* their medication. Children with ADHD are much more concerned that these medications may suppress their normal mood or personality and are then more likely to stop taking their medication and hide the fact from their parents.

Rexar also introduced a second change in formulation. It combined the amphetamine molecule with different salts. This second move did not change the function of Obetrol one bit, because before the medication gets to the brain, the body removes the salts. Rexar then placed Obetrol back on the market, with the same name, without FDA approval of the new formulation.

However, although the name Obetrol has faded from history, its legacy has persisted. Shire Pharmaceuticals acquired the rights to Obetrol in 1995, then immediately turned around and resubmitted the drug to the FDA. But this time, Shire did not ask for Obetrol to be approved for the treatment of obesity. Instead, Shire asked the FDA to approve it for the treatment of ADHD. Because Obetrol had already been approved as a safe and effective treatment for obesity, all Shire had to do was show that it was effective for treating ADHD, which the company had no trouble doing. The FDA approved Obetrol for the treatment of ADHD in 1996. Oh, and Shire Pharmaceuticals did one additional thing—the company dropped the name Obetrol and renamed it Adderall ("ADD for all"). And Adderall quickly became one of the most commonly prescribed medications to treat ADHD from the late 1990s, even to the present.

RITALIN OWES ITS EXISTENCE TO TENNIS

Leandro Panizzon was a chemist in the laboratories of the pharmaceutical giant CIBA. He had many responsibilities, but on the side, he was fascinated with the amphetamine molecule. He couldn't help but think that there was more to amphetamine than just weight control and head colds. He began tinkering with the molecule, altering a small part of it, and then another, but for a number of years his obsession went nowhere.

Marguerite, his wife, was an avid tennis player, and one day in 1944, he noticed that she was not on her game. She just didn't seem focused and was making errors common for beginners. He had just modified the amphetamine molecule yet again and had produced a new molecule, which he called methylphenidate. He felt that methylphenidate just might give her a little more energy and, at the same time, reduce her waistline. As was the habit in those days, chemists often tested their original discoveries on themselves, or occasionally on family members. He convinced Marguerite to try this new chemical substance. The effect was quick and dramatic. Both of them noticed a sudden improvement in her tennis game, and she lost a few pounds as well. Leandro had to come up with a new name for this substance, so he named it after his wife. His nickname for Marguerite was Rita, so he called this new chemical Ritalin.

In 1957, CIBA Pharmaceutical Co. began marketing methylphenidate as Ritalin to treat chronic fatigue, depression, psychosis associated with depression, narcolepsy, and to offset the sedating effects of other medications.

Remember that Dr. Bradley had first used amphetamine from the Benzedrine inhaler to treat his patients for severe headaches, but instead noticed a profound improvement in their attention and learning. This finding was ignored for more than twenty years, but by the late 1950s, ADHD (then called the hyperkinetic syndrome) was being described and diagnosed with increasing frequency.

Ritalin use increased in the 1970s and early 1980s, but prescriptions for Ritalin spiked between 1991 and 1999, increasing 500 percent.[14] As the diagnosis of ADHD was made with increasing frequency, and as physicians became more comfortable prescribing Dexedrine (amphetamine) and Ritalin (methylphenidate), many others were concerned that teachers were putting excessive pressure on parents to medicate their children with drugs that were potentially addictive because the teachers were too incompetent to teach. And parents were getting a not-so-subtle message from their physicians that they were being medically neglectful for not providing appropriate medical treatment for their children. Many of the schools were receiving federal funding, and congressmen were receiving complaints from their constituents. They were beginning to feel compelled to examine the issue and maybe limit the use of these medications in children. Pressure was building from all sides, and it seemed that the issue was ripe for a more public battle. Actually, the issue was ripe for an explosion. And that is exactly what happened.

RITALIN GOES MAINSTREAM

The year was 1970. I was a sophomore at the University of Kansas. The Vietnam War was at its height, and demonstrations on university campuses were common across the United States.

One of my classes was on the current literature that antiwar proponents were reading. Professor Hamilton was highly charismatic; and although he projected an air of objectivity, it was clear that he was more than liberally leaning. His classes were in high demand, and each class usually generated a great deal of enthusiastic debate.

On June 29, 1970, Robert Maynard wrote an article for the *Washington Post* titled "Omaha Pupils Given 'Behavior Drugs.'"[15] Dr. Hamilton made this article the focus of his next class.

The article got right to the point. The first sentence stated, "Between 5 and 10 percent of the 62,000 school children in this city in the American midlands are taking 'behavior modification' drugs (Ritalin and Dexedrine) prescribed by local doctors to improve behavior and increase learning potential." The article went much further and implicated one particular physician who prescribed the medications for most of the children. The article insinuated that the teachers, the school system, and this physician had collaborated to intimidate parents into giving these medications to their children.[16]

> This was part of a directed program by the school system in which some parental coercion to submit to drug therapy was involved, and that drugs were being given without adequate medical supervision resulting in pill swapping in school.[17]

To this day, I remember my reaction in that college classroom. I was outraged and indignant. But I did not participate in the discussion that ensued after the article was read. I remember sitting there thinking that this was wrong, that it could not be justified in any way, and that I had to do something to stop this medical abuse of children.

Apparently, my reaction was not unusual, and the reaction to this article was swift and furious. Numerous newspapers carried a summary of the article and then went on to write about the use of these medications in their communities.[18]

And the article caught the eye of a New Jersey congressman, Cornelious Gallagher. Less than four months after publication of the *Washington Post* article, Gallagher convened congressional hearings, with the following statement:

> I am well aware of the occasional frustrations which come from the fact that children simply do not sit quietly and perform assigned tasks. . . . For childhood is an exploratory time and the great energy of children propels them into situations which may look frivolous to

more restrained adults, but which are the sum and substance of the child's learning experience . . . Obvioulsy this unstructured passion for all the events in a child's world is regarded as unruly and disruptive, partiularly in overcrowded classrooms. I fear that there is a very great temptation to diagnose the bored but bright child as hyperactive, prescribe drugs, and thus deny him full learning during his most creative years.[19]

During the hearings, one mother testified:

The teacher started complaining about our little girl being too active, and soon the school nurse called me and suggested that I put her on tranquilizers. We objected as we do not believe in handing drugs out so freely. Soon the school started calling us up and complaining about her beahvior. They said she was restless and overactive, but not bad or disrespectful. Finally the school psychologist made an appointment with me and told me to put my daughter on Ritalin . . . I told her I didn't like the idea. . . . She made me feel as though I was a stupid, neglectful parent who was only doing my child harm by not giving her this Ritalin.

The reason that this incident has stayed with me is that it was instrumental in spawning my career as a developmental pediatrician. But the reason I mention it here is not autobiographical, but because it so strikingly illustrates what happens when statistics are misunderstood or taken out of context.

Many years later I learned that these figures misrepresented the facts. The statement that 5–10 percent of all Omaha Public School children were taking medication for behvaior control was completely and totally inaccurate. In fact, 5–10 percent of children *with special education disabilities* were receiving these medications.

Approximately 45 percent of children with ADHD have an associated learning disability as well. Thus, ADHD would obviously be overrepresented in a group of children with special education needs. As a matter of fact, the surprise is that the statement that 5–10 percent of children with special education needs are on stimulant medication would today, fifty years later, stand as a significant *underestimate*.

And rather than starting me on a crusade to ban the use of these medications in the classroom, I estimate that during my career as a developmental pediatrician, I have treated more than five thousand children with ADHD with stimulant medication. Obviously, something happened over the forty years, beginning with my righteous indignation as a young college student.

What changed? Once I finished my residency in pediatrics and my fellowship in developmental pediatrics, I started seeing children having trouble learning in school. After a full battery of tests including IQ tests, achievement tests, and processing tests, I would use medication only in the most severe cases. I was still skeptical about the use of medication, so I made arrangements with a pharmacist so that when I suspected ADHD, I would start medication in a double-blind trial. Upon my prescription, the pharmacist would give the patients six bottles, with seven pills in each bottle, one bottle for each of six weeks. Three of the bottles contained medication and three contained placebos. Both parents and teachers would fill out weekly questionnaires concerning learning and behavior. When I saw dramatic improvement in both behavior and learning only during the weeks when the child was on medication, then I would continue the medication with close follow-up.

Eventually, I would use these trials only when I had a doubt about the diagnosis or when two parents differed about the use of medication. Over time, when I continued to see improvement with few side effects from medication, I began to look more closely at the milder cases. Over time, I would see the children on medication thrive. Grades improved. Behavior problems that had not responded to counseling or behavior modification suddenly diminished . . . or vanished. And, most important, self-esteem skyrocketed. Children with ADHD had convinced themselves that they were "dumb." But with medication, they quickly began to see their inattention, not a lack of effort, as the problem.

How could I not continue medication when I saw a child's self-esteem flourish? This was not about making life easier for a teacher or parent. This was not about a lack of discipline at home. This was about the physical and mental health of a child who had been suffering before and now exhibited happiness and success in school and at home.

Chapter 4

IS ADHD REALLY REAL?

BUT WAIT! ISN'T ADHD OVERDIAGNOSED?

A few years ago, I visited my dermatologist for my annual checkup. He was not in the office that day, so I saw another dermatologist in the same practice. She came into the exam room, introduced herself, and then began to look at my chart.

"Oh, I see here that you are a physician. What kind of medicine do you practice?"

"I'm a developmental pediatrician. I see children with ADHD, autism, cerebral palsy, learning disabilities, that kind of thing."

"ADHD, huh? That's kind of overdiagnosed, isn't it?"

I hesitated for a second, then said, "Uh, let me answer that question by asking you a question. What is the prevalence of skin cancer in people over the age of sixty?"

"Well, about 40 percent of people over the age of sixty will get skin cancer at some point."

"Oh, that's really high. Skin cancer must be overdiagnosed then, isn't it?"

"No, those are accurate numbers. The rate of occurrence is high because people don't take care of their skin. They go out to the beach without sunscreen, don't moisturize their skin. . . . Oh, wait a minute, I see what you are trying to do."

The message here is that just because a disease or disorder is diagnosed in a lot of people, it does not mean that it is overdiagnosed.

Many people feel that ADHD is overdiagnosed. What they are really implying with this statement is that the actual prevalence of ADHD is higher than they would expect.

The prevalence of a disease is the percentage of people in a defined population that has that disease at any given time. So, what is the prevalence of ADHD? Most studies indicate that 6–8 percent of children have ADHD.[1]

The Centre for Research in Evidence-Based Practice at Bond University in Queensland, Australia, examined 175 different international studies that met criteria for high research standards. They found that the average prevalence of ADHD was 7.2 percent.[2]

In 2016 the National Survey of Children's Health conducted a survey of more than forty-five thousand children 0–17 years of age across the United States. They found that 9.4 percent of children in the survey had been diagnosed with ADHD. Some 62 percent of those children were treated with medication, and 47 percent were treated with behavioral therapy.[3]

The Center for Pediatric Psychopathology at the Massachusetts General Hospital in Boston examined twenty studies from the United States and thirty studies from other countries that used the same diagnostic criteria as in the United States. They found that the prevalence of ADHD in countries around the world was about the same as in the United States.[4]

Hundreds of studies have been conducted to estimate the prevalence of ADHD in the United States and across the world. Even though different populations were surveyed and different diagnostic criteria were used, the findings are surprisingly consistent. ADHD occurs in approximately 6–8 percent of children throughout the world.

That is an impressive number. Approximately seventy-four million children live in the United States,[5] and these studies all support the finding that ADHD affects approximately five million children in the United States alone. And that doesn't include the adults with ADHD.

Many people feel that this number is way too high. Some of them feel that doctors are overdiagnosing ADHD because it is so much easier to give a pill. Some of them feel that poor teaching or poor schools are responsible. Others blame the parents for not disciplining their children. Some people blame poor diets and food additives and TV and cell phones.

Many people believe that ADHD is overdiagnosed for many different reasons. And in some cases, children are misdiagnosed, and some of the explanations above are valid for some children. But ADHD is perceived to be misdiagnosed for two main reasons:

1. ADHD lacks an objective tool for making a diagnosis.
2. The symptoms of ADHD are normal behaviors that everyone exhibits, occasionally, some of the time.

Let's examine how these two statements may explain much of the concern that ADHD is overdiagnosed.

OVERDIAGNOSIS EXPLANATION #1: ADHD LACKS AN OBJECTIVE DIAGNOSTIC TEST

Imagine that you are eating dinner with your family, and your spouse tells you, "I heard today that Jim, our next-door neighbor, was just diagnosed with leukemia." And you respond, "That's terrible. But, hey, last week I was playing golf with Mark down the block, and he said that he was just diagnosed with leukemia, too. What a coincidence." Over the next few days, you learn that Susan across the street was diagnosed with leukemia about a month ago, and her husband is going through the same tests. They think that he might have leukemia as well. Over the next few weeks, you learn that of the seventy-five people on your block, eight have been diagnosed with leukemia in just four months.

What would be your reaction? You might think, *I don't know what's going on with those doctors, but obviously leukemia is being overdiagnosed.* Or, *Maybe it is because the treatment of leukemia requires expensive drugs that can increase the profits of the pharmaceutical companies, or maybe it is because they are not eating the right kinds of food?* No, I think your reaction might be more like, *Oh, my god, maybe there is something in the water, or maybe those power lines behind us are emitting some kind of radiation.*

The important difference between leukemia and ADHD is that leukemia is relatively easy to diagnose. Abnormalities in a common blood test done at most annual checkups can strongly suggest leukemia.

Further tests on the bone marrow allow a pathologist to place some of the white blood cells under a microscope and find characteristic changes in them that unequivocally make the diagnosis of leukemia. But for ADHD, no such test exists. There is no blood test, no genetic test, no X-ray, no EEG test, no MRI[6] that will "make the diagnosis of ADHD." MRI and genetic testing abnormalities have been found in some children with ADHD,[7] but these findings do not occur with enough consistency to accurately diagnose ADHD.

It is easy to be sceptical about the validity of the diagnosis when a diagnostic test is not available, but the lack of an objective medical test to confirm the diagnosis does not mean that the diagnosis is invalid. Remember that leukemia has been occurring for centuries and for most of that time, no objective test was available to make the diagnosis.

But ADHD is thought to be overdiagnosed for another reason.

OVERDIAGNOSIS EXPLANATION #2: ADHD IS A COLLECTION OF NORMAL BEHAVIORS THAT OCCUR IN EVERYONE, OCCASIONALLY

Symptoms of ADHD (Primarily Inattentive)
Difficulty paying attention
Trouble staying focused
Does not listen
Does not follow through on instructions
Disorganized
Avoids tasks requiring sustained mental effort
Loses thing
Easily distracted
Forgetful

Symptoms of a Stroke
Confusion
Difficulty walking
Paralysis on only one side of the body
Blurred or Double Vison
Slurred speech
Difficulty finding words to express oneself
Difficulty swallowing
Headache
Dizziness

Look at these two lists. The first is a list of behaviors most commonly seen in children with ADHD, primarily inattentive type. The second is a list of symptoms associated with a stroke. ADHD is clearly a very different disorder than a stroke, and you would expect the symptoms to be very different. They are. But ask yourself, what is different between the two lists, beyond the fact that the symptoms are different. The ADHD symptoms can all be considered "normal" behaviors in all people, if they occur occasionally and under certain circumstances. Everyone gets distracted, occasionally. Everyone loses things, at times. Everyone forgets things, on occasion. On the other hand, the stroke symptoms would be considered "abnormal" in any person of any age and in any circumstance. Would you ever consider the sudden onset of paralysis on one side of the body and slurred speech to be a "normal" behavior? Ever?

The *DSM-5* diagnostic criteria described in Chapter 1 rely on subjective observations of behaviors, and subjectivity leads to variability. I have seen many cases where the reading teacher will describe a child with many ADHD behaviors, but the math teacher will identify few ADHD behaviors in the same child. This difference in observations might be because the child does well in understanding math concepts but has difficulty reading and, therefore, has difficulty staying focused on something that he perceives as "too difficult." But it might also be because the teachers have different thresholds for being concerned with a particular behavior. At home, his mother may see many of these behaviors, because she spends a lot of time trying to keep her child focused on homework, while his father may be less likely to identify these behaviors as problems while they are throwing a football or playing in the backyard.

And that is what is at the heart of the belief that ADHD is overdiagnosed. ***All ADHD behaviors occur in everyone, sometimes.*** If they occur only occasionally and do not affect the overall learning or development of our children, we consider this just proof that we are all imperfect human beings. So how do we decide when distractibility is "occasional" and thus "normal" in one child, or abnormal and indicating ADHD in the other?

It is hard to believe that a collection of behaviors that occur in everyone from time to time can constitute a medical disorder. These "ADHD behaviors" occur on a spectrum. We can all agree that at one end of the spectrum occasionally forgetting something or occasionally having difficulty focusing is normal. But let us also accept the proposition that at the other end of the spectrum, when these behaviors occur frequently and when these behaviors significantly affect learning and social development, then we have a problem. Danny dedicated twenty-five pages of this book to demonstrate that at the extreme end of the spectrum the ADHD behaviors are too frequent and significantly affect learning so that they need further attention and cannot be ignored.

To further complicate this situation, some ADHD behaviors can be positive and productive, in certain circumstances and at certain times. For example, take impulsivity. Impulsivity could be defined as doing something without thinking about the consequences of that action. Is impulsivity a good trait or a bad trait? If you are a child standing in line to go out for recess, and the child next to you bumps into you, you can ignore that behavior, assuming that it was unintentional. Or you can push the child away. The second response would usually be considered impulsive, because you did not go through the thought process above. In that case, impulsivity would be considered socially inappropriate and would interfere with a child's ability to learn in the classroom and to form good social relationships.

However, consider a different scenario. You are driving your car, waiting at an intersection for a red light to turn green. It finally turns green, and you begin to apply your foot to the accelerator. However, at that same moment, an eight-year-old girl darts across the crosswalk, right in front of your car. What do you think at that moment? Do you think, *Oh, if I continue accelerating I am going to hit that girl. I need to transfer my foot from the accelerator to the brake.* No, most people would respond immediately, without thinking at all, and slam on the brakes. Everyone would agree that in this case, you do not have the luxury of time to think things through. Your ability to react quickly, impulsively, without thinking, saved the life of an eight-year-old girl.

Now, consider the symptoms of a stroke. Is there ever a time that you would lose part of your vision and consider that a productive behavior? Is there ever a time that you would consider paralysis of your right arm to be "normal"? Would you consider it normal and productive to be confused and unable to speak?

The difference between these two sets of symptoms is qualitative. The ADHD behaviors could be considered normal at some time or in some situations or at certain ages. The symptoms of a stroke normal? Never.

When the symptoms of a disorder are often normal behaviors, and when no medical test can unequivocally make the diagnosis, then it is perfectly understandable that people would doubt the validity of ADHD as a discrete diagnosis requiring medical treatment and assume the ADHD is no more than a collection of personality traits.

However, gradually, I came to the realization that that whole argument about whether ADHD is overdiagnosed just didn't matter. When I see an eight-year-old girl who is hyperactive, impulsive, inattentive, and disorganized, and when those behaviors are interfering with her ability to learn in the classroom, and when I have ruled out other causes of this ADHD behavior, only two scenarios are possible. Either the prevalence of ADHD in my office is 100 percent or it is 0 percent. It doesn't matter to me on that day, with that one child, at that moment, whether the prevalence of ADHD across the United States is 5 percent or 10 percent or 82 percent. I am addressing only one child at a time, and either she has ADHD (100 percent) or not (0 percent).

If she does have ADHD behaviors consistently and to the degree that it affects her learning, I can predict that she will have even more difficulty learning as the work gets more difficult and as the academic expectations become more demanding. Because of multiple long-term follow-up research studies, I can accurately predict that if her ADHD goes undiagnosed and untreated, she is at a higher risk to obtain grades in school significantly lower than her true cognitive potential, which will have a significant effect on her learning and self-esteem.

When the stakes are that high, and when the medications used to treat ADHD are effective 90 percent of the time with virtually no long-term, serious side effects, why would we deny a child the right to a happy, successful childhood and eventually a happy, productive life?

SO ADHD BEHAVIORS ARE NEUROLOGICALLY BASED. BUT COULDN'T ADHD BE A NORMAL PERSONALITY THAT EVOLVED OVER TIME?

In 1993 Thom Hartmann wrote a book titled *Attention Deficit Disorder: A Different Perception* in which he describes a very different way to visualize ADHD.

Distractibility is a hallmark of ADHD. Is distractibility a good thing or a bad thing? Most people would respond that it is a terrible thing, especially if you are a seven-year-old in a classroom of twenty-four children, trying to pay attention to the teacher's instructions. But suppose for a moment that that seven-year-old had been born 100,000 years ago? He would have been a caveman, living in a small tribe of maybe thirty people. You depend on each other, supporting each other with your different skills and talents. One of your jobs might have been to pick berries off a group of bushes near the cave. One day, you are bent over a bush, picking berries and placing them in a pouch. You hear a slight rustling in the bushes behind you. What should you do? You might say, "Start running," but if every time you heard a rustling in the bushes you ran back to the cave, you would never get the berries picked. Your tribe would never have breakfast, and you might get kicked out of the tribe. You would die young and childless.

On the other hand, when you hear rustling in the bushes behind you, a better idea might be to turn and look to see what caused the sound. If it was the wind, which was no threat, you could turn back and resume your job picking berries. However, if you turned and could see the movement of a tail attached to a saber-toothed tiger, you might decide to run, or instead, pull your knife to fight off the tiger. If you get back to the cave alive, then your distractibility saved your life. You would be praised by the other tribe members, you would live longer, you would have more children, and you would be much more likely to transmit your "distractibility" gene to the next generation.

So, at one point in our development as human beings, distractibility was an advantage, not part of a disorder at all.

What about impulsivity? Impulsivity is another behavior almost always present in children with ADHD. Impulsivity is defined as doing something without thinking about the consequences. Is *that* a good thing or a bad thing?

You are a six-year-old playing on a playground with other six-year-olds, and every time you want to get the attention of another child, you push her. That would not be seen as normal or productive behavior in this century. Everyone is impulsive at times, but if it occurs too frequently and interferes with your ability to live productively with other people in today's world, impulsivity can lead to poor social development, car accidents, and other risky behavior.

But what if that impulsive six-year-old had been born in Iceland two thousand years ago? As he grew into a teenager, he would undergo additional training by his tribe. If an enemy charges at him with a sword, he doesn't have time to ask himself, *Why is Sven charging at me? Maybe I should move out of the way and try to talk to him. Maybe I should yell at him. Maybe I should . . .* He has one-tenth of a second to respond. If his training has been effective, his response to draw his sword and fight off Sven would be the difference between living and dying. And if he lived, he could credit his impulsivity with saving his life. He would live a long life and father many children and pass that impulsivity gene to his children. Impulsivity then becomes a positive characteristic, at least in Iceland two thousand years ago.

When I first became aware of this argument, I thought it made good sense. Maybe ADHD is not a disease at all. Maybe it is just a difference in personalities. Some kids who would have been proficient in the world 100,000 years ago, or even 2,000 years ago, would meet multiple challenges in the twenty-first century that would dramatically interfere with their ability to learn and to live with other people in an orderly and productive society.

However, I struggled with this argument. Could ADHD just be considered personality traits at the extreme end of the spectrum of normal behaviors? And what is normal behavior? I remember my mother's oft-repeated comment fifty years ago when I was growing up: "Most people are normal."

But then I think of Danny. He may have been a leader of his tribe 100,000 years ago, but he lives in the twenty-first century. Our society is immensely different from what it was back then. Although his distractibility and impulsivity may have been very positive traits then, they are now only impediments to functioning well with others, in classrooms, in offices, and in social groups.

ADHD probably did evolve as a group of productive behaviors. But as our society has morphed and become incredibly more complex, children who were once potential leaders of their tribe are now sitting miserably in a classroom that makes it so difficult for them to learn that they give up. No one benefits from that scenario.

As a physician, once I have identified that a child is having great difficulty learning in the classroom and developing appropriate social relationships, and once I have attributed those difficulties to ADHD, I have three choices:

First, I could invent a time machine and send him back to live with cavemen or send him back to Iceland to enjoy the praise and power that would come with being a leader of his tribe. Unfortunately, neither I nor anyone else has been very successful with time travel.

Second, I could try to change the way we educate children all over the country. Children with ADHD are often quite intelligent and creative, but most schools say to their students, "We will teach you the way that has worked for us for hundreds of years. And to be successful at our school, you not only need to be intelligent and creative, but you also need to be structured and work hard for long, uninterrupted periods of time. You need to be polite and friendly, and, most important, you need to follow the rules. If you can do that, you will be successful in my classroom and in our school."

But what they don't say and what they may be thinking is "and if you can't, then we don't want you." So, I did attempt to change how children with ADHD are taught in the classroom. I purchased a small private school of a few classrooms with about fifty children with learning disabilities and developed it into a school that was, in my mind, a perfect environment for the ADHD child. We started with the assumption that if a child is not learning at our school, we don't blame him for being lazy. Instead of requiring a child to learn the way we teach, we instead blame ourselves for not finding a way to teach a child the way he learns. And that goal has been realized at Tampa Day School in Tampa, Florida. If all children with ADHD could be taught in such a school, then they could grow into adults who celebrate their differences and use them to find a career and lifestyle that is right for them. Unfortunately, it is hard to convince a school system that is different from county to county and state to state to remodel a school system with the same goals. Further, although such an educational approach does help a child to learn and to develop the skills to learn in college and on the job, it does not change the fact that his distractibility and impulsivity will become significant impediments in college and, especially, in the workplace.

My third choice is medication. Now that's a bold choice! I just told you that ADHD is not an abnormality, and now I want to medicate a normal child? That doesn't make sense. But it does. We have seen that ADHD is a "mismatch" between a child's attention span and the world and time in which she lives. If we can't change that world, then maybe we can change the way she pays attention and the way she learns in the classroom. And if medication reverses the way certain proteins work in the brain, the child with ADHD behaviors will now attend and focus and learn the way every other child does. And isn't that the goal? Yes, although it doesn't seem fair that a child without a disease, without an abnormality will need to take a medication for years.

But the only other choice is to let him continue to struggle and fail in the classroom despite his intelligence and desire to succeed like everyone else. The only other choice is to allow that constant struggling and failing in school to destroy his self-esteem, so that it is easier to give up than to continue to fight a battle without hope of success. The only other choice is to continue to expose him to the jokes and bullying and rejection of other children. I am not willing to do that. And that is why I choose to offer medication as an option. I will continue to recommend tutoring and special schooling and executive function training. But if those alternatives fail, then we have no other choice but to consider medication.

WHAT CAUSES ADHD?

It seems that many people have their own beliefs about the cause of ADHD. Some people feel that ADHD is caused by any one or combination of the following:

- Sugar
- TV
- Video games
- Cell phone and other computer screens
- Lack of sleep
- Lack of parental discipline
- Poor teachers
- And about fifty other explanations

And the truth is that in some cases, these factors play a role in producing some of the symptoms of ADHD. For example, a teenager may get into bed at 11 p.m., scroll through her phone, posting texts and pictures, until 2:30 a.m. She falls asleep but is shocked awake by an alarm only four hours later. She rolls over and goes back to sleep, only to have her mother open the door, flip on the light, and yell at her to get out of bed. That child **will** probably have trouble staying focused in the classroom. This book is not about this child. This book is about the many other children who have trouble with hyperactive behavior, trouble paying attention, distractibility and difficulty completing their work, starting as early as three years of age—despite the fact that they sleep nine hours each night, eat three healthy meals a day, have very focused, intelligent, organized parents; great teachers; and organized schools.

It can be difficult to distinguish whether certain behaviors (inattention, hyperactivity, difficulty organizing, etc.) are caused by problems in the child's daily life (environmental effects such as poor diet, parents arguing, lack of sleep, disorganized school or teacher) or whether these behaviors have a neurological basis. However, if a physician takes a detailed history, if she confirms that the criteria of ADHD are met; if she determines that these behaviors are present in two or more settings, have had a significant impact on learning or social skills, had their onset before twelve years of age, and have no other medical cause, then hundreds of research studies have determined that these behaviors very likely are neurologically based.

In 2007 the American Academy of Child and Adolescent Psychiatry published a comprehensive review of ADHD. It concluded, "Although scientists and clinicians debate the best way to diagnose and treat ADHD, there is no debate among competent and well-informed health care professionals that ADHD is a valid neurobiological condition that causes significant impairment in those whom it afflicts."[8]

WHAT IS HAPPENING IN THE BRAIN OF A CHILD WITH ADHD?

To understand the source of ADHD, it is first necessary to understand a little bit about how the brain works.

Let me ask you two questions:

First, do you know how many people presently live on Earth? If you said seven billion, you would be approximately right.

Second, do you use Facebook? If so, how many friends do you have? I would suspect that most of you reading this book would reply that either you don't use Facebook, or you have a few hundred friends. Your son or daughter might have 5–10 times that number.

Now, imagine that there are fourteen Earths. On each one of these Earths live seven billion people. That's approximately 100 billion people on those fourteen planets. Now, imagine that each of those 100 billion people has a Facebook account and that each of them has 10,000 friends. Now, imagine that every one of those 100 billion people on those fourteen Earths sends a message to every one of their 10,000 friends, all at the same time, and this process is repeated ten times every second. I would presume that whatever computers were involved in transmitting all these messages would melt down under the demands of such a system. And, yet, that is approximately what happens in the average developing child's brain.

Every child's brain is a collection of approximately 100 billion nerve cells, or neurons. Each neuron has extensive branches that link to thousands of other neurons. So, every one of those 100 billion neurons links with approximately 10,000 other neurons in the same way that the 100 billion people with Facebook accounts communicate with their 10,000 friends.

The point of connection between one neuron and another is called a synapse. At each synapse, neurons do not actually touch; the synapse is a minutely small space between neurons (Figure 4.1).

When one neuron sends a message to another neuron, an electrical impulse travels down the neuron until it reaches another neuron, ending at a synapse. In the synapse of the sending neuron are small packets of chemicals called neurotransmitters that are used to communicate with the receiving neuron. When the electrical impulse reaches the synapse, it causes a release of those neurotransmitters into the space of the synapse. The neurotransmitters then cross the synapse and attach to receptors on the receiving neuron. These receptors are like a lock, and the neurotransmitters act as keys to open the lock. The receptors are designed such that they will only allow a specific neurotransmitter to fit into the

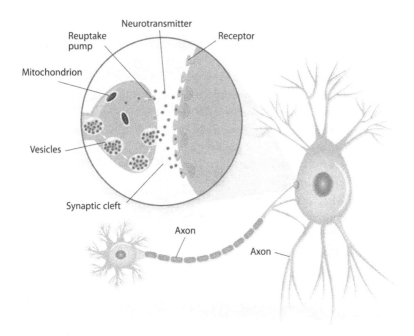

Figure 4.1 Neuron. © iStock / Getty Images Plus / ttsz; https://en.wikipedia.org/wiki/Neuron.

receptor. The receiving neuron then "gets the message." This process continues again and again with tens of thousands of other neurons.

You may have noticed a very big potential problem with this process. Once neurotransmitters have filled up most of the receptors, they block any new messages coming from the sending neuron. So, if this is the end of the process, then every nerve cell could only fire once in its lifetime, and never again. Within seconds after birth, the brain would become completely nonfunctional and would shut down.

Fortunately, the neurons have developed a final step. Within each synapse are transporter proteins. When they detect that a neurotransmitter is locked into a receptor neuron, the transporter protein attaches to the neurotransmitter and *removes* it. It kicks the key out of the lock. It then moves back to the sending neuron and injects the neurotransmitter back into the neuron. This recycling process saves energy (the sending neuron doesn't need to manufacture more neurotransmitters every time a neuron fires). More important, once this process is complete, neurotransmitters have been removed from all of the receiving neuron receptors, which allows the sending neuron to transmit another message.

Why is it necessary to delve into such detail about the anatomy of the brain and its chemical interactions? *Because ADHD happens in the synapse.* To understand why ADHD occurs in some people and what medication does in the brain, it is necessary to understand what is happening in the synapse.

Current research strongly indicates that ADHD occurs because of a difference in the way that the transporter proteins function in the brain. But these differences do not occur across the entire brain. In three different areas of the brain the transporter protein acts differently. We are going to focus on those three areas that appear to be responsible for most or all of the symptoms of ADHD (Figure 4.2).

The prefrontal cortex is a recently evolved area of the brain that is most developed in humans. It sits at the very front of the brain, just behind the eyes. The prefrontal cortex is responsible for planning and organization. When you decide that you had better start reading the book assigned in English literature class so that you can finish the book report on time, you are using your prefrontal cortex. The prefrontal cortex develops slowly in children and is not functioning fully until the mid-twenties.

The second area of the brain implicated in causing ADHD behaviors is the fronto-striato-cerebellar projections. These are longer

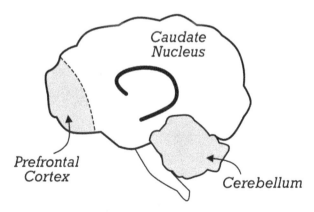

Figure 4.2   Areas of the brain affected by ADHD. Original Artwork - James Kelly.

neurons that allow communication between the prefrontal cortex and other areas of the brain, especially the cerebellum. These connecting neurons are responsible for the ability of the brain to attend to certain thoughts or activities and ignore other, nonrelevant thoughts and activities.

Finally, the caudate nucleus is located deep within the center of the brain. It plays a critical role in learning, especially allowing for the storing and processing of memories.[9] It uses information from past experiences to influence future actions and decisions.[10]

When you think about the behaviors seen in children with ADHD, it is not at all surprising that these areas of the brain are involved. Children with ADHD have more difficulty planning. They are often late, or they lose track of time (prefrontal cortex). They especially have trouble focusing and attending (fronto-striato-cerebellar projections) and have great difficulty retaining information that they have learned (caudate nucleus).

How do we know that these areas of the brain are most affected in children with ADHD? Some of the most convincing studies have examined the difference in the size of certain areas of the brain using MRI scans. A group of people with ADHD will be scanned and their scans can be averaged together. This scan is then compared against an average of the scans from people without ADHD. The size of each area of the brain is then compared.

Which areas of the brain have been found to be smaller in ADHD children? The prefrontal cortex,[11] the fronto-striato-cerebellar projections,[12] and the caudate nucleus.[13]

Neurotransmitters are the chemical messengers in the synapse that allow a message to be sent from one neuron to the next. Approximately two hundred neurotransmitters in the brain have been identified, and scientists suspect that many more have yet to be identified. The three areas of the brain implicated in the causation of ADHD are rich in two neurotransmitters, dopamine and norepinephrine.

Dopamine is the "reward neurotransmitter." When you do something that you enjoy, or when you do something that has a positive effect on the body, the brain releases dopamine in certain areas of the brain. That release of dopamine produces feelings of pleasure; and because these areas of the brain are also involved in learning, the brain learns that certain things (such as eating) should be repeated frequently.

Norepinephrine is also represented in these three brain areas as well. It is instrumental in learning and attending.

In children (and adults) with ADHD, the problem in these three areas is that the transporter proteins are *too* efficient. The neurotransmitters dopamine and norepinephrine are supposed to be released from the sending neuron and then attach to the receiving neuron, so that the receiving neuron can "get the message." After the message has been received, the transporter protein's job is to detach the neurotransmitter from the receiving neuron and move it back into the sending neuron. But if the transporter proteins work too quickly, the neurotransmitters dopamine and norepinephrine will be detached before they have a chance to stimulate the receiving neuron, and the message is not transmitted.

In people with ADHD, the receiving neurons in those three areas of the brain—those that mediate planning, organization, attention, movement, memory, and learning—are *understimulated* and not able to "pass along the message." The result is that the child will exhibit the classic symptoms of ADHD.

HOW DOES ADHD MEDICATION WORK?

ADHD medications are impostors. They have a molecular structure that mimics the structure of the neurotransmitters dopamine and norepinephrine, but they are not exactly the same. On the right side in Figure 4.3, you can see the molecular structures of the two neurotransmitters norepinephrine and dopamine. The two molecules are extremely similar in their molecular structures. The identical portion of the molecules are bolded.

Almost all medications used to treat ADHD have molecular structures that are very similar to each other and very similar to the two neurotransmitters (figure 4.3). Methylphenidate is the active ingredient in about half of the medications used to treat ADHD (e.g., Ritalin, Ritalin LA, Concerta, Daytrana, Metadate, etc.). Amphetamine is the active ingredient in the other half of the medications used to treat ADHD (e.g., Dexedrine, Adderall, Vyvanse). Both norepinephrine and dopamine play a critical role in focusing and maintaining attention.[14]

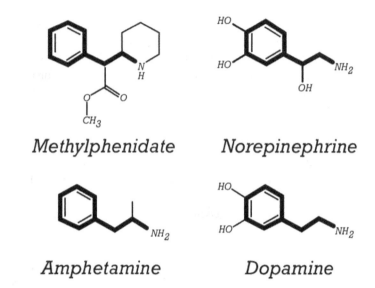

Methylphenidate   **Norepinephrine**

Amphetamine   **Dopamine**

Figure 4.3   Stimulant medication has similar chemical structure to brain neurotransmitters. Original Artwork - James Kelly; https://www.researchgate.net/figure/Chemical-structures-of-MPH-AMPH-and-of-the-neurotransmitters-NE-and-DA_fig1_316124761.

Because methylphenidate and amphetamine have molecular structures similar to the two neurotransmitters, they will bind with transporter protein receptors on the sending neuron, blocking reuptake of the neurotransmitters, causing the amount of neurotransmitter in the synapse to increase, allowing dopamine and norepinephrine more time to stimulate the receiving neuron and "move the message along."

Further, the unique structure of ADHD medications means that they will work primarily in the areas of the brain that use the dopamine and norepinephrine neurotransmitters. These areas of the brain are responsible for the characteristic behaviors of ADHD, hyperactivity, impulsivity, distractibility, and trouble learning and recalling memories.

Let's take this complex natural phenomenon and distill it down to its essential features.

Children with ADHD have three areas of the brain that are understimulated by a reduction of neurotransmitter activity in the synapse, produced by an over-efficient or overactive transporter protein. The prefrontal cortex is responsible for planning and organization, fronto-striato-cerebellar projections help a child maintain attention and ignore distractions, and the caudate nucleus is important in learning and creating memories. ADHD medications increase the activity of the neurotransmitters in these brain areas, and therefore enhance the function of these three brain areas, which result in a dramatic improvement in behavior and learning.

Chapter 5

COULD ADHD MEDICATION HELP MY CHILD?

HOW EFFECTIVE ARE ADHD MEDICATIONS?

Liz: I finally did it. I filled Danny's prescription two weeks ago, but I just couldn't bring myself to actually give him the medication. But a few days ago, his teacher told me that she had to correct him and redirect him so many times, that he broke into tears. So, I talked to Chris, and we agreed to give him his first dose of medication this morning, right before he left for Saturday morning baseball practice. Dr. Lawrence told us to start him on the medication on the weekend, so that we could see the effect of the medication or any side effects that might develop. He said that the medication might wear off about the time he comes home from school, and if we don't give the medication on the weekends, then Chris and I will never actually see him on medication and will never know how he is benefiting from the medication, or if he is having any side effects. So, I tried to avoid making a big deal. I handed him the pill and said, "Danny, you need to take this pill before we go to practice this morning."

"But, Mom, I already took my vitamin."

"No, Danny, this one's different. It's like a vitamin, but it's to help you focus in school."

"So, why do I need to take it today. I'm not going to school today, am I?"

"No, but you have to start taking it a few days before school, so you have a chance to get used to it."

"Ugh, OK, I hope it tastes better than my vitamin." He put the pill on his tongue, swallowed the water that I handed to him. "Gotta go find my mitt," and he was gone. I was actually surprised at how easy that was.

Ten minutes later, the three of us were in the car, driving to the park where his team practices. I must admit that I kept turning around and looking at Danny, to make sure that he was OK, that he wasn't zoning out or growing horns. But he looked fine.

"Mom, why do you keep looking at me?"

"Oh, just because I think you're cute."

"Ah, Mom, STOP!"

When we arrived, I turned around again to remind Danny to bring his mitt (because he almost always forgets it, and then I have to run back to the car). I started to say something but was cut short by an amazing sight. Danny opened the door and stepped out of the car with his mitt under his left arm.

The rest of practice was full of more surprises.

They played a shortened practice game. Danny is a fairly good hitter, when he focuses. His first time up at bat, he hit a ball over the left outfielder's head that bounced off the wall. He rounded first base, headed toward second, not slowing down, looking like he was going for a triple. But the ball had bounced off the wall and right into the hands of the outfielder, and he shot the ball to third base. I started to groan, because I knew what was going to happen. It had happened too often before. He was going to get tagged out at third.

But as Danny ran, he must have been watching his coach just behind third base. His coach saw the ball coming toward third and had his hands raised as if trying to push Danny back to second base. Danny immediately noticed, stopped dead in his tracks, turned around, and dove back to second base just in time.

I was amazed. He was actually watching his coach!?

"Phew, that was close," Chris said. I had almost forgotten that he was sitting next to me.

When practice was over, coach called a short meeting. All the kids stood in a semicircle around the coach. He was talking about the first game of the season next weekend. He read the starting line-up, and Danny was going to start at shortstop. Danny smiled.

As the kids started to scatter, coach called us over. "Boy, Danny had a great day, don't you think?"

I started to respond, but Chris was all excited, "You bet. A double, two singles, and that amazing home run," he responded with a big smile.

"Well, that, too," said coach, "but I was referring to the way that he was listening. He followed directions from the third-base coach. And I talked to him earlier about using a different batting stance that we had worked on last week, and he followed that throughout the game. He was paying attention and asking appropriate questions.

I started to respond, "Well, we tried something . . ."

Chris interrupted me. "Yeah, we've been working on his batting stance."

"No, it's not that he is hitting the ball well," said coach. He's always been good there. It's just that he was more "with it" today. I don't know, he's almost like a different kid."

The ride home was unusual. Chris was smiling while he was driving, probably thinking about Danny's home run. I was smiling because we weren't arguing after practice like we usually do. And Danny was smiling, for obvious reasons.

"Great practice today, Danny," said Chris.

"Yeah. Did you see my home run? Knocked it outta the park."

When we got home, Danny jumped out of the car, put his mitt back on the shelf where it belongs, and hung up his jacket. Chris and I sat in the car, talking. He wanted to talk about Danny's potential baseball career. But I wanted to talk about the big elephant in the car, his medication. He did seem more focused, more in control of himself. He wasn't running around the field when coach was trying to give directions. He wasn't interrupting coach. He followed the third-base coach's directions.

I didn't want to say it out loud, and I didn't want to spoil Chris's good mood. But could it be that Danny had such a great practice because of the medication? Could medication work that fast, after one dose, and make that much difference?

The answer is, "Yes, absolutely." Most of the medications used to treat ADHD are spinoffs of the two medications we have discussed up to this point, amphetamine and methylphenidate. Although multiple medications are used now to treat ADHD (see the medication table at the end of this book), each "new" medication is mostly a different method (liquid, chewable, short acting, long acting, etc.) for administering the same two medications.

But there is something about all ADHD medications that makes them very different from most other medications.

When penicillin was discovered, it was hailed as a medical breakthrough, sometimes referred to as the "magic bullet." But even as effective as penicillin was, as are the multiple new antibiotics currently available to physicians, it still took days before you could see their effect. If a patient has a bacterial pneumonia and antibiotic treatment is initiated, it still takes 2–3 days before he might begin to breathe more easily and 2–3 weeks before he could discontinue medication.

Antibiotics are designed to cure the infection. Once cured, you can stop the medication . . . forever. ADHD stimulant medications are the opposite. Methylphenidate and amphetamine are absorbed from the stomach into the bloodstream and can be detected in the brain as soon as 15–20 minutes after swallowing a pill. Positive changes in behavior can be seen as soon as 25–30 minutes, on the first day of treatment.

However, stimulant medications also wear off quickly, so that the effects of the medications will disappear anywhere from four to twenty-four hours after a dose (depending on the medication preparation). Once the medication has worn off, the child's neurological function and behavior revert to the way they were before medication was taken. ADHD medications work as long as there are sufficient blood and brain levels, and they stop working when the blood level drops. ADHD medications are highly effective, almost amazingly so, but they do not "cure" ADHD.

However, what I just said about how quickly the ADHD medications work is not completely true. In most cases, when physicians initiate an ADHD medication, we usually start with a dose lower than we might presume is the optimum dose. This is done to determine if side effects develop before a higher dose is given. So, in most cases, after ADHD medication is started, the child is observed for a few days. In many cases, side effects will not be evident on this low dose, but not much beneficial change may be observed either. As a result, the dose will be increased. The important message here is that once a child is on the proper dose for his or her age and weight, the effect of a single dose will be almost immediate.

HOW COULD ADHD MEDICATION HELP MY CHILD?

The decision to start any medication for any medical condition is a trade-off between benefits and side effects. A medication may reduce or eliminate the offending symptoms, but almost every medication comes with the risk of unwanted side effects. If a medication is highly effective at relieving your symptoms and if the side effects are minor and infrequent, then you will start the medication enthusiastically. On the other hand, if a medication reduces your symptoms only minimally but the side effects are serious or even life threatening, then you would run from that medication.

As we discussed earlier in this book, many people discount the existence of ADHD as a real medical condition. And many people feel that the side effects of these medications are frequent and serious. If you approach ADHD with those beliefs, then you probably will refuse medication for your child. So, what I am going to say next will either surprise you or provide you with hope that an end to your child's significant difficulties in behavior and learning is within reach.

The most commonly used ADHD medications are highly effective in diminishing or eliminating the disabling symptoms of ADHD, with minor side effects that can be minimized, and with virtually no serious side effects.

The remainder of this chapter is devoted to explaining what you can expect to see if your child has ADHD and is treated with medication. A later chapter will discuss potential side effects in detail, so that you can decide whether to use medication by contrasting the potential benefit with the potential side effects.

Three different lines of evidence together provide highly convincing confirmation of the effectiveness of certain medications to treat ADHD:

1. *Core behaviors* are the primary symptoms of ADHD (e.g., hyperactivity, impulsivity, distractibility, and difficulty focusing, attending, and listening) and ADHD medications are highly effective in minimizing or even completely eliminating the core behaviors. The beneficial effects and side effects can be seen almost immediately, as early as the first day on medication if the right dose is given.
2. *Long-term effects into adulthood.* Children with ADHD usually grow up to be adults with ADHD, but if children and adults with ADHD are appropriately treated, they are more likely to succeed as adults.

3. *Neurological effects on brain structure and function.* ADHD is caused by a difference in the way the brain functions. ADHD medications improve learning and behavior by enhancing the function of the brain at the synapse. But recent research findings on the physical structure of the brain have produced some astonishingly surprising findings that change the outcome for ADHD treatment dramatically.

CAN ADHD MEDICATIONS HELP MY CHILD'S CORE ADHD BEHAVIORS?

Core behaviors are the primary symptoms of ADHD. These behaviors were detailed at the beginning of this book. Physicians make a diagnosis of ADHD when a preponderance of behaviors are present. These behaviors include hyperactivity, impulsivity, distractibility, difficulty attending and focusing. Most of the research on the effectiveness of ADHD medications has been a study of the effects of these medications on the core symptoms of ADHD.

Lilly is a six-year-old girl who was referred to me by the family pediatrician because of her difficulty listening and because of her "resistance to behavior management strategies." At home, she is described as "stubborn." At school, the teacher said that she "typically has good behavior," although she is active and has difficulty listening and focusing. In group activities, she would sit in a chair but would be off "doing her own thing." The teacher filled out the behavioral questionnaire.

Notice that the teacher provides clear evidence of attentional difficulties, excess activity, and impulsivity (Figure 5.1). The mother's questionnaire was similar. A psychoeducational evaluation found average to superior cognitive abilities and no evidence of a learning disability. Because of her young age, and to help clarify the diagnosis, I asked our school psychologist to interview her teacher and to observe Lilly in the classroom. The teacher confirmed that Lilly had frequent difficulty following directions and "tends to be in her own world." The teacher said that she was not concerned about her overall development, but she felt that her performance in the classroom was not representative of her full potential because she had such difficulty sitting and engaging in activities for an extended period of time.

Behavior Questionnaire (Teacher)

Florida
Children's Center
3670 Henderson Boulevard
Tampa, Florida 33609
(813) 353-0211

CHILD'S NAME:
PERSON FILLING OUT FORM:
DATE OF OBSERVATION PERIOD 09/17/99
MEDICATION (OR WEEK NUMBER) none

Please mark how each of the following describes this child. Do not spend too much time thinking about each question. Mark the column that feels right.

	Never	Some times	Often	Always
1. Does not pay close attention to detail			✓	
2. Makes careless mistakes		✓		
3. Has difficulty maintaining attention for longer periods of time			✓	
4. Does not listen			✓	
5. Has difficulty following instructions			✓	
6. Does not finish what is started (schoolwork or chores) (not due to refusal or failure to understand instructions)			✓	
7. Seems unorganized			✓	
8. Reluctant to do challenging tasks requiring prolonged mental effort (like schoolwork, homework or chores)				✓
9. Loses things necessary for tasks or activities (e.g., toys, school assignments, or books)			✓	
10. Distractible		✓		
11. Forgetful			✓	
A-total				
12. Fidgets or squirms in seat			✓	
13. Leaves seat in classroom or in other situations in which remaining seated is expected (for example, mealtimes)				✓
14. Runs about or climbs excessively when she/he knows she/he should not		✓		
15. Has difficulty playing quietly		✓		
16. Is "on the go" or acts as if "driven by a motor"			✓	
17. Talks a lot				
H-total				
18. Blurts out answers before questions have been completed			✓	
19. Has difficulty awaiting turns			✓	
20. Does things without considering the consequences				✓

	Never	Some times	Often	Always
21. Interrupts or intrudes on others (i.e., butts into conversations or games, or talks out of turn)			✓	
22. Has difficulty developing or following a plan for schoolwork or other activities			✓	
I-total				
23. Loses temper		✓		
24. Argues with adults	✓			
25. Refuses to obey rules or commands	✓			
26. Deliberately annoys people		✓	✓	
27. Blames others for his or her mistakes or misbehavior			✓	
28. Is touchy or easily annoyed by others		✓		
29. Seems angry		✓		
30. Spiteful or wants revenge	✓			
31. Hits adults	✓			
32. Hits other children	✓			
O-total				
33. Seems sad, unhappy or depressed			✓	
34. Cries or whines easily	✓			
35. Seems nervous or irritable		✓	✓	
36. Facial tics or twitches		✓		
37. Decreased appetite N/A				
38. Drowsy or sleeping during the day		✓		
39. Seems "like a zombie"	✓			
40. Seems to have lost the "spark" in his or her personality		✓		
41. Headaches N/A				
42. Stomachaches	✓			
SE-total				

Adapted from The Diagnostic and Statistical Manual of Mental Disorders, 4th Edition, American Psychiatric Association, Washington, D. C., 1994

December 1997
Walt Karniski, M. D.
Florida Children's Center

Figure 5.1 Teacher questionnaire describing Lilly's behavior prior to ADHD diagnosis.

Physical examination was normal, with no evidence of any medical conditions that might be interfering with her ability to focus and attend. Parents were found to be fairly consistent and appropriate in their discipline strategies at home, and no home environmental difficulties were identified. Lilly was enrolled in a social skills class with other children

Behavior Questionnaire (Teacher)

CHILD'S NAME:
PERSON FILLING OUT FORM
DATE OF OBSERVATION PERIOD   10/04/99   SR Ritalin
MEDICATION (OR WEEK NUMBER)   yes   12 mg

Florida
Children's Center
3670 Henderson Boulevard
Tampa, Florida 33609
(813) 353-0211

Please mark how each of the following describes this child. Do not spend too much time thinking about each question. Mark the column that feels right.

	Never	Some times	Often	Always
1. Does not pay close attention to detail				
2. Makes careless mistakes		✓		
3. Has difficulty maintaining attention for longer periods of time		✓		
4. Does not listen		✓		
5. Has difficulty following instructions		✓		
6. Does not finish what is started (schoolwork or chores) (not due to refusal or failure to understand instructions)	✓			
7. Seems unorganized		✓		
8. Reluctant to do challenging tasks requiring prolonged mental effort (like schoolwork, homework or chores)		✓		
9. Loses things necessary for tasks or activities (e.g., toys, school assignments, or books)	✓			
10. Distractible		✓		
11. Forgetful		✓		
A-total				
12. Fidgets or squirms in seat		✓		
13. Leaves seat in classroom or in other situations in which remaining seated is expected (for example, mealtimes)		✓		
14. Runs about or climbs excessively when she/he knows she/he should not		✓		
15. Has difficulty playing quietly	✓			
16. Is "on the go" or acts as if "driven by a motor"		✓		
17. Talks a lot		✓		
H-total				
18. Blurts out answers before questions have been completed	✓			
19. Has difficulty awaiting turns		✓		
20. Does things without considering the consequences				

	Never	Some times	Often	Always
21. Interrupts or intrudes on others (i.e., butts into conversations or games, or talks out of turn)		✓		
22. Has difficulty developing or following a plan for schoolwork or other activities				
I-total				
23. Loses temper	✓			
24. Argues with adults	✓			
25. Refuses to obey rules or commands	✓			
26. Deliberately annoys people			✓	
27. Blames others for his or her mistakes or misbehavior	✓			
28. Is touchy or easily annoyed by others			✓	
29. Seems angry	✓			
30. Spiteful or wants revenge	✓			
31. Hits adults	✓			
32. Hits other children	✓			
O-total				
33. Seems sad, unhappy or depressed serious				
34. Cries or whines easily	✓			
35. Seems nervous or irritable			✓	
36. Facial tics or twitches	✓			
37. Decreased appetite NA				
38. Drowsy or sleeping during the day (Morning)	✓			
39. Seems "like a zombie"		✓		
40. Seems to have lost the "spark" in his or her personality				
41. Headaches NA				
42. Stomachaches In school	✓			
SE-total				

Adapted from The Diagnostic and Statistical Manual of Mental Disorders, 4th Edition, American Psychiatric Association, Washington, D. C. 1994

December 1997
Walt Karniski, M. D.
Florida Children's Center

Figure 5.2   Teacher questionnaire describing Lilly's behavior after treatment for ADHD with stimulant medication.

her own age, and the same difficulties were observed in the social skills class.

After this extensive evaluation, a diagnosis of Attention Deficit Hyperactivity Disorder, Combined Type, was made. I met with the parents to discuss the diagnosis and recommended treatment with stimulant medication. They understood, had appropriate questions, and after some hesitation, they agreed.

Lilly was started on a low dose of a sustained-release preparation of methylphenidate. Three days later, her teacher filled out the same questionnaire again (Figure 5.2).

The improvement in attention is obvious. The majority of the attention behaviors, hyperactive behaviors, and impulsive behaviors were still present but dramatically reduced in frequency, without side effects (questions 33–42). As a matter of fact, these behaviors that are often seen as side effects were more prominent when Lilly was OFF medication than ON medication, such as nervousness. Lilly was seen as *less* nervous ON medication.

Lilly's mother stated that they received "a great deal of positive feedback" from her teacher. Her after-school gymnastics teacher was not aware that she had started medication, but she commented that Lilly showed an "incredible improvement in her ability to follow directions."

Many people have claimed that ADHD is a diagnosis invented by doctors and pharmaceutical companies. There has even been more argument about the use of stimulant medication to treat this "invented" disease. However, if you ask Lilly and her mother whether ADHD is a true disorder, I am sure that they would have much to say about the validity of the diagnosis of ADHD and the medication treatment. And Danny and his mother from the notebook experience in the early pages of this book would not tolerate the concept that ADHD is an invented disorder.

WHAT DOES RESEARCH TELL US ABOUT THE EFFECTIVENESS OF ADHD MEDICATIONS?

I am pleased that Lilly's ADHD responded so well to medication, but a single, successful case does not prove the overall effectiveness of ADHD medications. To determine that, we need to look to the research. Fortunately, we don't have to look very far.

ADHD medications have been studied extensively. In 1998, the American Medical Association convened a group of the top researchers in ADHD. The American Medical Association Scientific Counsel wrote

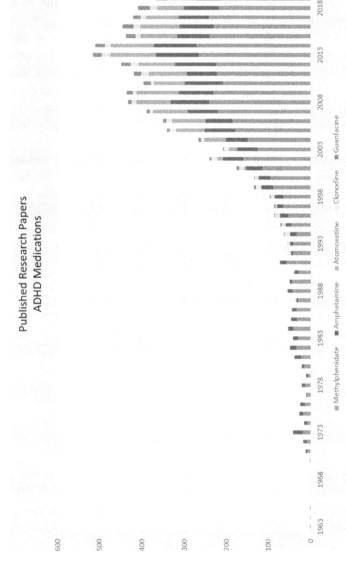

Figure 5.3   Number of research papers published on ADHD medications.

a complete review of the diagnosis and treatment of ADHD. In that review, they summarized the status of ADHD research and recommendations for treatment. They concluded by stating:

> Overall, ADHD is one of the best researched disorders in medicine and the overall data on its validity are far more compelling than for many medical conditions.[1]

The chart shows the number of research papers published each year from 1970 to 2019.[2]

The number of research papers on ADHD medications has been increasing from the early 1970s, with a gradual decline since 2014 (Figure 5.3). But the most important thing to notice is that since 2005, 300–500 research papers have been published *each year* concerning medications used to treat ADHD.

The most frequently studied medications for the treatment of ADHD were methylphenidate and amphetamine, collectively referred to as stimulant medications. Methylphenidate has been studied 2–3 times more often than amphetamines. Clonidine is one of the early non-stimulant medications studied for its usefulness in ADHD. Guanfacine is very similar to clonidine, but it has received increased scrutiny because it appears to have fewer side effects than clonidine. Finally, atomoxetine has been studied as a non-stimulant ADHD medication. Each of these medications will be discussed in much more detail later.

Not only have an enormous number of studies been published, but each of these used different populations (only children, only adults, only boys or girls, only adolescents) or different methods (using only parent rating scales, or only teacher rating scales, or direct observation of behaviors in a classroom). So how do we compare these studies and draw important conclusions about each medication's effectiveness?

Fortunately, a simple statistic can be used to compare the effects of these medications across many different methodologies and patient populations. This statistic, appropriately, is called the **effect size**. The effect size is a number that ranges from 0 at the lowest and has no upper limit. However, for most research studies, the effect size ranges between 0.5 and 1.0. An effect size of 0 means that there was essentially no difference between a medication and a placebo ("sugar pills"). An effect size of 0.1–0.4 is considered a small difference, an effect size of 0.5 to 0.8 represents a moderate difference, and an effect size greater than 0.8 is considered to indicate that the difference between the beneficial effect of two medications is very large.

Effect Sizes of ADHD Medications		
		0.0 0.1 0.2 0.3 0.4 0.5 0.6 0.7 0.8 0.9 1.0 1.1 1.2 1.3
		Small Effect Moderate Effect Major Effect
methylphenidate	0.8-1.2	———————
amphetamine	0.8-1.2	———————
atomoxetine	0.4-0.8	———————
clonidine	0.3-0.6	———————
guanfacine	0.3-0.6	———————

Figure 5.4   Effect sizes of ADHD medications.

Hundreds of studies have consistently confirmed that the stimulants (methylphenidate and amphetamine) are by far the most effective medication treatments for ADHD. These studies reveal that the stimulants have an effect size of 0.8–1.2, indicating that the stimulant medications have been shown to be highly effective for the treatment of ADHD (Figure 5.4).

Five **non-stimulant medications** have been found to be effective for the treatment of ADHD (clonidine, guanfacine, atomoxetine, viloxazine, and bupropion). Although these medications are moderately effective for the treatment of ADHD, they are not nearly as effective as the stimulants. As a result, when most children are diagnosed with ADHD, they are almost always started on a stimulant first (unless they have additional neuropsychiatric diagnoses or comorbidities). The non-stimulants are then used if side effects prevent the use of stimulants.

In one particular study, the authors reviewed the effectiveness of ADHD medications in 133 studies with 10,068 children and adolescents and 8,131 adults. For the core symptoms of ADHD (hyperactivity, inattention, etc.) clinician and teacher rating scales indicated that all ADHD medications were found to be effective, including methylphenidate

(Ritalin, Concerta, Metadate, and others), amphetamine (Dexedrine, Adderall, and others), atomoxetine (Strattera), lis-dex-amphetamine (Vyvanse), bupropion (Wellbutrin), clonidine (Catapres, Kapvay), and guanfacine (Intuniv and Tenex). The same study found that methylphenidate medications had significantly fewer side effects and were better tolerated than amphetamines.[3]

CAN ADHD MEDICATIONS HELP WHEN MY CHILD GROWS UP?

The hyperactivity and impulsivity of ADHD gradually diminish as children get older, whether or not they are treated with medication. This has led to the conclusion that most children outgrow their ADHD. If you ask young adults diagnosed with ADHD as a child, only 8 percent will self-report symptoms that would support a diagnosis of ADHD in adulthood. However, 46 percent of their parents will confirm the persistence of behaviors consistent with the diagnosis of ADHD. And if the symptoms are reworded to indicate behaviors more likely seen in adults (e.g., job performance instead of school performance), 90 percent still meet criteria for diagnosis, indicating that ADHD clearly persists into adulthood in most cases.[4]

Children with ADHD will continue to be disorganized as adults. They are often late for appointments and put off things to the last minute. Although their hyperactivity may have been diminished, they still say and do things impulsively. In younger children, we expect these behaviors to affect learning and development of appropriate peer relations. But as adults, these behaviors affect work performance, relationship with spouses and children, and even personal finances. ADHD has a profound impact on just about every facet of adult life.

What follows is a summary of the numerous studies that have been performed to understand the long-term effects of ADHD on the lives of the individual with ADHD and his or her friends and family. Before you read this, be cautioned that this summary can be overwhelming, even frightening. No child will show all of these behaviors as adults. Some children will engage in only a small number of these problem behaviors. And some will not show any evidence of any of these behaviors at all.

Finally, remember that many of these studies are comparing the difficulties that occur in children and adults *who have not been treated* versus those *who have been treated*. As a matter of fact, many of these studies have shown that when adults with ADHD take medication on a regular basis, they are much less likely to exhibit these adverse behaviors.

Education: It should come as no surprise that children with ADHD have difficulties in school. They receive lower grades than children without ADHD.[5] They are more likely to be retained,[6] and eight times more likely to be expelled.[7] They are more likely to have frequent disciplinary actions at school[8] and less likely to finish high school and college.[9] However, children with ADHD who take stimulant medication are much less likely to experience these educational difficulties.[10]

Employment: ADHD children grow up, and more often than not, they continue to have difficulty focusing. Their hyperactivity and impulsivity may have diminished, or even have disappeared, but they continue to be unorganized. They are forgetful. These symptoms affect every aspect of their adult lives, especially at work. ADHD adults are three times more likely to have been unemployed compared to non-ADHD adults.[11] They change jobs frequently,[12] are more likely to have poor job performance, quit a job impulsively, or have been fired.[13] They often earn a lower salary (one study found the average salary of an adult with ADHD to be $41,500, whereas adults without ADHD had an average salary of $52,000).[14]

Finances: Adults with ADHD are more dependent on family members for their finances, experience more difficulty paying bills, have fewer savings accounts, use credit cards more, and are more likely than adults without ADHD to borrow money at high interest rates.[15]

Family and Social: ADHD adults are more likely to have social difficulties than non-ADHD adults.[16] They report less satisfaction with their social relationships,[17] have fewer friends[18] and more difficult relations with their parents, spouses, and children.[19] They move more frequently.[20] ADHD adults are more likely to parent a child at a younger age.[21] They are twice as likely to be separated or divorced[22] and more likely to have remarried.[23]

Health: Physical health is affected as well. ADHD adults are 1.2 times more likely to be obese than non-ADHD adults.[24] They have significant sleep problems (separate from the side effects of medication that can also produce sleep difficulties).[25] ADHD adults are more likely to die young, partially due to the fact that they still act and think impulsively, and these impulsive actions lead to more frequent and more serious accidents.[26] Children with ADHD are more likely to have suicidal thoughts than children without ADHD, even in children as young as ten years of age, but children who have been treated with medication for their ADHD are *less* likely to have suicidal thoughts or behavior.[27]

Sexual Activity: Adults with ADHD have higher rates of sexual adjustment difficulties.[28] They are four times more likely to have contracted a sexually transmitted disease (STD),[29] although this risk is minimal in adults who were taking medication for their ADHD. ADHD adults are more likely to have a child born outside of marriage.

Driving: When you examine the driving records of young adults with ADHD, you will find another reason for the earlier deaths in ADHD adults. They are more likely to have had traffic violations and more likely to have had a suspended license.[30] ADHD adults are 2–6 times more likely to have had a car accident.[31] When they do have an accident, the damage to the car is greater than accidents that happen with non-ADHD adults, indicating more serious accidents.[32] Adolescents who were treated with stimulant medication were 38 percent *less* likely to have an accident during times when they were receiving their ADHD medication.[33]

Illegal Activities: ADHD adults are twice as likely to have been arrested[34] and fifteen times more likely to have been incarcerated for longer periods of time.[35] They are 3–5 times more likely to have been convicted of a crime,[36] although there was a 38 percent reduction in crime in ADHD adults who were taking medication for their ADHD.

Substance Abuse: ADHD adults are more likely to smoke and to begin smoking at younger ages.[37] They are more likely to use alcohol at a younger age and more likely to abuse alcohol as adults. ADHD adults who are not taking ADHD medication are 2–3 times more likely to abuse drugs.[38] Many people believe that the stimulant medications used to treat ADHD are addicting. In fact, the opposite is true. Multiple research studies indicate that when children and adults have been treated with stimulant medication, they are *less likely* to abuse drugs in the future.[39]

If you have a child who has been diagnosed with ADHD, it may be painful to read this exhaustive list of adverse outcomes without causing you to worry that in the future your child may experience many of the same difficulties. I can try to reassure you by telling you that no child exhibits all of these adverse outcomes. Some children with ADHD have excellent social skills, or they are very bright, or highly creative, and these strengths can partially make up for a short attention span, distractibility, and impulsivity. But the fact is that the diagnosis of ADHD in childhood still increases the risk of these adverse outcomes. The diagnosis does not predict that every child with ADHD will have these difficulties as adults, but it does imply that the risk is much greater.

Can you do anything to reduce or even eliminate that risk? Yes. The good news is that you can dramatically reduce the risk of these adverse outcomes.

Most of these adverse outcomes occur less frequently in adults who were either treated with stimulant medication as children or as adults, or both. The studies of adolescents driving are the best example. Adolescents with ADHD who were treated with medication had fewer vehicle accidents and traffic violations than those who were not treated. Many of the adverse outcomes not only occurred less often in the treated group, but **the treated group had adverse outcomes at the same rate as those adolescents who did not have ADHD.**

When I have talked to some parents or some professionals in the field about these research findings, many of the same arguments come up. A discussion still ensues about whether ADHD is overdiagnosed and overtreated.

But here is the bottom line: If a child has a short attention span, distractibility, and impulsivity to the point that these behaviors are adversely affecting school performance or peer relations, or both, then that child has a greater likelihood of developing the adverse outcomes itemized in the previous few pages, *even if he was not diagnosed as having ADHD*. It is the impulsivity that leads to a car accident when an adolescent quickly changes lanes without checking behind him. It is the short attention span that leads to being fired because her boss feels that she is not getting the work done on time.

It doesn't matter how often ADHD occurs in the overall population. What matters is what happens to *your* child. What matters is that a short attention span, distractibility, and

impulsivity produce adverse outcomes in childhood and in adults. But here is the good news: Treatment with medication significantly decreases the frequency of those adverse outcomes. Treatment with medication focuses attention and reduces distractibility and impulsivity. Medication treatment for ADHD reverses the risk for almost every one of the adverse behaviors listed in the previous pages. If ADHD adults were treated with medication as children, they are less likely to have the work-related difficulties, the financial difficulties, the health difficulties, the car accidents, and almost every one of the problems listed above. And if ADHD adults continue to take medication as adults, they are even less likely to experience these difficulties.

If you analyze each of these adult outcomes, you will realize that they represent a very significant impact to society. One study found that $13 billion are lost annually in the United States due solely to job loss in ADHD adults.[40] Add in the more frequent car accidents and more divorces and more STDs and more children born outside of a two-parent home and more drug abuse, and you have a major health crisis. I would challenge you to find a medical diagnosis that is more damaging to the lives of our children and young adults than Attention Deficit Hyperactivity Disorder.

But, remember, it doesn't have to be this way for your child. These risks can be safely minimized if you become knowledgeable about medication treatment of ADHD. When making a decision about whether to start medication in your child, understand that treatment can be the key to a happy, productive life for your child.

CAN ADHD MEDICATIONS HAVE LONG-TERM EFFECTS ON THE STRUCTURE OF MY CHILD'S BRAIN?

I have been asked frequently about the long-term effects of ADHD medication. But the question is usually asked in such a way that it implies that medication has long-term *adverse* effects.

"Yes, I understand that ADHD medication may help in the classroom, but what happens when a child has been on these medications for years?"

Because ADHD continues into adulthood, medication is often continued into adulthood. What is the effect of taking stimulant medication for so long? In the forty years that I have been treating children with medication for their ADHD, I have been concerned about this question. Could I unknowingly be harming a child's heart, liver, or kidneys by continuing treatment for years? I have read books on ADHD and thousands of research studies. I have attended medical conferences. I have tried to stay very up to date on the latest research findings, all to make sure that I am practicing medicine consistent with the most recent research. And in the past few years, I have been stunned to learn that the structure of the brain in adults who were treated with ADHD medications as children shows very real and long-standing changes.

But they are not what you think.

When we discussed the cause of ADHD, certain areas of the brain were identified as being different in children with ADHD compared to children without ADHD (prefrontal cortex, caudate nucleus, and fronto-striato-cerebellar projections). The most common finding was that these areas of the brain were smaller in size. But more recent studies using sophisticated brain imaging techniques have revealed some startling new findings. When the brains of adults diagnosed with ADHD as children are scanned using these new techniques, those who were untreated with medication showed the same thinner cortices and smaller volumes as the previous studies. However, these newer studies showed that *patients who were treated with medication had* **less** *cortical thinning than patients who were untreated. Many studies no longer showed any differences between those patients who were treated for their ADHD with stimulant medication and patients without ADHD.*[41]

These findings strongly suggest that stimulant medication, given over time, may reduce or even eliminate some of the brain differences that may be responsible for the behaviors and symptoms of attention-deficit/hyperactivity disorder. Of course, these findings do not prove that ADHD is "cured" by taking stimulant medication. But they do address the question that a father of an ADHD child asked at the beginning of this section:

"Yes, I understand that ADHD medication may help in the classroom, but what happens when a child has been on these medications for years?"

Not only is there absolutely no evidence to support the fear that ADHD medication could cause long-term harm, but these findings suggest instead that medication may dramatically reduce the adverse behaviors of ADHD by reshaping brain structures.

ARE THERE ANY NON-MEDICATION TREATMENTS THAT CAN EFFECTIVELY TREAT ADHD?

Despite the hundreds of scientific studies that show stimulant medication as the most effective treatment for both children and adults with ADHD, resistance to using medications that exert their effect on the brain of a developing child persists. As a result, many different non-medication treatments have been proposed, including:

- Megavitamins and mineral supplements
- Anti–motion-sickness medication (to treat the inner ear)
- Treatment for candida yeast infection
- EEG biofeedback (training to increase brain-wave activity)
- Applied kinesiology (realigning bones in the skull)
- Reducing sugar consumption
- Optometric vision training (asserts that faulty eye movement and sensitivities cause the behavior problems)

Unfortunately, no scientific evidence shows that these interventions help reduce the socially and academically unproductive behaviors in children with ADHD. None of these interventions are recommended, and they should be discouraged.

But what about behavioral management counseling? Wouldn't it make more sense to try counseling before diving into medication?

In the late 1990s, a multimodal treatment study of ADHD was conducted. Hundreds of children with ADHD were followed at six different sites throughout the country. These children were divided into four groups, based on the therapy that they were to receive:

1. Intensive medication management alone
2. Intensive behavioral treatment alone
3. A combination of both intensive medication management and behavioral treatment
4. Routine community care (the control group—standard care by their pediatrician and community providers)

After following these children for years, the study concluded:

- Intensive medication management alone was superior to behavioral therapy alone.
- The combination of intensive medication management and intensive behavioral treatment was superior to both intensive behavioral treatment alone and to routine community care alone in reducing ADHD symptoms. The study also showed that these benefits last for as long as fourteen months.
- Overall, the data shows that for children with straightforward ADHD without other associated conditions (anxiety, obsessive compulsive, mood problems) who have a positive response to medication, psychosocial or behavioral intervention may not provide much added benefit.[42]

The overall conclusion of this extensive study over many years, across multiple sites, and with hundreds of children with ADHD is:

> *Nearly one-fourth of the subjects randomized to receive behavioral treatment alone required treatment with medication during the trial because of a lack of effectiveness of the behavioral treatment. It seems established that a pharmacological intervention for ADHD is more effective than a behavioral treatment alone.*[43]

CAN ADHD MEDICATIONS HELP MY CHILD?

To summarize, three different lines of evidence support the conclusion that ADHD medications, and especially stimulant medications, are highly effective for the treatment of ADHD:

Approximately 300–500 studies of the stimulant medications used to treat ADHD are conducted each year. These studies overwhelmingly support the finding that ADHD medications effectively treat the core symptoms of ADHD (hyperactivity, impulsivity, short attention span, distractibility, difficulty focusing, lack of organization, etc.). Long-term follow-up studies of children diagnosed with ADHD show that they are more likely to have multiple adverse adult outcomes, affecting their health, relationships, family life, financial life, substance abuse, and crime. Treatment with stimulant medication significantly reduces the likelihood of these adverse outcomes. Finally, brain imaging studies provide strong evidence for a neurological basis of ADHD, and that neurological basis appears to be at least partially reversed by long-term use of stimulant medication.

So, is medication right for your child? You and your doctor will have to decide, based on what you feel is best for your child. But when you do, base your decision not on the opinion of your friends and family members, but on the science.

The science strongly supports that avoiding medication when the diagnosis of ADHD is clear only puts your child at risk for a difficult future. I have followed many children for 15–20 years and into early adulthood. I can confirm from my clinical experience that these conclusions are not only valid, but they are serious. I may sound like I am overzealous for the use of medication, but it is only because I have seen the outcome, over years, in thousands of children with ADHD. We are fortunate to have such an effective treatment for ADHD, with no known long-term side effects. Can you afford to abandon the evidence?

Chapter 6

WHY ARE THERE SO MANY DIFFERENT MEDICATIONS FOR THE TREATMENT OF ADHD?

ONE PRESCRIPTION, FIVE MEDS

Liz: *Danny and I are sitting in one of the exam rooms in Dr. Lawrence's office. This time I am prepared. I downloaded two video games to my phone and gave it to Danny right after the nurse left. He is now engrossed in some game, shooting alien spaceships out of the sky. I usually only let him play educational games on my phone, but I needed to make sure that he would be "contained" today and not so wild like he was last time.*

Chris and I had a long talk last night, and he finally agreed to let Danny try medication. I thought as Danny got a little older, his ADHD behaviors might "ease up," but, in fact, the opposite has occurred. His distractibility and his difficulty focusing are now affecting his grades. But Mrs. Miller's comments on Danny's last report card were the final straw.

"Danny's understanding of math concepts is amazing. He understands the concepts better than any other child in the class, and he is advanced by at least three grades. However, I have to give him a D on this report card because he has not done his work. He gets A's on all his tests, but he doesn't turn in much homework, so with F's in homework, and A's on his tests, his grades average to a D. I am worried that his superior potential will be compromised by his inability to stay focused and get the work done. And that would be very sad. He is so bright, but he still has to do the work to get the grades."

I think it was this note that finally convinced Chris. When we talked last night, instead of blaming Danny's "laziness" like he has done in the past, Chris admitted that this must be difficult for Danny.

When Dr. Lawrence walked into the room, Danny didn't look up, and he didn't respond at all when Dr. Lawrence told him hello. He just kept playing his video game.

Dr. Lawrence looked at his notes for a minute, then looked up and smiled. "So, a couple of weeks ago, you brought in the questionnaires that you and Chris filled out together and another one from his teacher. We obtained some testing, and that, combined with your history and the results of the questionnaire, clearly indicate a diagnosis of ADHD. We talked about both medication and non-medication treatments, but you said that you wanted to talk to Chris before you accepted a prescription. Is that about right?"

"Yes, it is. So, Chris and I talked again last week, and he and I both feel like we would like to try medication and try to 'fix this' before it gets any worse."

"Remember that we talked about this before. Medication does not 'fix' the problem. Medication will probably help Danny considerably, but it won't 'cure' his ADHD. As soon as his medication wears off, the distractibility and impulsivity will return. But medication can make a huge difference in the classroom."

I was chastised for my "fix it" comment, and I understood what he meant.

"I understand. So, what are you recommending?"

"Well, I would like to start him on a medication called Ritalin. It can be very effective if Danny takes a dose in the morning and a dose around lunchtime." Dr. Lawrence started to discuss how to give the medication and the possible side effects. However, I had to interrupt him.

"Dr. Lawrence, Chris and I have heard some real horror stories about Ritalin. Chris told me that he would agree to starting Danny on medication, but anything other than Ritalin."

"OK. Well, luckily, we have other options. We could start him on Adderall. It is a similar medication and has the same benefits and side effects. One dose in the morning, and one at lunch." He pulled out his prescription pad.

I was afraid to object again, especially after the "fixing" comment. But I had to.

"How does a lunch dose work? Do I put the pills in his lunch box? I don't think he would remember to take them."

"No, the school won't let him take any medication to school, even Tylenol. It must all be given by someone in the office, preferably a school nurse."

"But Dr. Lawrence, he goes to a small school, and they don't have a school nurse. They do have a nurse who comes once a week, but what would happen on the other days?"

"Well, there is another option. I could give you a prescription for Concerta. It also works like Ritalin and Adderall, but a single dose can last 9–10 hours. You could give it at home, and it would last throughout the school day."

"OK. Let's try that," I said, wondering why he hadn't started with this medication in the first place, but I was afraid to ask.

He wrote the prescription, and in a few minutes, we were out the door.

But it wouldn't be as easy as I thought. I stood in line at the pharmacy, feeling guilty the whole time because I was drugging my child, but I eventually got the prescription and headed home. The next morning, I decided to give him a dose of the medication, but when I opened the pill container, I saw a solid capsule. Danny wouldn't be able to take this. He usually chews his pills, or they come in a liquid. He can't swallow a whole capsule, unless I can break it open and sprinkle it on his cereal. So, I called Dr. Lawrence's office, and after a twenty-minute hold, I spoke to his nurse. She said that she would check with Dr. Lawrence and call me back.

An hour later she called back after talking to Dr. Lawrence, and he recommended another medication, Quillivant, which is a liquid. Finally, we're getting somewhere. So, I drove over to Dr. Lawrence's office, picked up the prescription, and made another trip to the pharmacy, glad that we were finally ready to go. But it was not to be. They told me that Quillivant was not covered by our insurance.

So, I made another trip to the doctor's office. Dr. Lawrence agreed to see me without an appointment. He gave me a prescription for Metadate CD, and he said that this medication was almost the same as Ritalin, Concerta, Adderall, and Quillivant. Metadate CD came in a capsule with little beads that I could see through the transparent pill. Dr. Lawrence said I could easily twist open the pill, but he told me to sprinkle it on a spoonful of pudding or ice cream (not in his milk or in his cereal, because the beads would sink to the bottom, and he would end up getting too low a dose). He said that Danny could swallow the little beads without chewing them.

So, back to the pharmacy I went. They then told me that insurance would cover this medication, but I would need a "prior authorization." The pharmacist told me that the insurance companies use "prior authorization" as another step to deter you from getting that medication because it is more expensive.

I spoke to Dr. Lawrence's nurse again, and I explained that the pharmacy said that we would need a "prior authorization" (she seemed familiar with this exception). She said that she would talk to Dr. Lawrence and let me know. This time she called me back the next day. She said it took three faxes to the insurance company, but they finally covered the medication. I had to go back to the office (for a third time) to get the new prescription. The nurse said that ADHD medications are "controlled substances" and could not be called in. She said I had to take a paper prescription to the pharmacy.

Well, finally! We got the medication, and Danny was able to swallow it without any difficulty. But what a hassle! Why are there so many different medications for treating ADHD?

WHY ARE THERE SO MANY DIFFERENT ADHD MEDICATIONS?

By the time I started training as a developmental pediatrician in the early 1980s, three medications had been approved by the Food and Drug Administration (FDA) for the treatment of ADHD: Ritalin, Dexedrine, and Cylert. Ritalin was the brand name for methylphenidate, Dexedrine was the brand name for dextro-amphetamine, and Cylert was the brand name for pemoline. Cylert was not as effective as the other two, and production of Cylert was discontinued in 2005 because of rare but severe cases of liver damage.[1] So, for years, only two medications were available to physicians for the treatment of ADHD, Ritalin (methylphenidate), and Dexedrine (dextro-amphetamine).

Fast-forward to today. At the time of this writing, the FDA has approved at least forty-six medications for the treatment of ADHD. By the time this book is published, there will undoubtedly be more. Each of these forty-six medications is listed in Figure 6.1.

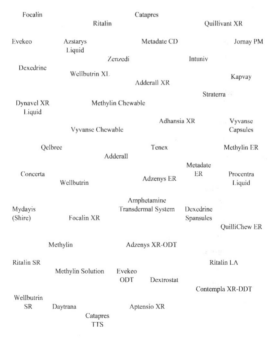

Figure 6.1   Medications approved for the treatment of ADHD.

Kind of overwhelming, isn't it? How can anyone expect you as a parent to understand the differences and similarities of these medications? You can't. That's your doctor's job, right? Most pediatricians will be very knowledgeable about many of these medications, but they can't know about the detailed workings of all of these medications. I have specialized in the treatment of ADHD for forty years, and when I started working on this book, a few medications were on this list that even I had never heard of.

It is not your job to select the right medication for your child, but wouldn't it help if you knew enough to ask the right questions?

But pharmaceutical companies don't want you asking these questions, because if you do, you might uncover an enormous secret. **These medications have some valid medical differences among them, but far more similarities than differences.** It is important to understand the medical differences among these medications, and we will discuss the important differences in just a few pages. But it is also important to understand that pharmaceutical companies have major financial incentives to have multiple medications with only subtle differences.

Figure 6.2 again lists each of the same forty-six medications currently approved by the FDA for the treatment of ADHD (see next page). The first section lists twenty brand-name medications, from Ritalin to Azstarys. But here is the surprising thing. **Every one of these twenty medications is methylphenidate.** Among each of these medications are differences: Some are short acting (3–4 hours) while others are long acting (8–12 hours). One even comes as a skin patch that can last twenty-four hours or less, depending on how long it is applied! Some are pills that can be cut to deliver a more specific dose; others are capsules, which cannot be cut, but some of the capsules can be opened and sprinkled on food, to make it easier for young children to take. Even better, some are liquid, which can render the fine-tuning of the dose even more accurate. And the chewable or liquid preparations can be critical if a child has trouble swallowing a pill.

But remember, each of these medications is methylphenidate. When they get into the body and migrate to the brain, it is impossible to tell which brand name the medication came from, because what the brain sees is the same. It is all methylphenidate.

Now look at the second section in Figure 6.2. Sixteen brand-name medications are listed here, from Dexedrine to Adderall to Vyvanse. But notice that all sixteen of these medications are a mixture of

Brand Name	METHYLPHENIDATE	Generic
Ritalin		methylphenidate
Ritalin SR		methylphenidate
Ritalin LA		methylphenidate
Adhansia XR		methylphenidate
Aptensio XR		methylphenidate
Concerta		methylphenidate
Metadate CD		methylphenidate
Metadate ER		methylphenidate
Methylin		methylphenidate
Methylin ER		methylphenidate
Methylin Chewable		methylphenidate
Methylin Solution		methylphenidate
Focalin		dextro-methylphenidate
Focalin XR		dextro-methylphenidate
Daytrana		methylphenidate
Quillivant XR		methylphenidate
QuilliChew ER		methylphenidate
Contempla XR-DDT		methylphenidate
Jornay PM		methylphenidate
Azstarys		dextro-methylphenidate
Brand Name	**AMPHETAMINE**	**Generic**
Dexedrine		dex-amphetamine
Dextrostat		dex-amphetmaine
Dexedrine Spansules		dex-amphetamine
Zenzedi		dex-amphetamine
Procentra Liquid		dex-amphetamine
Adderall		dex-amphetamine (75%) levo-amphetamine (25%)
Adderall XR		dex-amphetamine (75%) levo-amphetamine (25%)
Adzenys ER Liquid		dex-amphetamine (75%) levo-amphetamine (25%)
Adzenys XR-ODT		dex-amphetamine (75%) levo-amphetamine (25%)
Dynavel XR Liquid		dex-amphetamine (75%) levo-amphetamine (25%)
Mydayis (Shire)		dex-amphetamine (75%) levo-amphetamine (25%)
Evekeo		dex-amphetamine (50%) levo-amphetamine (50%)
Evekeo ODT		dex-amphetamine (50%) levo-amphetamine (50%)
Vyvanse Capsules		lis-dex-amphetamine
Vyvanse Chewable		dex-amphetamine
Amphetamine Transdermal System		
Brand Name		**Generic**
Tenex		guanfacine
Intuniv		guanfacine
Catapres		clonidine
Catapres TTS		clonidine
Kapvay		clonidine
Straterra		atomoxetine
Wellbutrin		bupropion
Wellbutrin SR		bupropion
Wellbutrin XL		bupropion
Qelbree		viloxetine

Figure 6.2   Medications approved for the treatment of ADHD.

dexamphetamine and levo-amphetamine. We will talk about the difference between these two substances in a moment, but all of these medications are amphetamine.

Remember the origin of these two medications. Amphetamine was synthesized from the ephedra plant in 1887. Then in 1944 the amphetamine molecule was tweaked a little, and voila! Methylphenidate was born. The two molecules have not changed substantially since then. Although they both have very similar chemical structures and both work in the brain in virtually the same way, they have some important differences.

Thirty-six stimulant medications are listed in these two sections, but they really only represent two active ingredients, amphetamine and methylphenidate. But because of the way that these two medications work in the brain and because the beneficial effects and adverse side effects of the two medications are so similar, they are collectively referred to as stimulant medications.

Ten additional ADHD medications differ significantly from the stimulants in chemical makeup and have different benefits and different side effects. They are referred to as non-stimulants.

So why are there so many ADHD medications? There are two main reasons.

WHY ARE THERE SO MANY ADHD MEDICATIONS?

Reason #1: Because That's Where the Money Is

The first reason is simple to understand. There are so many new ADHD medications because ***that's where the money is!***

ADHD affects about 7 percent of the population. There are seventy-three million children in the United States, so that works out to about five million children with ADHD (although they are not all diagnosed or treated). When medication is prescribed and when it is effective, as it usually is, that's a whole lot of prescriptions. And when the medication is effective, it is common for children to stay on medication for at least ten years. If only 1 percent of the 244 million adults remain on medication, that is an additional 2.5 million, for a total of 7.5 million people receiving at least one of these ADHD medications. At $100 per person per month, that works out to about $90 billion over ten years. And that's just in the United States alone.

Because these medications have been around for so long, their safety and efficacy have been proven multiple times over. A pharmaceutical company is under much less pressure to spend the time and money to develop a "new" stimulant because FDA approval is almost a foregone conclusion. And, finally, these medications are relatively easy and inexpensive to produce.

What pharmaceutical company could resist that lucrative temptation?

WHY ARE THERE SO MANY ADHD MEDICATIONS?

Reason #2: Evergreening

The Food and Drug Administration (FDA) is responsible for protecting the public health by ensuring the safety, efficacy, and security of human and veterinary drugs, biological products, and medical devices; and by ensuring the safety of our nation's food supply, cosmetics, and products that emit radiation.[2]

The FDA is responsible to ensure that a new medication does what the pharmaceutical company that produces it says it does. Pharmaceutical companies are required to produce clinical studies that demonstrate that the new drug is effective. So, if a new medication is developed to treat ADHD, the company must produce studies that clearly demonstrate that people with ADHD who take the new drug have reduced ADHD symptoms that significantly exceed any effect from a non-active substance (a placebo).

The pharmaceutical company is not required to demonstrate that the new medication is without side effects, but that the side effects are minor and infrequent compared to the benefits, so that the medication can be considered safe. And the pharmaceutical company does not need to show that its medication is better than medications already approved. It just has to show that it is more effective than a non-active sugar pill.

The FDA uses many tools to accomplish these goals, but probably the most effective is *unannounced on-site inspections*. The FDA will inspect the drug-producing equipment and the cleanliness of the facility. More important, inspectors will examine computer records of testing the company has done to ensure the safety and effectiveness of the medications produced there. Most important, the inspectors want to be certain that the data used to prove both safety and efficacy are accurate. More than twenty thousand approved drugs are currently being used in the United States,[3] so this is a huge task.

However, once the pharmaceutical company has produced all the required data and studies, and once it has passed the inspections, the company receives an immense reward.

It has been estimated that it costs a pharmaceutical company more than $1 billion to bring a new brand-name medication to market.[4] This number includes the cost of drugs that failed efficacy and safety studies, because one does not know at the start whether a prospective new medication will be a blockbuster success and generate billions of dollars in profit or a complete bust.

Imagine that the Burkarn Pharmaceutical Co. spends $1 billion to develop a new medication to treat high blood pressure. It jumps through all the regulatory hoops set up by the FDA and passes every inspection without any violations. Studies show that the medication is highly effective in reducing blood pressure without serious side effects. After the medication receives FDA approval, Burkarn releases the medication five years after it began. The company is happy to finally be in a position to gain back the money it spent on drug development and make a hefty profit as well.

Three months after releasing the new medication and after physicians start prescribing it extensively, Burkarn Pharmaceutical Co. learns that Hijack Pharmaceuticals, a small company in New Delhi, India, has learned how to copy the same medication. Further, Hijack plans to sell its generic copy at one-tenth the cost of the brand-name medication that Burkarn sells.

If you were the CEO of Burkarn Pharmaceuticals, wouldn't you be furious that your company spent $1 billion to produce this new medication, only to watch a small generic company in India reap the financial rewards? You might have a very strong tendency to avoid investing company resources in new drug development and move to producing the "easier" generics.

Early on, the FDA quickly realized that this situation could lead to a complete cessation of new medication development. Only the patients would suffer. So, the FDA decided to hand developers of new brand-name medications a huge incentive to continue producing new medication treatments. Once a company demonstrated that the new medication was effective and safe, it would receive two valuable protections. First, it would receive a patent on that medication. A patent protects the intellectual property of the pharmaceutical company. But an even bigger incentive goes along with the patent, and that is "exclusivity." Exclusivity means that for a specified period of time, the pharmaceutical company that develops a new medication will be the only company allowed to produce, market, and sell that medication. When the exclusivity period expires, generic companies are then allowed to step in and produce a generic of the original new medication. Exclusivity periods are often 5–7 years, but can be extended to 12 years or more under many different circumstances.

The effect of these protections is to incentivize companies to produce more new medications to treat or cure more diseases and disorders. The FDA knows that if it did not grant exclusivity, the pharmaceutical company would have little incentive to invest $1 billion in development of a new drug.

But this approach has a dark side. If a pharmaceutical company has no competitors for its new medication, what do you think they will charge for the new blockbuster drug? That's right. A lot. That is partially the reason that new antiviral drugs for hepatitis (a severe infection of the liver) can cost $80,000 to $90,000 for a twelve-week treatment. The FDA does not exert any price controls. So, without a competing drug of equal effectiveness, a pharmaceutical company can basically charge whatever it wants—one of many reasons for the extremely high cost of drugs in the United States.

When a brand-name medication gets close to the end of the exclusivity period, the company is well aware that in a few years it will lose exclusivity on that medication—and, in turn, lose the huge revenue stream that has been boosting its profits for the past 10–15 years.

But brand-name companies will not resign themselves to such a significant loss of revenue, so they have developed an ingenious scheme to prolong their lucrative profit. This scheme is called **evergreening** (because it keeps the **green** stuff [money] coming in for**ever**).

Evergreening is the process of modifying an existing FDA approved brand-name drug just enough so that the modified drug can be seen as a new drug in its own right, but not so much that it changes the effectiveness or safety profile of the drug.

Turns out that this is not so hard to do. Here are some of the ways that this is done:

The original molecule can be changed slightly by adding another atom or group of atoms to it. This change results in a new molecule that has exactly the same chemical properties and the same effect in the human body as the original molecule. The brand-name pharmaceutical company will have to show that the "new" medication is both effective and safe. But this is not hard to do, because in essence, the drug has not changed and will work as it did before. When the company submits its new studies to the FDA with this "new" molecule and new name, the FDA treats it as a new brand-name medication. When the FDA does approve the "new" drug, it grants a new exclusivity period. This new and extended exclusivity period means that generic manufacturers cannot jump in to copy the drug for another at least 5–7 years, although this time period can often be extended to 10–15 years.

The pharmaceutical companies still have to convince doctors to prescribe this "new" medication instead of the old, but that is not hard to do. The pharmaceutical companies have large marketing divisions that will come up with a new twist that makes the "new" drug seem superior to all the other drugs out there, even though in reality, there is little difference in the safety or effectiveness of the new drug. By gaining an extension of its exclusivity, the pharmaceutical company can continue to charge the higher price that a generic would have threatened and be assured of maintaining its revenue stream without interruption. This approach has been used extensively to account for almost all of the many amphetamine medications.

But a pharmaceutical company has many other ways to "evergreen" its brand-name drugs.

Both medications (methylphenidate and amphetamine) will produce improvement of the ADHD symptoms within 25–30 minutes after swallowing a pill, and the medication will remain effective for another 3½–4 hours. Therefore, 2–3 doses might be required per day.

So, a "newer" extended-release medication that lasts eight hours can help a child with ADHD throughout the day and will be seen as a big improvement from the original short-acting immediate-release medication. As a matter of fact, this change is responsible for many of the "newer" methylphenidate ADHD medications (Ritalin LA (7–8 hours), Focalin XR (7–8 hours), Metadate CD (8–9 hours), Aptensio XR (8–9 hours), Adhansia XR (10–12 hours), Cotempla XR (8–9 hours), Concerta (10–12 hours), Jornay PM (11–12 hours), and Daytrana Skin

Patch (10–24 hours, depending on how long the patch is applied). The same approach has been used with the amphetamine medications (Dexedrine Spansules (7–8 hours), Adderall XR (8–9 hours), Dynavel XR (8–9 hours), Vyvanse (9–10 hours), and Mydayis (15–16 hours).

The active ingredient in each of these medications is still identical to the active ingredient in the original medication (methylphenidate or amphetamine), and the "new" medication is just as safe and effective as it was before, but now for a longer period of time. But each of these "new" medications is considered a brand-name medication.

Another way that a drug can gain brand-name status is to change the delivery system or the way the medication gets into the body. Some ADHD drugs are in pill form that can be cut to deliver a more specific dose. Some are in a capsule that can be opened and sprinkled on food (Metadate CD). To make a medication easier to swallow and to allow more fine-tuning of the dose, the FDA has approved liquid preparations (Methylin, Quillivant XR, Procentra, Dynavel XR, Adzenys ER), chewable tablets (Methylin, QuilliChew ER, Vyvanse), and orally dissolving tablets (Cotempla XR-ODT, Adzenys ODT, Evekeo ODT, Adzenys XR-ODT). One medication (Daytrana) is in a skin patch that can give the patient the ability to determine how long the medication will last by removing the patch at specific times.

An astonishing 78 percent of all medications that receive new patents in the United States are not new drugs at all but existing drugs that have been changed, altered, or modified in slight ways, but enough to qualify as a "new" drug.[5] And 70 percent of the best-selling drugs in the United States have received extensions of their exclusivity periods.[6] This practice is occurring more frequently each year.

A study by the Drug Spending Research Institute of the Pew Charitable Trust recently reported that the United States spends more than $450 billion a year for prescription medications. The reformulation of ADHD drugs from their immediate-release medications to an extended-release medication resulted in a delay of the production of a *generic* extended-release medication that cost Medicaid $6 billion from 2008 to 2016.[7] Not to mention that the patients were denied access to some of these medications because the increased cost caused insurance companies to limit the number of ADHD medications that they cover. And this does not take into account the increased costs to individuals for increased copayments or increased out-of-pocket costs when an insurance company does not cover a more expensive extended-release medication.

Gaming the system to extend exclusivity periods is not a problem isolated to just a few medications or a few pharmaceutical companies. Instead, it is a widespread practice—and it is legal.[8] With the best of intentions, the FDA established this system to encourage development of new medications on the one hand, and then eventually to lead to lower prices. However, this system is broken. It **has** led to development of more than forty medications used to treat ADHD, and although each medication has unique features, none of these medications is "new." All of these medications are the result of pharmaceutical companies and their lawyers playing an elaborate game to extend their period of exclusivity and protect their profits. Evergreening is legal, but it does not function as intended.

Nevertheless, this system has been of great benefit to children and adults with ADHD. The many different preparations of methylphenidate and amphetamine offer options to ADHD patients that did not exist previously.

CAN GENERIC ADHD MEDICATIONS BE SUBSTITUTED FOR BRAND-NAME MEDICATIONS?

Liz: Last night was like dating again. Chris took me to Manarios, one of the nicest restaurants in town, and we had a wonderful dinner. But a strange thing happened while we were ordering. The waitress came over, welcomed us, and then told us about the specials. She handed us the menus and then asked, "Can I bring you some water?" It was 92 degrees out, so a glass of fresh water sounded good. "Yes, please."

"OK, we have many different water preparations. Sparkling Springs comes from a small clear-water spring in central Florida. A glass is $2. We also have Purity. This water comes from the Purity River, located in northern Portugal. It has a slight licorice presence. A bottle will give you four glasses, and the cost is $43.50. The final preparation is Liquid Diamond. This premium water comes from the melted icecap in Antarctica. Its aftertaste will remind you of a cross between mint and cocoa. It comes in a beautiful bottle with a small diamond in the cork. This is my favorite."

"The Liquid Diamond sounds good. How much does a bottle run?"
"We just got a shipment from Antarctica this morning, so I can give you a bottle for the low price of $395. Can I bring you a bottle?"
"That sounds nice. But I think just a glass of tap water would be fine. How much does that cost?"

Would you pay $395 for a bottle of water? I doubt it. But do you know that you probably are doing the same thing with your ADHD medication? The exact same practice takes place in the pharmaceutical industry and affects the price you pay for your medication, as well as the quality of the medication you consume.

I suspect that most of the people reading this book will know the brand name of at least one medication used to treat ADHD. Thirty years ago, few people knew what methylphenidate or dextro-amphetamine was, but almost every parent who brought a child to my office had heard of Ritalin. Ritalin and methylphenidate are the exact same medication, with methylphenidate the name of the generic substance that is active in the brand-name Ritalin. Hundreds of research studies have shown methylphenidate to be highly effective for the treatment of ADHD (see Chapter 5). Multiple follow-up studies have shown methylphenidate to be very safe as well, with virtually no serious or long-term side effects. Like most other medications, some side effects are common with methylphenidate treatment (decreased appetite, insomnia, irritability, suppressed mood, headaches, stomachaches) (see Chapter 8). However, all of these side effects resolve within twenty-four hours after discontinuation of methylphenidate. And yet despite this record of safety and effectiveness, Ritalin developed a reputation as a medication that was cursed. Magazine and newspaper articles railed about a national epidemic of school-age children being medicated for a disease "invented" by pharmaceutical companies. The articles would presume that pharmaceutical companies had collaborated with unscrupulous physicians to medicate children for vast profits. Visions of children sitting unresponsive in classrooms, like zombies, were mentioned frequently.

So, it was not surprising that when parents came to my office, most were aware of Ritalin and wanted to avoid its use for their child at all costs. One father told me, "I know my child has ADHD and it is seriously affecting his learning. And I know that he needs some medication to help him focus and concentrate, but I don't want him on Ritalin. I don't want to turn him into a zombie. We would consider using another medication, like Concerta, but not Ritalin." Little did he know that Ritalin and Concerta were the exact same medication, methylphenidate. Concerta is an extended-release form of methylphenidate and is a better way to treat ADHD, but it is still methylphenidate. So, this father would not allow his child to be treated with one medication that he felt was dangerous, but he was perfectly willing to allow his child to be treated with another medication that was exactly the same but in a different form. I don't blame this father for his fear of Ritalin. Unfortunately, no one had discussed the low risk of side effects compared to the dramatic benefit that almost always occurs with an accurate diagnosis and appropriate treatment. And no one had ever explained to him the similarities and differences of these medications.

Most of the forty-six medications currently approved to treat ADHD are made from the same two active ingredients that have been available for the past eighty years (methylphenidate and amphetamine). Do we really need forty-six medications to treat ADHD?

WHAT IS THE DIFFERENCE BETWEEN A *GENERIC* MEDICATION AND A *BRAND-NAME* MEDICATION?

There are many different types of coffee beans, but two beans represent more than 95 percent of the coffee consumed in the United States. The most common bean is Arabica, grown in many different parts of the world, such as the Jamaican Blue Mountains, Colombia, Costa Rica, Guatemala, and Ethiopia. Another coffee bean is Robusta. It comes from a different plant, it is more bitter in taste, and it has a higher concentration of caffeine.

One coffee company might take the Arabica bean, grind it, put it in a can with a red label, and call it Folgers. Another company might take the same bean, grind it, put it in a can with a blue label, and call it Maxwell House. A third company might take that exact same bean, grind it, put it in a bag with a white and green logo, and call it Starbucks. But they are all Arabica coffee. Each coffee company might use Arabica beans from different countries, or use a different roasting technique, and these variations might produce a coffee with a subtle difference in flavor, but they are all Arabica coffee. They all taste like coffee. They will all produce similar feelings of arousal and alertness.

Methylphenidate is like Arabica coffee. It is the generic medication used to produce Ritalin, Metadate, Concerta, Focalin, and Daytrana, which are brand names, much like Folgers, Maxwell House, and Starbucks. Each medication is different because of differences in how long it is effective. Ritalin lasts 3–4 hours, Metadate 7–8 hours, Concerta 9–10 hours, and Daytrana can last as long as 24 hours. But the active ingredient in each of these medications is methylphenidate and methylphenidate only.

Alternately, amphetamine might be like Robusta coffee. It is a different generic medication from methylphenidate, but it has a similar chemical structure and a similar effect on the brain. It is used to produce Dexedrine, Adderall, Vyvanse, and many other medications.

So, to produce a brand-name medication for the treatment of ADHD, the pharmaceutical companies will produce a medication that is different enough from the original Ritalin and Dexedrine to warrant classification as a brand-name medication.

Brand-name drugs are "protected" from generics during the exclusivity period, but generics have some perks as well. The biggest is that the generic pharmaceutical company does not have to invest the huge amount of money required to produce a new medication from scratch. It has been estimated that it costs more than $1 billion to bring a new brand-name drug to market.[9] This includes the cost of paying the scientists to identify substances that might lead to a new treatment, developing methods to produce the substance in the lab, performing studies in animals that demonstrate that the new substance is without serious side effects, and most important, designing, performing, and paying for studies to prove that the medication is at least as effective as current medications on the market for the same disease process.

However, the generic company is responsible to demonstrate that its generic drug is both *pharmaceutically equivalent* and *bioequivalent* to the brand-name drug it is copying.

Two drug products are considered *pharmaceutical equivalents* if they contain the same amount of the same active ingredient in the brand-name drug[10] and deliver similar amounts of the active drug ingredient over a similar dosing period.

A generic drug is *bioequivalent* to a brand-name drug if it can be shown that there is no significant difference in the rate or extent to which the active ingredient is absorbed into the body and becomes available at the site of action. For ADHD medications, that would mean that a generic must be absorbed through the stomach (or the skin for one medication) and get into the brain at about the same time and last about as long as the brand-name medication.

If a potential generic medication is determined to be both *bioequivalent* and *pharmaceutically equivalent*, it is considered to be *therapeutically equivalent* to the brand name. That means that it can be expected to have the same clinical effect and safety profile. Although there are other criteria, including purity of the medication, manufacturing methods, and so forth, once a medication is shown to be therapeutically equivalent, the medication becomes an approved generic.[11]

Unfortunately, it is not as simple or straightforward as it sounds. *Equivalent* does not mean identical. I have to admit that when I first started reviewing this process, I naively assumed that to prove that a generic medication was therapeutically equivalent, the FDA would take some of the generic pills and use them in a study to prove that both the brand-name medication and the proposed new generic medication produce virtually the same clinical effects on a patient without producing any more side effects than the brand-name medication. For example, I assumed that the FDA would want to demonstrate that an antiseizure drug reduced the frequency or severity of seizures, similar to the brand-name medication.

But that is not what happens. The FDA hardly ever does any of the actual testing to demonstrate bioequivalence and pharmaceutical equivalence. So, who does? The generic pharmaceutical company is required to do all the testing described above and then submit its results to the FDA. What? Isn't that like the fox guarding the henhouse? Absolutely.

The FDA relies on the testing that the pharmaceutical company does. The only tool the FDA has to ensure the safety and efficacy of our generic medications is periodic, on-site inspections. If the generic company is located in New Jersey, that is not a big problem. The FDA inspection team will show up on a Tuesday morning at eight, completely without notice or warning. The inspectors will check for cleanliness and ensure that the company is using state-of-the-art manufacturing techniques. They might even get into the large vats where the medications are created to check for cleanliness. They may spend hours, even days inspecting computer files, looking for unexplained incongruities or data that has been altered.

These unannounced inspections are essential to the approval process, but they are not the same as if the FDA were testing the drug themselves. But here it gets even more complicated . . . and more dubious.

Approximately 40 percent of generic drugs prescribed in the United States are produced in India. Some 80 percent of the active ingredients in all drugs, whether brand name or generic, are made in India and China.[12] By its own rules, the FDA is supposed to inspect generic manufacturing plants every two years. However, some companies may not see an inspector for ten years, especially if the plant is overseas, where the likelihood of deadly deception is far greater.[13]

Performing an inspection of a drug manufacturing facility in India is much more problematic than performing the same inspection in a plant in the United States.

The first big difference is that when the FDA sends an inspection team to that pharmaceutical plant of Hijack Pharmaceuticals, until very recently, it was common practice to alert the company months in advance. The pharmaceutical company would pick up the inspectors in limousines, make reservations for them in the finest hotels and upgrade those rooms to elaborate suites. The companies would encourage the inspectors to bring their spouse, and the company would then subsidize shopping sprees for them.

When the inspectors arrive at the site, they would be met by high-up executives who would then escort them through the facility and show only what the executives wanted the inspectors to see.

In her book *Bottle of Lies*, Katherine Eban[14] describes one such inspection. In January 2014, the FDA was scheduled to inspect the Toansa plant in India, which produced a generic of Lipitor, a highly effective medication for reducing cholesterol. Earlier, glass fragments had been found in some of the generic Lipitor from that plant. Instead of immediately banning sales of medications produced in that plant to the United States, the FDA insisted that company improve its manufacturing methods.

This inspection was announced in advance. However, unknown to the company, the FDA inspection team made plane, hotel, and car reservations and purposely showed up a few days early, on a Sunday morning. Even though the plant was supposed to be closed on Sundays, inspectors found a great deal of activity in the quality control laboratory. One FDA inspector opened the door to the lab and walked in. Nobody greeted him, and most did not even know that he had come into the room. He saw dozens of plant employees sitting in front of computers, with documents scattered around the room. He noticed an open notebook lying on a desk with a list of documents that needed to be destroyed, altered, or forged. All of these activities were supposed to be completed before the FDA inspectors were expected to arrive.

Many pharmaceutical companies produce generic medications of a quality almost exactly identical to the brand-name medications but might cost one-tenth.[15] They are safe and effective. However, some pharmaceutical companies do whatever they can to cut corners and reduce costs to increase profits. Generic companies have been found to substitute lower-cost and lower-purity ingredients. They then forge test results so that the generic is falsely identified as being as pure as the brand name. In some cases, generic companies have been found to buy the brand-name drug, crush it, and perform bioequivalence tests on the brand-name drug, but then report that the test was done on the generic. It then looks as if the generic is exactly the same as the brand-name medication.

In the most severe cases, a few generic companies simply fabricated and invented data to demonstrate that a drug was safe without actually performing any tests at all.[16]

Some generic pharmaceutical companies will create two or three different generics. The company will produce one generic made from the highest quality ingredients in a plant that is sterile and state of the art. In a separate plant, it will create a second generic to the same brand-name medication, but produce this generic in a plant that is filthy and uses substandard ingredients with poor quality controls. It will then send the high-quality generic to the United States and European Union. The second generic might have far less active ingredient and, therefore, be less effective. It will send these medications to African nations that have no regulatory controls. The generic pharmaceutical companies know that they can get away with it, because they will let the U.S. inspectors inspect the high-quality plant but keep the second plant under wraps.

All of these cunning side steps result in tens of thousands of deaths worldwide and hundreds of thousands of patients taking a drug that is no better than candy for a severe and painful illness. One company produced two different AIDS generics, one for the United States and one sold to Doctors without Borders and UNICEF to be used in Africa where AIDS was devastating the populations. When confronted with this disparity, the plant manager responded, "Oh, those markets in Africa and Asia? They don't ask for proof of safety."[17]

Although it is easy to criticize countries that do not have agencies to enforce quality controls, the United States is not perfect. In the United States, the FDA requires exacting documentation that drugs are safe and effective. But when they find drugs that are clearly substandard, they continue to allow them into U.S. pharmacies and hospitals while telling the offending pharmaceutical company to clean up its act. In one case, the violations were so egregious that criminal charges were brought, but it took nine years before the FDA stopped the import of those drugs to the United States.[18]

Understand that many pharmaceutical companies in India and China produce high-quality medications. Both countries have the scientific knowledge and scientists needed to do so. Some pharmaceutical companies in China and India (and the United States) cut corners or produce poor-quality medications out of pure greed. The obvious solution to the problem of poor-quality generics is to do more frequent, *unannounced* inspections, and when violations are identified, to halt the importation of *any* drugs produced by that plant until the violations are remediated. Regulators cannot be in bed with the companies and plants that they regulate. Neither can the United States rely on India or China to investigate their own. Regulators in India define bioequivalence far less stringently than does the FDA.[19] Dr. G. N. Singh, director of the India equivalent of the FDA, admitted, "If I have to follow US standards in inspecting facilities supplying to the Indian market, we will have to shut down all of those."[20]

However, the problem of generic drugs is not going away anytime soon for another reason: generic medications are always much cheaper than the brand name.

Approximate brand-name costs and generic medication costs are listed for each of the forty-six ADHD medications in Chapters 10, 11, and 12. For years, the U.S. Congress has been pressuring the FDA to allow more generics into the country to reduce drug prices. And, of course, some of those congressmen receive campaign contributions from the pharmaceutical companies.

This information is not meant as an exposé of foreign generic medication manufacturers. Most generics are, indeed, bioequivalent to the brand-name medications. And in the face of the hundreds of medications submitted to the FDA as new brand-name medications or as generics of brand-name medications, the FDA does a monumental job to ensure the safety of the 4.5 *billion* prescriptions written in the United States each year.[21]

So how is this information relevant to your child's situation? Many patients in the United States use generic forms of their medication, and these generics are usually just as effective as the brand-name drugs, at one-tenth the cost.

If your doctor diagnoses ADHD in your child, then writes a prescription for an ADHD medication for the first time, it will be clear within days whether or not that medication is helping. But what if your child has been on a brand-name ADHD medication for two years, and your insurance company and pharmacy substitute a generic on your next refill? Three weeks later, at the parent-teacher conference, his teacher tells you that he seems to be goofing off in the classroom. You may not realize that the deterioration in your child's attention or mood started right after you filled your last prescription, which contained a generic of the medication that he had received for the past two years.

Doctors do not usually know if their patients are receiving the brand-name medication or the generic from their pharmacy (unless they specify brand name when writing the prescription). In many cases, neither does the patient know. If a doctor writes a prescription for Adderall XR, and the pharmacy fills it with brand-name medication and then later switches the prescription to a generic as it becomes available, this may be done without the knowledge of the doctor and, often, the patient. But even if the doctor *was* informed of the change, he would have no reason to change the dosing of the prescription, because the FDA assured him the generic medication is bioequivalent to the brand name. The result can be more frequent and severe side effects. A doctor can write "brand name only" on the prescription, but often will not do so, because the insurance company will not cover the brand name or will cover it at a much greater cost.

My practice is always to start a patient on brand-name medication, if possible. With ADHD medications, if a patient pays for the medication out of pocket, the difference in price might be a few hundred dollars a month, not the tens of thousands of dollars for many other medications. I would tell the patient's family to start with the brand name; assuming that we see a positive response to the medication, we can adjust the dose until an optimal response is reached. When the child is stabilized on that dose (which can be done quickly for most ADHD medications), then we can switch to the generic. If the family continues to see the same positive effects from the generic as with the brand name, that's great. Then we can continue the less expensive or insurance-covered generic. However, if we see an immediate deterioration in the ADHD symptoms, we may have to consider a higher dose of the generic, or switch back to the brand name.

No one is asking you to decide whether to use a brand-name or generic medication. **In most cases, generic medications can provide the same benefits as the brand name.** But the next time you pick up a prescription refill, and the pills are pink instead of white, or they are smaller than before, or they are oval when they were round, pay attention to how your child is doing with that generic medication and let your doctor know that he is now receiving a generic.

Chapter 7

WHICH MEDICATION IS RIGHT FOR MY CHILD?

FOUR MEDICATION CHARACTERISTICS THAT DIFFERENTIATE ALL ADHD MEDICATIONS

We have learned that two different but similar stimulant medications (methylphenidate and amphetamine) are the most effective treatment for ADHD. And we have learned that the pharmaceutical companies have made changes in the characteristics of these two medications to produce thirty-six brand-name stimulant medications. In addition, there are ten non-stimulant medications. So, once your physician has diagnosed ADHD in your child, how does she know which one of these medications to prescribe? That is probably one of the most important questions posed and answered by this book.

Four characteristics of these medications will determine which one is best for your child:

1. Medication Duration Time (How long throughout the day is a medication effective?)
2. Delivery Mechanism (How does the medication get from the bottle to the brain?)
3. Medication Mirror-Image Molecules (A medication can exist in two forms that are mirror images of each other—how do these forms contribute to the efficacy of a medication?)
4. Medication Cost and GoodRx

MEDICATION DURATION TIME

Most medications are swallowed. After a medication is swallowed, there is a lag time before it begins to take effect in the brain (usually, but not always, one-half hour to an hour). The period of time from the moment the pill is swallowed to the time when it loses its effectiveness often varies between four and twelve hours, and for this discussion, it will be referred to as the duration time (abbreviated as *Time* in the tables). After a medication performs its intended function, it is released from the brain and is metabolized, usually by the liver or kidneys, and expelled from the body.

Without any modifications, the two stimulant medications (amphetamine and methyophenidate) are effective for only about 3½ hours. As a result, multiple daily doses will be needed to maintain the therapeutic effectiveness throughout the school day when it is needed the most.

With a short-acting medication such as the original Ritalin (methylphenidate), it is hard to keep medication blood levels stable. Schools usually require that a child see the school nurse to get medication during the day. Requiring three doses a day on a school day will often mean sporadic times during the day when the child's medication is low in the bloodstream and other times when it is high. This medication variability can cause emotional lability and irritability; it is discussed in more detail in Chapter 8 on side effects.

Most of the alterations that pharmaceutical companies have made to the methylphenidate medications extend the therapeutic effect to eight hours (Ritalin LA, Metadate CD), ten hours (Concerta), and in one case, twenty-four hours (Daytrana). **These newer extended-release medications produced a profound impact on the way that stimulant medications are now used in children with ADHD.** Your child no longer needs to see the school nurse around lunchtime to get his second dose of medication at school. Because these extended-release medications wear off more gradually, the medication has a "smoother" release into the bloodstream and into the brain. This gradual release of medication over a longer period of the day eliminates the roller-coaster variability in mood caused by a medication wearing off rapidly, every 3–4 hours. And it reduces the probability of an emotional "crash" that occurs at the end of the day. (See Chapter 8 on side effects for a more detailed explanation of this effect.)

Having multiple medications that last different lengths of time gives your doctor the ability to tailor the medication for your child. If a medication wears off too soon, your child will have trouble with siblings at home, following instructions, and doing homework. On the other hand, if a medication lasts longer than expected, then your child may have major difficulties with appetite at dinner or falling asleep.

A medication duration time of 10–12 hours usually means greater stability and effectiveness with fewer side effects. That means that a dose given at 6:30 a.m. will last until 4:30–6:30 p.m. It wears off before dinner, so that appetite and sleep are less likely to be negatively impacted by the medication. In many cases, a dose of the same medication in a short-acting pill lasting 3–4 hours can be given at dinner to help with homework done in the early evening. By altering the time that a medication is given and by using both immediate release and extended release, a medication can be "customized" to each child's specific needs and schedule.

If you go to the website of the pharmaceutical company that produces the medication, you will often notice that their estimate of the medication duration is usually a few hours longer than I am reporting in the text of this book or in the tables at the end of the book. For example, the pharmaceutical company reports that Vyvanse is effective for up to fourteen hours, whereas in my experience, it lasts 9–10 hours. An examination of the research studies does show that fourteen hours after a morning dose, children with ADHD who had taken Vyvanse were, indeed, doing better than children with ADHD who had taken a placebo (sugar pill). Although the difference was still statistically significant, the benefit was smaller, and the amount of medication remaining in the child was clearly becoming less effective. My estimate of duration time is based upon what parents are seeing at home, or on the soccer field, or with an after-school tutor. My estimates refer to how long the medication provides *optimal* benefit, whereas the pharmaceutical company is reporting what can be seen in an ideal setting, like what you might see in a research study, but not necessarily in a classroom.

My estimates will often be lower than estimates from the pharmaceutical company for another reason. Studies that the pharmaceutical company performs are usually done in adults, adolescents, and children. Children metabolize both methylphenidate and amphetamine faster than adults,[1] and younger children metabolize these two medications faster than adolescents. If more adolescents and adults were included in their studies, then the average duration of Vyvanse in their studies would be greater than in children alone.

I followed one ten-year-old patient with ADHD who had shown a very positive response to Concerta 36mg without significant side effects. After seeing the positive effects of the medication for his son, his father recognized (with his wife's encouragement) that he might have ADHD as well. He went to see his own physician, who agreed with the diagnosis and started him on Concerta 18mg with the expectation that they would need to increase the dose. However, the father responded so well to 18mg (and his wife agreed) that he stayed on this low dose for years. This father weighed three times what his son weighed, and yet he was receiving one-half the dose of his son.

The message here is that everyone responds to different medications and different doses differently. One person may absorb the medication rapidly and completely, whereas the next person may absorb the dose of medication more slowly and may absorb only half the medication. Your child might respond well to a certain dose of a medication, but the next child might require twice that dose to achieve the same benefit.

DELIVERY MECHANISMS

Here are some of the ways that medications can be modified, either to extend the duration time or to make it easier for a child to take the medication:

- A mixture of immediate-release and coated extended-release beads
- Skin patch
- Liquid
- Orally dissolving tablet
- Chewable tablet

These options potentially decrease side effects by providing a more gradual onset and offset of the medication and increasing the probability that the child will actually get the prescribed medication, because it is easier to swallow in a liquid or an orally dissolving tablet. It also allows a pharmaceutical company to make a minor modification to an inexpensive medication and turn it into a new, expensive, brand-name medication. That is why cost will be highlighted for each of these medications to be discussed.

MEDICATION MIRROR-IMAGE MOLECULES

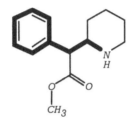

Methylphenidate

Figure 7.1 Methylphenidate. Original Artwork - James Kelly.

Everything in the universe is made up of molecules, and a molecule is made up of atoms, the basic elements in the universe, connected together. Figure 7.1 is a picture of the methylphenidate molecule.

But this picture is slightly misleading. The methylphenidate that is produced in the lab and then used in brand-name products (such as Ritalin, Daytrana, Concerta, etc.) is an equal combination of the methylphenidate molecule above and its mirror image. This is true for many substances in nature, and our body has learned how to interact with both the left-sided molecule and its counterpart, the right-sided molecule.

These mirror-image molecules are referred to as stereoisomers. Most medications are a combination of their mirror image in a 50

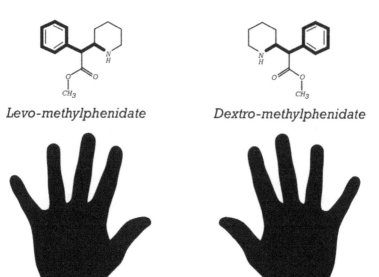

Levo-methylphenidate   Dextro-methylphenidate

Figure 7.2   ADHD medications come in two chemical structures that are mirror-images of each other, called stereo-isomers. Most of the effect from stimulant medications is produced by the right-handed version (dextro) of the molecule. Original Artwork - James Kelly.

percent–50 percent ratio. And this is true for both methylphenidate and amphetamine as well. The right-sided methylphenidate is referred to as *dextro-methylphenidate* and the left-sided methylphenidate is *levo-amphetamine*. The right-sided amphetamine is referred to as *dextro-amphetamine* and the left-sided amphetamine is <u>levo</u>-*amphetamine*.

Why does this matter? Well, it turns out that for methylphenidate, it doesn't matter very much. The right-sided stereoisomer, dextro-methylphenidate, is responsible for most or all of the positive effects, while the left-sided stereoisomer has little to no effect in the brain.[2] Dextro-methylphenidate is doing all the work; levo-methylphenidate is just along for the ride. Almost all of the methylphenidate medications contain dextro-methylphenidate and levo-methylphenidate in a 50 percent–50 percent ratio, so the distinction between the effects of the two stereoisomers is irrelevant, with one exception. Focalin is the only methylphenidate medication that consists of dextro-methylphenidate only. If dextro-methylphenidate is responsible for all the benefit, eliminating the ineffective mirror-image molecule (levo-methylphenidate) should decrease the side effects without changing the effectiveness of the medication.

The amphetamine medications are a completely different story. Some of the amphetamine medications consist only of dextro-amphetamine (Dexedrine, Dextrostat, Procentra, Zenzedi, and Vyvanse). This is fine, because dextro-amphetamine is responsible for most of the positive effects of these medications. But in 1996, Adderall was approved as an ADHD treatment, which seemed to change all the rules. Adderall consists of both stereoisomers, but instead of the 50 percent–50 percent combination seen in the methylphenidate medications, Adderall is designed to consist of 75 percent dextro-amphetamine and 25 percent levo-amphetamine. Why does Adderall use a different ratio of stereoisomers? Neither the scientific research community nor the pharmaceutical company has ever been able to determine any benefit to this ratio. More to the point, no benefit to inclusion of levo-amphetamine has ever been determined.

Overall, dextro-amphetamine is 2–10 times more effective than levo-amphetamine. So levo-amphetamine does provide some benefit but far less than the benefit provided by dextro-amphetamine.[3] On the other hand, levo-amphetamine is responsible for more appetite suppression and more cardiovascular side effects (increased heart rate and elevated blood pressure),[4] although these elevations are mild.

So why would a pharmaceutical company produce a new medication to treat ADHD by taking an established medication (dextro-amphetamine) and adding a second substance (levo-amphetamine) that is less effective and has more side effects?

One independent research study concluded, "Dextroamphetamine has generally been found to compare favorably with methylphenidate in ADHD; it acts through release of newly synthesized dopamine. Levo-amphetamine is present as a minor component in a combination product (Adderall), but the rationale for inclusion of the levo isomer remains unclear."[5]

Indeed, when I asked a representative of the pharmaceutical company that makes Adderall why the two stereoisomers were included in Adderall in a 3 to 1 ratio, his response was, "It was a business decision." What he meant was that because Obetrol, the precursor to Adderall had already been approved by the FDA, and Obetrol and Addedrall were identical medications, all that was necessary was to change the name from Obetrol to Adderall—and instead of marketing Obetrol as a treatment for obesity, Adderall would be marketed as an effective treatment for ADHD. And it is effective, highly effective, but thirty years later, we still do not have a good understanding of what the different ratios of dextro-amphetamine and levo-amphetamine in Adderall do.

What all of this means is that the only difference between many ADHD medications is the ratio of dextro-amphetamine to levo-amphetamine. For example, the ratio of dextro-amphetamine to levo-amphetamine in Dexedrine is 100 percent to 0 percent, whereas as this ratio in Adderall is 75 percent to 25 percent, and for Dynavel XR liquid it is 76 percent to 24 percent. But for all practical purposes, this means that these medications are not really different at all. A medication's effectiveness will be determined by how much dextro-amphetamine is present. Levo-amphetamine will only increase the side effects.

As a result, your doctor's decision to use some of these medications or not may be made on the basis of other medication characteristics, such as cost, or how easily the child will take the medication (skin patch, liquid, orally dissolving tablet) rather than on some arbitrary ratio of these mirror-image molecules.

It is not a question of the right versus the wrong medication. It is a matter of the right medication versus the left medication.

MEDICATION COST AND GOODRX

Some of the forty-six ADHD medications will be covered by your insurance plan. However, it is highly likely that many of these medications will not be covered by insurance. Some of the medications listed below are very inexpensive, even without insurance ($27 for a one-month supply of generic Ritalin), whereas others are very expensive ($500 for a one-month supply of Daytrana skin patches without insurance). Further, the covered medications will change from year to year. To complicate this even further, each insurance company will have different "tiers" for their medications, and your co-payment will be different for each tier. The even bigger problem is that we have no easy way to find the relative costs of all of these different medications. In order to provide some basis of comparison, I have relied on GoodRx.com.

GoodRx has negotiated discounts for almost all medications with the major pharmacies across the country. You can download its app from GoodRx.com at no cost. Type in the medication name and dosage, and the app will show you the cost of your medication at each pharmacy near you. The cost listed is what you would pay out of pocket with a GoodRx coupon, instead of using insurance. In many cases, you can find substantial discounts. In my own experience, I have noticed cases where a medication *is* covered by insurance, but the co-pay was greater than the cost of the discounted medication listed by GoodRx. To pick up the medication, all I had to do was show the pharmacist the coupon on the app, and the pharmacy charged the reduced cost. For one medication, I was able to save more than $200 by paying out of pocket as opposed to submitting the prescription through the insurance company. Finally, if the insurance company price is lower than the GoodRx app price, you just pay the co-pay and proceed without the app.

Chapters 10, 11, and 12 will contain detailed descriptions of each of the ADHD medications, including approximate average costs. In these chapters, I have used GoodRx to provide an approximate cost comparison for you. For each medication, four costs are provided:

1. Brand name average cost if paid in cash (without insurance)
2. Brand name average cost by using the GoodRx discount
3. Generic average cost if paid in cash (without insurance)
4. Generic average cost by using the GoodRx discount

Prices of medications at pharmacies can change on a daily basis, but these changes usually, but not always, are just a few dollars. Further, prices might be very different depending on what part of the country you live in and which pharmacies are near where you live. (You may be reading this book years after it was published and when these prices were verified. The prices listed here offer a basis for comparison only, and you should check GoodRx or other similar sources for more accurate and timely information.)

Here is why these comparison costs might be helpful. Your physician recommends a medication for the treatment of your child's ADHD, but you check with insurance and learn that it does not cover the medication. You tell your physician, who tells you that he could recommend a relatively equal alternative. The originally recommended medication and the second medication both contain methylphenidate, but the only difference is that Medication A lasts eight hours and costs $80 and Medication B lasts nine hours and costs $300. Is it worth it to you to get an extra hour of medication from Medication B, which costs $220 a month ($2,640 a year) more than Medication A?

WHEN MEDICATION IS INDICATED, WHICH MEDICATION SHOULD BE STARTED FIRST?

In one of the most comprehensive reviews of ADHD medication to date,[6] 133 separate research studies conducted in more than ten thousand children and more than five thousand adults were systematically reviewed for both the effectiveness of these medications and side effects.

Methylphenidate and amphetamine were superior to other non-stimulant medications, such as Strattera (atomoxetine), Catapres (clonidine), and Tenex (guanfacine) in treating the cardinal symptoms of ADHD. Although methylphenidate and amphetamine are effective in children, amphetamines were slightly better at managing the ADHD symptoms than methylphenidate. On the other hand, methylphenidate was better tolerated and caused fewer side effects than amphetamine (especially increased blood pressure and weight loss due to decreased appetite).

In adults, the opposite was true. Amphetamine was more effective than methylphenidate and caused fewer side effects.

In the end, the authors concluded:

> Overall, ADHD drugs were more effective and better tolerated in children and adolescents than they were in adults; the cause of this discrepancy is unknown. Accounting for all included outcomes, our results support methylphenidate in children and adolescents, and amphetamines in adults, as the first pharmacological choice for ADHD.[7]

The National Institute for Health and Care Excellence and the European Network for Hyperkinetic Disorders recommends that when using medication to treat ADHD, methylphenidate should be attempted first.[8]

In my clinical experience, I have found that although the amphetamine medications are just as effective as the methylphenidate medications in children, the amphetamine medications are more likely to cause irritability when wearing off, depress appetite, and elevate blood pressure. As a result, I almost always start with a methylphenidate medication in children. And although amphetamines are a little more effective in adults, I almost always start with methylphenidate in adolescents, because it is less likely to be abused or diverted to friends and roommates, especially in college.

WHAT SHOULD I SAY TO MY CHILD BEFORE STARTING MEDICATION?

Liz: *I could see Danny through the kitchen window. He got off the bus and came running to the house, waiting until the last second to check and see if any cars were coming before crossing the street.*

"Mom, Mom, guess what?," he yelled after slamming the door.

"What happened, Danny? Is everything OK?," and then I knew everything was fine when I saw the huge grin on his face.

"I got an A on my math test!"

"Danny, that's great! I know how hard you studied for it."

"Yeah, and Mrs. Miller said I should think about joining the Math Club, but I don't know about that."

"Well, guess what? I bought some cupcakes today. How about you and I get a couple and celebrate."

After he devoured the cupcake and the glass of milk, we were sitting for a minute, not talking, and I felt that maybe now would be a good time to bring it up.

"Danny, tomorrow is Saturday, and don't forget that you have baseball practice in the morning."

"Yeah, I know."

"And remember that I said you need to start taking some medicine tomorrow."

"What medicine? I'm not sick."

"But remember when we saw Dr. Lawrence last week? He wants you to start taking this new medication."

"But what for? I'm not sick," he said, his voice rising.

"Danny, you are not sick. You're perfectly fine. You are incredibly smart, and school should be really easy for you. But it seems to be really hard for

you to keep your mind focused on what is going on at school. Mrs. Miller said that you are one of the smartest kids in the class, but your grades are C's and D's."

"But I just told you. I got an A on my math test."

"I know, and that's really great. But yesterday, Mrs. Miller said that *you forgot to turn in your book report. You spent so much time last week, reading the book and then writing the report, but since you didn't turn it in, she assumed that you didn't do the work. But you did."*

"So, what's all that got to do with medicine?"

Dr. Lawrence said that you have trouble keeping your mind focused. Kind of like what happened last week when Dad was driving, but he forgot his glasses."

"Yeah, and he almost got in an accident. Could've run into that big truck *if we hadn't all yelled. And you dropped your ice cream cone on the floor." Danny was laughing now.*

"But that accident almost happened because Dad wasn't wearing his *glasses and couldn't see well; he couldn't focus without his glasses. So, Dad had trouble keeping focused while driving, and you have trouble focusing on schoolwork."*

"So, I have to wear glasses now?"

"No, honey, there are no glasses to help with focusing in school. But *there is this medicine that can help your mind focus, so that you can ignore Michael laughing and the other kids moving around in their chairs and the bird flying by the window."*

"I don't want to take medicine. I'll try harder, I promise."

"Danny, I think you are already trying as hard as you can. For some people, paying attention is easy, but a lot of people need help focusing on what the teacher is saying, just like Dad needs his glasses to drive safely.

"And I know you want to be a great swimmer, just like Michael Phelps."

"Yeah, he won twenty-three gold medals. No one's ever done that."

"But did you know that he had a problem called ADHD? He had big *trouble focusing, too . . . and he took the same medicine."*

"Really?"

"Really."

I reached into my purse and put a bottle of medicine on the table in front of Danny.

"And Danny, I take medication every day, too. Not for focusing, but *sometimes my heart skips a beat, and my medicine helps my heart beat regularly. BaBoomp. BaBoomp."*

Danny smiled. "Or, BaBoompa. Loompa. Doompa."

"Yes, like that."

"Like wearing glasses?"

"Yes, just like wearing glasses."

He sat for a minute, not moving, not talking. Then I noticed a wisp of a smile on his lips.

"OK, I guess we can give it a try. Like Michael Phelps. BaBoompa!"

Here are three simple rules for talking to your child about ADHD medication:

1. **Stay Focused on Your Child's Interests:** Tailor your explanation to the age and interests of your individual child. Tell stories about things that have happened to other family members, but even though you may need to simplify your explanation for a younger child, keep it honest. In the example above, the mother brought in a story about Danny's dad and his need for glasses while driving. It doesn't have to be an elaborate story, just one that he can feel close to. And then she talked about Michael Phelps, a person Danny could relate to because of their mutual interests in swimming. Using a celebrity or sports figure helps your child identify with a real person who has ADHD. He feels that if Michael Phelps can do it, then he can do it. And then she discussed her own medication, without making it scary. This makes it feel like they are "in this together."[9]

2. **Stay Honest:** Don't say that the medication is a vitamin. Don't put a time limit on the medication: that is, don't tell him he has to take it only until the end of the school year, implying that he will not need medication next year. Keep it honest. ADHD is here to stay. As he gets older, he still will need medication. If you tell him that his ADHD medicine is a vitamin, at some point he will find out that that's not true, and he will question everything you have ever told him about ADHD and medication.

3. **Stay Simple:** Danny's mother did not go into detail about what would happen if her heart stopped beating, which would only frighten Danny. And she didn't explain what the medication is

doing in the brain. Instead, she turned it into something honest but simple to understand.

Here are some well-known people who have struggled with ADHD:[10]

- Simone Biles, gymnast
- Justin Timberlake, pop star
- Adam Levine, singer from *The Voice*
- Emma Watson, actress from Harry Potter movies
- Michael Phelps, Olympic swimmer
- Scott Kelly, astronaut
- Terry Bradshaw, NFL player, and member of the NFL Hall of Fame
- Michael Jordan, basketball star

Some people have even proposed that the following had ADHD, based on historical information:[11]

- Vincent Van Gogh, artist
- Abraham Lincoln, president
- Thomas Edison, inventor
- Albert Einstein, physicist

Chapter 8

STIMULANT MEDICATION SIDE EFFECTS

Almost every medication causes side effects. Side effects to stimulant medications are frequent, but none are serious or permanent or life threatening.[1] You can use the information in this section to identify which side effects are occurring and when they occur. And you can use this information to discuss with your doctor a way of either minimizing the side effects or eliminating them altogether.

THREE TYPES OF SIDE EFFECTS

Side effects come in three general varieties—dose related, time related, or idiosyncratic. When attempting to manage side effects, it is extremely important to determine which type of side effect you are dealing with.

A *dose-related* side effect means that **the more you give, the more you get.** If the side effect does not occur on a low dose of medication, it may come out later as the dose is increased, and as the dose is increased further, the side effect may worsen. The best example of this is the reduced appetite produced by stimulant medications. On a low dose of medication, your child may eat fine, but as the dose is increased, you may find him eating only half his lunch and then avoiding it altogether as the dose is increased again. You may be lucky and never experience a dose-related side effect, but it will almost always occur if you give enough medication. Sometimes you may find that even though an increased dose of medication will be more effective for treating ADHD, the additional benefit gained is not worth the side effect, and you may then decide to use the lower dose instead or switch to a different stimulant medication.

A **time-related** side effect occurs only at certain times during the day but occurs consistently at that time. A good example of this type of side effect is the irritability that often occurs when stimulant medication wears off. The time of day when a side effect occurs may provide the clue that you and your physician need to develop a solution to eliminate the side effect.

An **idiosyncratic** side effect is not related to dose and not related to the time of day, but because of some, often unknown, characteristic of the child, one child will experience the side effect whereas most others will escape it, no matter what the dose and no matter when the side effects occur.

APPETITE AND GROWTH

Hunger is a complex feeling controlled mostly by the brain. Although the stomach does send messages to the brain by the way of certain hormones, your brain decides when you are hungry. Appetite is affected by obvious things, such as the energy needs of the body and the time of the last meal, but it is also affected by state of mind. For example, if someone is very hungry, but then suddenly becomes very scared or upset, he may quickly lose his appetite.

Remember that amphetamines were prescribed to overweight adults from the 1940s through the 1970s with the express purpose to *reduce* appetite. That was the main reason for taking the medication back then. That is why Adderall was initially called Obetrol (short for obesity control). But in children with ADHD, appetite suppression is an unwanted side effect of medication.

Decreased appetite is both a dose-related and a time-related side effect that occurs in approximately 30 percent of children treated with stimulant medication.[2] As the dose is increased, appetite will decrease, and the effect is greatest at a time when the medication is at its peak. Research supporting this 30 percent figure is always performed in children who are receiving an *average* dose. Increase the dose of medication, and appetite will decrease in *almost every child.*

Which Stimulant Medications Cause a Loss of Appetite?

All stimulant medications can decrease appetite in almost any child if the dose is high enough. But amphetamine is more likely than methylphenidate to cause appetite suppression.[3] Appetite suppression occurs two and a half times more often in children treated with methylphenidate[4] than in untreated children and six times more often in children treated with amphetamines.[5] The non-stimulants (clonidine, guanfacine, atomoxetine, and bupropion) usually have little or no negative effect on appetite.

Does the Time of Medication Dosage Affect Appetite?

When immediate-release Ritalin was being prescribed every four hours, appetite suppression was not much of a concern. Because medication is usually taken in the morning and because stimulants take 30–45 minutes to take effect, medication will not affect appetite at breakfast, so long as breakfast is finished before medication begins to take effect. The morning dose would wear off before lunch, so appetite at lunch would not be affected either. Then a dose given after lunch would wear off around 4:30 p.m. so that appetite would have returned for dinner as well.

Appetite suppression has become a bigger problem as physicians have stopped using multiple doses of short-acting Ritalin and now routinely use longer-acting medications such as Concerta and Vyvanse. A dose of Concerta given at 6:30 in the morning will reach its peak level in the blood about 5–6 hours later. That is good for a child's attention span, but it means that appetite will be at its lowest right around lunch. However, this is not always a concern. If a child eats a normal breakfast (because her medication has not yet taken effect) and a normal dinner (because her medication has worn off), most children will naturally eat a little more at these two meals to make up for what they did not eat at lunch. As a result, they will often consume approximately the same number of calories and nutrients that they did before medication, and growth will then be unaffected.

Does Stimulant Medication Affect Growth?

If stimulant medication has an effect on growth, it does so through its effect on appetite. Therefore, if a child's appetite is not decreased by stimulant medication, then his or her growth should not be affected by stimulant medication.

Children who are treated with stimulant medication do experience some modest effect on weight but much less effect on height. These growth effects are greater in the first few years of stimulant medication treatment, but most studies find that children receiving stimulant medication eventually reach their normal, predicted adult height.[6]

It is not unusual to see a child lose a few pounds the first few months after starting medication. More often, the child seems to not gain weight as fast as he was previously. Even when a child loses weight from stimulant medication, it is far less common for height to be affected.

If a child does lose weight after starting stimulant medication, do not presume that the weight loss is harmful. It is extremely important to use growth charts when measuring both weight and height, and you should ask your doctor to show you your child's growth chart. If a child is overweight before starting stimulant medication, it is common for that child to lose weight after starting stimulant medication until a more appropriate weight is reached. A child may start medication at the ninetieth percentile and then drop to the fiftieth percentile (which is average) or even lower. At this point, in most cases, normal growth will resume.

What Can Be Done to Prevent Appetite Suppression?

If you are starting to give medication for ADHD for the first time, be gently warned. Appetite suppression is common for the first 2–3 weeks after starting medication. Do not panic, and do not discontinue medication, because in most cases, appetite will improve after your child has been on medication for a few weeks as the brain adjusts to the medication.

Children with ADHD might have trouble eating because they are so distracted in the morning before medication kicks in. Breakfast does not mean grabbing a protein bar when you are running out the door. I know that you do not often have time in the morning to prepare a three-course meal, but make sure that breakfast is both a meal and is healthy. Bacon and sausage can be prepared the night before and heated in the microwave in the morning. Frozen waffles can be toasted in 2–3 minutes. Be sure that you are not rushing out the door at the last minute so that even if your child is hungry, he may not eat. Or make sure that he is not always watching TV or playing a video game while eating so that he is distracted from his food.

Pack a healthy lunch, or if lunch is served at school, you could send something additional that the child likes (frozen strawberries, an apple, a protein bar, maybe even a cookie).

Most parents prefer to give stimulant medication as early as possible in the morning so that it will begin to take effect earlier to help the child be more compliant about getting ready for school, but these children are then more likely to have appetite suppression at breakfast. Other parents might give medication after breakfast so that it has no chance to affect appetite and will last longer into the afternoon. Each child requires a unique solution.

The most important thing you can do is pay attention to the time that medication is given and when it wears off relative to the time of meals, and then let your doctor know what you have noticed. Often a minor adjustment, such as giving medication after breakfast, can help significantly.

Medication Vacations

Many physicians recommend a "vacation" from stimulant medication on weekends, and many parents wholeheartedly embrace this strategy. The thinking is that a few days off medication on the weekend will allow a child to gain back any weight or sleep lost during the week, but it doesn't quite work that way. A few weeks after starting medication for the first time, the brain adapts to being on medication, much like our eyes adapt to the dark, and appetite usually improves. But if you avoid medication over the weekend and start back on medication Monday morning, it is as if that child is starting on medication all over again every Monday morning. Because he is never on medication for more than five days in a row, the brain does not have a chance to adapt. **I have found that children who do not take medication on weekends actually have *more* appetite suppression on Mondays when they start back on medication.** Not to mention the fact that most children with ADHD should stay on their medication on weekends, because that is when they play most with other children and when they learn social skills.

Physicians may also recommend a "vacation" from medication during the summer. Does learning stop during the summer? During summers, children will be in camp, visiting grandparents, tutoring, and many other activities. Medication improves their ability to learn in those situations as well. I would contend that what we learn on the weekends and during the summer is even more important than what we learn in school. And teenagers will be driving more during weekends and summer. Every adolescent with ADHD should always be on medication while driving.

If a child is denied medication during the summer, he or she will almost always have *more* difficulty with appetite (and sleep) when starting back on medication as they return to school in the fall. If you elect to suspend medication during the summer (not recommended), be sure to resume medication at least two weeks before school starts to allow the brain to adapt to it before the start of the school year.

Generally, I am opposed to medication vacations. The one day I would consider allowing a child to forgo his medication is Thanksgiving.

Is There a Special Diet to Deal with This Problem?

Avoid the temptation to push high-fat foods. Some parents will stop at McDonald's after picking up their child from school and will get a milk shake and fries. Because most children's medication is wearing off about this time, they will usually eat. But because these foods are high in fat (especially the more harmful saturated fats), appetite is again reduced after eating. Fats produce satiation (a feeling of fullness) that can then last for hours. So, the child comes to the dinner table feeling full and not particularly hungry. The final result is that with the after-school snack and decreased dinner, your child gets about the same number of calories that he would have if he had eaten a smaller, healthier snack after school and a normal dinner.

Will Dietary Supplements Help Prevent Weight Loss in Children with Appetite Suppression?

A dietary supplement can be used to help ensure a healthier approach to gaining weight in a child with appetite suppression due to stimulant medication. Liquid supplements usually have a milk base and are prepared to provide a balanced nutritional supplement (Carnation's Instant

Breakfast, Ensure). Protein bars are another option. However, if you use a supplement, pay attention to the sugar content. Look for a supplement that is higher in protein and lower in carbohydrates.

A supplement can be given at any time of the day, but it is best to give it *after* a meal. There is no sense in giving a supplement to take the place of a regular meal. Let the child view the supplement as dessert. On the other hand, if the child is not eating any lunch, encourage her to at least eat a protein bar. For the liquid supplements, you can partially freeze them, put them in a blender, and make a milk shake. Add some chocolate sauce and/or peanut butter.

What Should I Say to My Child about Eating?

You would think that you could explain to your child, "Even though you don't feel very hungry, you know how important it is for you to eat. You won't grow up to be the athlete that you want to be, unless you eat. So go ahead and eat something even though you don't feel like it." This approach usually fails. Appetite is a very powerful drive, but when it is absent, it is virtually impossible to talk oneself into feeling hungry.

Above all, don't nag or get angry. We have lost the art of using the family dinnertime to let everyone catch up on each other's day or to discuss the "issues of the day." The life of a child with ADHD includes plenty of difficulties; you don't want to add another one at dinner, constantly nagging your child to eat. If he is not hungry, don't force the food. Listen to your child. Maybe he would be more likely to eat certain foods. If your child eats the school lunch, you might check to see if he would prefer that you packed a lunch if he could specify that certain foods be included. However, it is a good idea to check what he is actually eating. Ask him not to throw away food that he does not eat but to bring it home. And this is a good time to promise that you will not be angry if he does bring home some or all of his lunch (and then stick to this promise).

And if a child does not eat a full dinner, put it away. If his appetite returns later in the evening, microwave his dinner and let him eat later. Just don't let him avoid dinner and then eat only dessert instead.

Younger children may not care much about a loss of a few pounds. Older children might be more concerned, especially those who are involved in sports.

If Growth Is Affected, Should Medication Be Stopped?

Appetite suppression is not a problem if it does not affect growth. If a child does have a mild reduction in weight, it is not necessary to stop the medication. Remember, you can always add weight later in life (and we almost always do). Failure to grow in height is another matter. Height growth occurs primarily by an increase in the length of the long bones of the body. Once the growth plates within the bones close near the end of puberty, then further increase in height cannot occur. Girls usually reach their adult height by fifteen years of age and boys by seventeen years of age. Thus, even if appetite suppression does occur in an adolescent, height will not be affected by stimulant medication after adult height has been reached.

Stimulant medication does not usually produce any permanent effect on height, but if a child shows no height increase over a six-month period on medication, then strong consideration should be given to stopping the medication and trying a different stimulant. If that does not help, you could try a non-stimulant. Appetite is usually unaffected by clonidine, guanfacine, and atomoxetine (Strattera). However, don't forget that non-stimulants are effective in treating ADHD behaviors, but not nearly as effective as stimulants.

The growth suppression side effects of stimulant medication must be weighed against the benefits. If a child has shown very significant improvement on medication and alternative medications have been tried without success, but appetite suppression is still a concern, consider reducing the dose of medication. Surprisingly, sometimes a child will do just as well on a lower dose but with improved appetite.

I can't emphasize enough that although appetite suppression is very common with stimulant medication, in the forty years of my medical practice, I rarely, if ever, had to completely stop medication due only to appetite suppression.

SLEEP

Most people spend one-third of their lives in what Shakespeare called "innocent sleep."

> Innocent sleep. Sleep that soothes away all our worries. Sleep that puts each day to rest. Sleep that relieves the weary laborer and heals

hurt minds. Sleep, the main course in life's feast, and the most nourishing. —William Shakespeare, *Macbeth*

But when our children do not sleep, we worry. We worry about their health (Grandma said that lack of sleep stunted your growth). And we worry about their ability to handle the tasks of the next day. And just as important, if our children do not sleep, often, neither do we.

With all that we have learned about the human body in the past century, we still do not know much about why people sleep. We do know that sleep is critical to both learning and memory. During sleep, our brain filters wakeful experiences and decides whether those experiences should be retained as memories or forgotten.

Sleep has a complex relationship with ADHD. The most effective treatment for ADHD, stimulant medication, can cause insomnia (difficulty falling asleep), although about a third of children with ADHD have significant sleep disturbances even before medication is started.[7]

Can Stimulant Medication Help a Child Get to Sleep?

Some of the sleep difficulties that exist in children with ADHD **prior to** starting medication include increased movement during sleep, reduced rapid eye movement sleep, nighttime awakening, restless leg syndrome, bed-wetting, nightmares, difficulty awakening in the morning, and significant daytime sleepiness.[8] **Surprisingly, some of these preexisting problems may actually improve on stimulant medication.**

Some children with ADHD will have a very difficult time getting to sleep at night, even before medication is started, because they have a difficult time settling down. They relive the entire day in their minds, or are constantly distracted by things in the room, getting out of bed, playing with toys, asking for water, or going downstairs to see what everyone else is doing. Sometimes, just enough medication will be left in the body at bedtime so that they can calm down enough to fall asleep. If this is the case, stimulant medication may actually help a child get to sleep at night.

One of my patients was a child with classical ADHD who also had problems with bed-wetting and nightmares. I started him on the Daytrana skin patch, and the improvement at school and with his behavior at home was remarkable. On one follow-up visit, this young man told me that one night they accidentally left the patch on. That night, he said, he had his best night of sleep ever. He did not wet the bed, did not have nightmares, and felt more refreshed in the morning.

I have found that for some sleep problems, such as bed-wetting and nightmares, a very small dose of short-acting methylphenidate can help dramatically. A child might be receiving 36 mg of Concerta in the morning, but a very small dose of short-acting methylphenidate (often no more than 2.5 mg) can result in more normal sleep at night. Any trial of a small night-time dose should be attempted on a weekend, in case medication prevents your child from falling asleep until very late.

How Does Stimulant Medication Cause Insomnia?

When a child with ADHD and hyperactivity is treated with stimulant medication, hyperactivity subsequently disappears, suggesting that stimulant medication is sedating. But remember that these medications are stimulants, like caffeine—the exact opposite of a sedative. If you drink a cup of coffee before bed, you probably will have difficulty falling asleep. The stimulants do not sedate but, instead, increase alertness and wakefulness.

Insomnia is one of the most common side effects of stimulant medications (methylphenidate and amphetamine). It is both a time-related and a dose-related side effect.

The severity of the insomnia is directly related to the amount of these medications in the bloodstream and, thus, in the brain. Some stimulant medications last for a fairly short period of time (Ritalin, Adderall last for about 3–4 hours). Other medications last much longer (Vyvanse, Adderall XR, Concerta last 10–12 hours). As a result, the longer-acting medications are more likely to have an impact on sleep. The shorter-acting medications can cause insomnia as well, especially if they are given later in the evening to help with homework. Some children may be treated with a long-acting medication in the morning that wears off just before dinner (so that the child can eat better). But that same child might take a short-acting pill after dinner so that she can complete her homework. A dose taken at 7 p.m. will last until 11 p.m. or later and is, therefore, more likely to cause insomnia. The bottom line is that if stimulant medication remains in the brain, it can cause difficulty falling asleep.

Which Stimulant Medications Cause Insomnia?

Although all stimulants affect sleep, the amphetamines, especially Vyvanse, are more likely than methylphenidate to cause insomnia.[9] An extended-release preparation is obviously more likely to produce insomnia than a short-acting preparation of the same medication, because some medication may still be present at bedtime. If you know how long a medication is effective, it is easier to adjust the time of dosage to prevent or reduce the insomnia from stimulant medications.

How Does Medication Dosage Affect Insomnia?

In addition to being a time-related side effect, insomnia caused by stimulant medication is also a dose-related side effect.[10] The more you give, the more you get. As a matter of fact, almost all children will experience some insomnia from these medications if the dose is high enough. The goal is to give just enough to achieve the optimal effect with minimal insomnia. This goal, however, is not always easy or even possible. For example, 10 mg of Adderall XR might produce a mild improvement in the ADHD symptoms, and your child falls asleep easily at 10 p.m. If the dosage is increased to the next possible amount, 15 mg, then the improved attention might be even better, but now the child may not fall asleep until midnight. You are then left with a choice. Accept the sleep difficulties and learn to manage them, reduce the dose back to 10 mg and accept less well-managed attention, or change to a different stimulant medication.

How Does the Time of Dosage Affect Insomnia?

Sometimes, even a single dose of medication *in the morning* can produce significant insomnia. How can that be? When stimulant medication wears off at the end of the day, ADHD behaviors will usually return. However, at that time a little bit of medication remains in the brain. Although that amount may not be enough medication to treat the ADHD behavior, it may still be enough to cause insomnia. If your child is sensitive to the insomnia effects of the medication, then it may be necessary for the blood level to drop even further before he can fall asleep. Unfortunately, this means that in some children, there will necessarily be a "down time" during which the medication is no longer effective, but your child still cannot get to sleep. It might take some doing, but it is often possible to adjust the dose of medication or the time of medication dosage so that this "down time" is minimal.

Can Lack of Sleep Cause ADHD?

Sleep is critical to maintain alertness and attention during the day. Studies have shown that when people are deprived of sleep, activity in the prefrontal cortex is decreased.[11] Remember that the prefrontal cortex is one of three areas that show reduced activity in children with ADHD. The question is, "Does ADHD cause sleep problems, or do the sleep problems cause ADHD?" The answer is that poor sleep habits can cause difficulty attending but do not cause ADHD. Sleep deprivation can cause a child to have trouble paying attention during the day, but ADHD is so much more than trouble focusing and attending. The sleep difficulties are a symptom of ADHD, not its cause.

How Much Sleep Do Children Need?

This is not an easy question to answer. Some children need more sleep than others, and children overall need more sleep than adults. Children often get less sleep than they need for lots of reasons. Some parents simply do not require that their children get into bed early enough. Some kids watch TV until they fall asleep. Others spend hours browsing social media on their phones, even after getting into bed and lights out. Sometimes a family's lifestyle is so hectic that not enough time remains for the sleep that children need.

As a guideline, until about ten years of age, children need 10–11 hours of sleep a night. As children get older, they seem to do fine with less sleep; a child older than ten might need only 9–10 hours of sleep. Before a child starts taking stimulant medication, it is important that you know at least how much sleep your child is getting, so that you can tell your physician how much his sleep has changed once he starts taking medication.

What Can Be Done to Avoid the Insomnia That Stimulant Medication Produces?

The most obvious answer to this question is to make sure that your child gets into bed earlier, but this might be the wrong thing to do. Insomnia caused by medication may express itself in two ways. For some children, medication will prevent them from falling asleep until a certain time, no matter when they get in bed. For example, before medication, one child might fall asleep at 9 p.m., and when he starts taking medication, he might fall asleep at 10, no matter if he gets into bed at 9 or 9:30. Insisting that this child get into bed at 8:30 will only increase the time that he tosses and turns. On the other hand, another child might take twenty minutes to fall asleep before he starts taking medication, no matter when he gets into bed. After starting medication, he might take an hour to fall asleep. This child might benefit from getting into bed earlier because if it still takes him an hour to fall asleep, he will now fall asleep earlier. However, the first type of insomnia is more common.

If your child does have trouble getting to sleep because of stimulant medication, don't panic, and don't stop his medication. Insomnia is most problematic right after starting stimulant medication. Sleep for many children improves after about 2–3 weeks on medication.

You can do a number of things to help avoid insomnia from stimulant medication. First, ensure that you are doing all you can to promote an environment that is most conducive for sleep. A bedtime routine is essential, and consistency is paramount:[12]

- Avoid naps during the day.
- Children should sleep in their own beds, not the parents' or a sibling's bed.
- Stick to a routine. Make sure your child starts getting ready for bed at the same time every night and gets into bed at the same time every night. You might want to set 9 as the time for him to be in bed and 9:30 as "lights out," and you can read to him or let him read for a half hour before turning the lights out.
- Discontinue all screen time an hour before bedtime (computer and games, phones, tablets, TV).
- Soothing music is a better alternative, with the emphasis on soothing. Obviously, avoid heavy metal music, but rap music (with appropriate lyrics) might actually "talk" a child to sleep. Dare I suggest classical music? Make sure that if music is allowed, turn down the volume.
- Above all, make sure that there are no sounds coming from other parts of the house that will cause a child to get up and explore. If

an older child is staying up later in an adjacent room, make sure that child is quiet.

- Sometimes a fan in the room will produce enough "white noise" to shut out sounds from other parts of the house and prevent the distractions that keep children awake. Or you can use a sound maker that creates "white noise" such as the sounds of waves at the seashore or a light rain.
- If a child has not eaten much at dinner because of the appetite suppression from medication, then a bedtime snack might help.

The good news is that sleep problems from stimulant medication decrease over time for children who have been on stimulant medication for a number of years.[13]

Medication Vacations

Medication vacations were discussed in detail in the section on appetite. Many physicians recommend a vacation from medication on the weekend or during the summer, to let a child "catch up" on sleep. But medication vacations should be avoided, and medication should be given during weekends and summer without fail. The brain can adapt to being on medication, much like our eyes adapt to the dark, but this usually takes 2–3 weeks. When children start back on medication in the fall, it is like they are starting medication all over again. Many times, when medication is not given on the weekend, a child will have greater difficulty falling asleep Monday night after starting back on medication. Summer medication vacations are even worse. Both sleep and appetite side effects can be diminished by using medication as consistently as possible, including weekends and summer.

You Have Tried These Recommendations, and Your Child Is Still Having Trouble Falling Asleep. What to Do Now?

Weigh the different "costs" and "benefits" of medication. If your child has made dramatic improvements in behavior and in school from medication, and she is only taking twenty minutes longer to fall asleep, maybe that is a small price to pay. On the other hand, do not neglect the possibility that some tinkering with the time that the medication is given (under your physician's direction) will improve things.

Once you have decided that the insomnia is resulting from the medication, and you feel that some change is necessary, do the following:

- **Change the Time That Medication Is Given:** Examine the time that the medication is given in relation to the time that your child goes to sleep. Can the medication be given a little earlier in the morning so that it wears off earlier in the evening, allowing your child to fall asleep earlier? Can a short-acting medication used after dinner for homework be given earlier?
- **Change Medications within the Same Class:** Consider switching to a different version of the same medication. If your child is on Concerta (methylphenidate), which lasts 10–12 hours, switching to Metadate CD (also methylphenidate), which lasts 7–8 hours, might be a better alternative. Of course, this strategy also means that the medication benefits may not extend to the evening hours that might be essential for homework. You might have to give up some benefits of medication so that your child can get to sleep, but this is better than stopping medication completely.
- **To an Extended-Release Medication in the Morning, add an Immediate-Release Medication at Dinner:** Say that your child is taking Concerta in the morning, but that dose of medication is causing difficulty falling asleep at night, because it is one of the longest lasting methylphenidate preparations. You could switch to a shorter-acting extended-release medication such as Metadate CD, then add immediate-release methylphenidate right before dinner. It will take a half hour for the immediate-release medication to take effect, so that it will not take effect until after dinner is finished. The benefits will extend through homework time but then should wear off right before bedtime.
- **Switch to a Different Medication Class:** If a child is experiencing sleep problems on an amphetamine during the day, try switching to a methylphenidate medication. If your child is experiencing sleep problems with methylphenidate, consider switching to an amphetamine, such as Adderall or Vyvanse. However,

amphetamines are more likely to cause insomnia than methylphenidate, so this second alternative might be less helpful.

- **Add a Second Medication:** Consider adding a second medication before bedtime to help with sleep.

Should Another Medication Be Used to Counteract the Insomnia?

After all the above alternatives have been tried, some parents are left with the following dilemma: One stimulant medication works so much better than the others, but it causes your child to toss and turn at night for hours. What should be done?

At this point it is appropriate to consider adding a second medication before bed. There are both over-the-counter medications and prescription medications that can "take the edge off" or cause a child to calm down so that he can fall asleep.

Antihistamines

Two medications are sold in almost any drugstore without a prescription, diphenhydramine and brompheniramine. These medications are both antihistamines. They are most often used as a decongestant and have been used safely in children for years for colds and allergies. You are probably familiar with the brand names Benadryl and Dimetapp, but there are many others. Benadryl (diphenhydramine) especially has been packaged as a sleep aid under a number of brand names. But do not add one of these over-the-counter medications on your own. Talk to your physician first. If you do try one of these medications, remember this:

- **Use the smallest amount necessary** to get your child to sleep. It is sometimes more convenient to use a liquid, and start with the standard dose for your child's age (follow the directions on the bottle). Then each night, give a little bit less until you find the least amount that is needed.
- The **generics** work just as well and are usually half the cost.
- Do not use any of the over-the-counter "**combination medications**." It is a common practice for pharmaceutical companies to mix an antihistamine with acetaminophen

(the ingredient in Tylenol) or other medications. This simply elevates the cost and exposes your child to a medication that he doesn't need. Avoid any other name that indicates that a combination is being used (e.g., Tylenol PM). Check the label for "active ingredients."

- **Avoid extra-strength preparations.** These preparations usually just double the dose (and triple the price).
- An antihistamine should be discontinued every 3–6 months to see if it is still needed.

Melatonin

Melatonin, another over-the-counter medication, has been shown to be effective for sleep. Melatonin is a naturally occurring hormone that encourages sleep. It is released by the pineal gland, in the very middle of the brain. Darkness causes the pineal gland to produce melatonin, and light stops the production. Through this process, melatonin controls the sleep-wake cycle.

One study found that 14 percent of children with ADHD were taking melatonin.[14] Melatonin is generally well tolerated with few side effects. On the other hand, melatonin has been studied only sporadically in children.[15]

Here are some things to remember when using melatonin:

- **Do not give melatonin to a child without discussing it with your pediatrician first.** There is some suggestion that melatonin may affect the immune system, so it should not be used in any child who is immunocompromised.[16]
- **The ideal dose in children is unknown.** Some studies recommend 2.5–3 mg in children, and 5 mg in adolescents,[17] but check with your pediatrician first.
- **Give melatonin consistently every night.** Consistency is important with melatonin, so that the brain can come to "expect" the dose at a specific time.
- It is important to **give melatonin about the same time each night**, usually about an hour before bedtime. Over the long run, melatonin may help establish a healthier sleep pattern.

- **Purchase melatonin from a pharmacy.** You are more likely to get a higher-grade formulation. Do not purchase through the internet.

Clonidine, Guanfacine, and Atomoxetine

Clonidine, guanfacine, and atomoxetine are three non-stimulants that are effective for the treatment of ADHD (see Chapter 12). However, none of these three medications is as effective as the stimulants. As a result, these medications are not usually used to initiate treatment. Nevertheless, these medications provide a critical benefit for many children with ADHD, because they can extinguish many of the common side effects that stimulants cause, including the irritability that can occur as stimulant medication wears off in the afternoon, tics, some obsessive-compulsive behaviors, and insomnia. They can be used instead of a stimulant or combined with a stimulant.

Clonidine and guanfacine are not sedatives, but in either case, the addition of one of these medications about an hour before bedtime can provide a calming effect that allows a child to fall asleep easier. They are safe, with no serious side effects. The most common side effect is a mild drop in blood pressure.

A child with ADHD might have trouble falling asleep because he is so active. An anxious child with ADHD might have difficulty falling asleep because the leaves on the trees moving in front of the streetlight cause disturbing patterns on the ceiling. A child with compulsions might have trouble falling asleep because he could not go through his usual night-time routine. In all of these scenarios, clonidine or guanfacine can provide just enough calming to quell the hyperactivity or the anxiety or the compulsions. Finally, a small amount of an evening dose may still be present the next morning, enough to provide calming without sedation, so that getting ready for school before the stimulant begins to take effect is a little easier. The doses needed for this purpose are usually quite low and if given during the day, that dose would not be expected to cause any sedation. This is not an uncommon strategy; in one study,[18] approximately 10 percent of children with ADHD were receiving clonidine for sleep, in addition to a stimulant.

When insomnia occurs from a stimulant, atomoxetine (Strattera) can be used the same way, with a dose about 1–2 hours before bedtime.[19] However, more often, atomoxetine may be used during the day **instead of** a stimulant, so that the insomnia does not occur. One of the problems with atomoxetine is that it can take a few weeks before it becomes effective. Remember that although atomoxetine is effective at treating the primary symptoms of ADHD, it is not nearly as effective as the stimulants.

Should I Have My Child Referred for a Sleep Study?

Some doctors specialize in sleep disorders, and they usually perform a sleep study (polysomnography) in almost every patient with sleep difficulties. These studies are usually performed in the lab and record brain-wave activity, the oxygen level in the blood, heart rate, and breathing, as well as eye and leg movements.

I have found that sleep studies are not very helpful in children with ADHD.

In children with ADHD who have a history of sleep difficulties, a sleep study will almost always be abnormal. The report will reveal a lot of movement during sleep, disordered breathing patterns, night-time awakening, and even subtle changes in brain-wave patterns. The conclusion is usually that this child has a sleep disorder, associated with his ADHD. But then we already knew that. Further, sleep studies cost thousands of dollars and are not usually covered by insurance. Follow the strategies in this section, and a sleep study usually will not be necessary.

EMOTIONAL LABILITY (TIME RELATED)

Liz: It was 3:20, and the rain had turned from a light sprinkle to a downpour. Danny would be getting off the bus in a few minutes, so I grabbed an umbrella and picked up a small bag of potato chips and went out the door. As I reached the corner, the bus was pulling up. The door opened, and the kids started streaming out. Danny was one of the last ones out. I smiled and waved, but he kept his head down and didn't see me. When he realized how hard it was raining, he jumped down the last step and started to run toward our house. As he turned, he bumped into another boy, but this didn't stop him. He took off running without an apology.

"Hey, Danny, over here," I yelled. "Danny." He turned, saw me, and ran over to get under the umbrella.

"Kind of wet, huh?"

He grunted, "Yeah, guess so."

"Well, I brought you some water and potato chips. Here you go." He took them from me, opened the bottle, and began slurping.

"Well, what about a thank-you?"

"Yeah, thanks," he said without much enthusiasm.

We arrived at our garage door a few minutes later, and Danny ran in without saying anything. He dropped his jacket and book bag to the floor and ripped open the potato chips.

"So, how was your day?"

Silence.

"Danny?"

"What?"

"How was your day?"

"Fine."

"Well, what did you learn today?"

"Nothing."

"You must have learned something. I can't imagine that Mrs. Miller would just let you sit there all day."

"Mom, stop asking me these stupid questions." He threw the bag of potato chips on the floor, stomped out of the room, and went up to his room, slamming the door behind him.

I went upstairs and quietly stood outside his door. I wasn't sure whether I should open the door and confront him for being rude, or whether I should just let it pass.

Danny had started on Ritalin for his ADHD about a week ago. One in the morning and one at lunch. Mrs. Miller said that the effect was dramatic. Danny was happy, engaged, and learning in school. She said that he was focused in the classroom, always had the correct answer when called upon, and his grades now reflected the intelligence that had been hiding within. She said that he was like a different kid, more confident and at ease. And the other kids had noticed as well. They were beginning to seek him out on the playground. As a result, he just seemed . . . happier.

Which was very curious, because at home, he seemed to be constantly irritable, arguing at the least little thing. Granted, he wasn't running around like before, he wasn't as active and impulsive, but he was so irritable. Chris had noticed as well, as it seemed to get worse around 4 or 5, right about the time Chris would get home from work. Last night, after Danny had gone to bed, Chris and I had had another argument about the medication.

"I don't know, Liz; I don't think this medication is working. And Danny just seems mad all the time. I asked him to take out the trash yesterday, and he yelled at me. He has never done that before. He said the trash wasn't his, so he shouldn't have to take it out. I think it's time to stop this medication."

I was still outside Danny's door. I knew I couldn't let his rudeness pass, so I turned the doorknob. It was locked. "Danny, could you please open the door?"

Nothing.

"Danny, please . . ."

"Go away," he yelled.

"Danny, did something bad happen at school today?"

"Go away. Get outta here."

"Danny, please open the door." I waited about fifteen seconds and turned to go downstairs. I heard a click, and the door slowly opened. Danny was standing there, looking at his wet shoes.

"Danny, what's wrong?"

Again, he said nothing. He stood there for a while, then rushed toward me. He wrapped his arms around my legs and began sobbing. "Danny, what's wrong? You know I love you and don't like to see you so upset. What happened? What's wrong?"

Ritalin was the first brand name of methylphenidate approved by the FDA for the treatment of ADHD in 1954. It is highly effective for treating the symptoms of ADHD, but like any medication, it has side effects. Even though Danny has had a negative change of personality at home, his mood has improved at school. He is doing so much better retaining what he has learned. He is getting along with the other kids. But why is he so angry?

Everybody's emotional state changes throughout the day. Things can be going well, but then you open the mail and find out that you owe a little more on your taxes. This makes you irritable because you were expecting a refund. Then your best friend calls and invites you to dinner, and you feel better again. You start to make lunch and realize that you are out of mayonnaise. These minor events represent the little ups and downs that we experience throughout the day.

Emotional lability is different. Emotional lability is a term used to describe mood swings that are sudden, usually due to some small disappointment, often without an obvious cause, and usually with an exaggerated emotional response.

Emotional lability is a fairly frequent *effect* of taking Ritalin, but it is not a direct *side* effect of the medication itself. Instead, this anger and irritability reflect how Ritalin is often prescribed, not a direct effect of the medication itself. It is included here because most parents and even some physicians believe that it is a side effect.

The following explanation will take a few pages, but it is important to understand this aspect of the ADHD medications, because *timing* is the key to understanding just about everything with ADHD medications. This explanation will use Ritalin as an example, but this explanation is relevant for any of the short-acting, immediate-release medications (Methylin, Focalin, Adderall, Dexedrine, DextroStat, and Evekeo). This issue will come up with just about every subsequent medication we will discuss, so stay with me on this.

Ritalin takes effect quickly. You begin to see the benefits within 20–30 minutes after taking a dose. But Ritalin doesn't last very long, usually wearing off about four hours after it is taken. As a result, most of the time Ritalin is prescribed twice or even three times a day. Most parents give the medication around seven in the morning. And because it wears off before lunch, the school nurse is asked to give the child another dose, just before lunch. Sometimes a third dose is prescribed when a child gets home from school so that she can get her homework done.

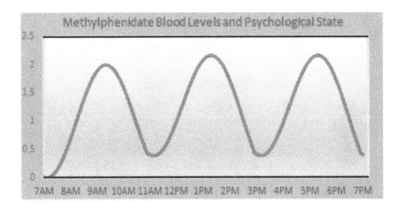

Figure 8.1, Methylphenidate Blood Levels and Psychological State: This depicts the hypothetical blood level of methylphenidate over one day, after administration of three doses of methylphenidate at 7 a.m., 11 a.m., and 3 p.m.

Figure 8.1 depicts what is happening. The horizontal axis represents the time of day, and the vertical axis represents the blood levels of methylphenidate (the generic ingredient that is in Ritalin) at each hour of the day. The wavy line represents how much medication has been absorbed by the body, and you can see the effects of the three doses as they are absorbed. The first dose rises rapidly, reaches a peak about two hours after a dose, and wears off quickly thereafter. The second dose, if given early enough, will be added to the amount already in the body from the first dose, so that the peak effect of the second dose is a little higher than from the first. And then a third dose is often given after school, so that your child can do homework before dinner, or see a tutor, or go to baseball practice.

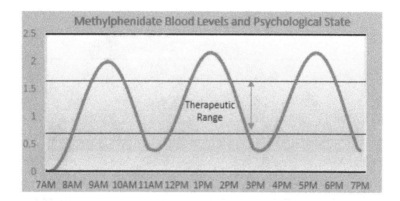

Figure 8.2, Methylphenidate Blood Levels and Psychological State: Blood levels of medication above the lower horizontal line result in a beneficial, therapeutic effect, whereas levels above the upper horizontal line produce side effects. The blood level between the two horizontal lines is referred to as the therapeutic range.

Now I will add two horizontal lines to this graph (Figure 8.2). The lower horizontal line represents the amount of medication needed to have a positive effect on the ADHD symptoms. When the methylphenidate blood levels are below this amount, the medication has little beneficial effect. If the blood level rises above this horizontal line, the medication will be effective and do what it is supposed to do.

A blood level above the higher horizontal line represents the methylphenidate level that produces side effects. The range ***between*** the two horizontal lines is called the **Therapeutic Range**. Ideally, we would prefer to have all our medications stabilize between these two horizontal lines, so that we can realize the benefit of the medication without a side effect.

Each person will metabolize a medication differently, and the medication curve will vary greatly by person, by dose, and by medication. However, it is easy to see that the situation above is not ideal. This child is spending some time during the day when the medication is highly effective without side effects. But he is also spending periods of time throughout the day where side effects are prominent and other times when the medication is not effective at all.

Notice how often the medication curve and the two horizontal (therapeutic range) lines cross. To delineate these times more clearly, let's draw a vertical line every time the medication curve crosses a horizontal line.

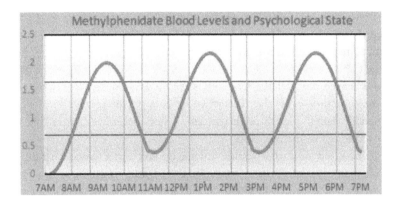

Figure 8.3, Methylphenidate Blood Levels and Psychological State: The vertical lines indicate every occurrence where the medication curve (methylphenidate blood levels) intersects with either of the two horizontal lines (efficacy and side effects). The vertical lines indicate the time at which a psychological state change would be expected to occur.

Something very important is happening at each vertical line. At 7 a.m., a child takes a dose of Ritalin, and the body starts to absorb the medication into the bloodstream almost immediately. Just before 8 a.m. (first vertical line), the amount of Ritalin that has reached the bloodstream is within the therapeutic index, and the child is realizing the benefit of the medication. However, as more medication is absorbed, the methylphenidate level rises. By 8:45 a.m., the methylphenidate blood level has risen above the side effect line, and the child is beginning to exhibit side effects (second vertical). One of the common side effects of a higher dose of Ritalin is suppression of mood. As the medication reduces impulsivity, that lack of impulsivity might be seen as a reduction in spontaneity. As the blood level rises further, the child's mood may become more somber and quieter, and he is less likely to contribute to the classroom discussion. By

10 a.m. (third vertical), the methylphenidate blood level has dropped a little, so that the amount of medication is again within the therapeutic range.
Side effects diminish while the benefits continue. However, by 11 a.m.
the blood level has dropped further, and the medication is producing no
benefit at this lower level (fourth vertical). So, a second dose might then
be prescribed at 11 a.m. Danny has to go to the nurse's office to get his
medication, and he doesn't like taking it. Sometimes a teacher will remind
him, sometimes the nurse will come to him, and sometimes Danny just
forgets. Needless to say, Danny does not get his medication every day,
and when he does get the second dose of medication, he does not get it
at the same time every day. But when he does get the second dose, what
happens? Danny goes through the same emotional roller-coaster that he
went through in the morning.

If a child is having trouble staying on task and focused on homework (and most of the time he will), a third dose of medication might
be given when the child gets home to help with homework, and the
roller-coaster ride repeats a third time.

What happens at each vertical line? Danny experiences a change in
his psychological mental state. Mental state refers to a dominant mode
of the brain reacting to its environment. We have many different mental
states (love, fear, pleasure, pain, etc.).

Each vertical line represents a change in mental state. Most of the
time, we establish a relatively constant mental state, and we stay in that
state until something causes us to change. These changes in mental state
are very disruptive to a child. And notice that the end of the second
cycle kicks in about the time he gets home. Teachers may see benefit,
but all the parent sees is a very irritable child. This is often referred to as
medication rebound.

So, what happens when Danny's mother meets him at the bus stop
in the afternoon? Danny has been in his irritable, somber mode for the
past forty-five minutes, and his medication, now four hours out from
when he took it, is becoming ineffective. And that is why the teachers
are describing one child, and the parents are seeing another.

So, if a parent tells me, "Doc, I know my son has ADHD, and
I know that he needs medication, but I don't want him on Ritalin
because it causes mood swings," I want to scream. *Of course*, it causes
mood swings. He is moving from one psychological mental state to
another, every hour or so. That would cause mood swings in anyone.

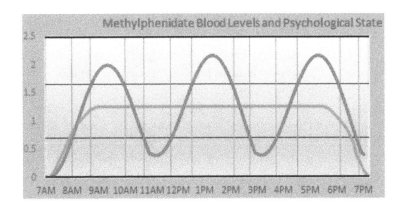

Figure 8.4, Methylphenidate Blood Levels and Psychological State: The slow, horizontal curve indicates the blood levels of an "ideal" medication, which would produce efficacy without producing side effects and without mood swings.

But what if we could produce a medication that generates more stable blood levels? This new medication would start like Ritalin and take effect early, but the big difference would be that when this new medication reached the therapeutic range, it would stay in that range throughout the day, without the ups and downs of the short-acting medication (Figure 8.4). A more stable medication, lasting longer, without the ups and downs of short-acting Ritalin, and wearing off more gradually at the end of the day, would prevent the changes in psychological state that made Danny so irritable when he got off the bus.

Many of the "newer" medications are designed to do just that, with varying degrees of success. Each medication uses either methylphenidate or amphetamine, but each medication uses a different approach to achieve that goal. The benefits and differences in each of these medications will be discussed in detail (Chapters 10–12).

If your child develops emotional lability after starting on stimulant medication, consider the following:

- If emotional lability was present prior to starting medication, is it the same, worse, or better on medication? If the emotional lability occurs as often and with the same intensity as before medication, then medication could not have caused it.

- If the emotional lability happens more often on medication, or when it occurs, it is more intense, then stimulant medication is the likely culprit. A change in the dose of medication might help. Alternatively, the dose might need to be given earlier or later.

- If the emotional lability occurs less often on medication, then the emotional lability may be part of the ADHD, and the improvement is an indication that the medication is working. No change is needed, but in this case an increase in dose might reduce emotional lability even further.

- Does the emotional lability occur only when medication is wearing off, as in Danny's case? Most of the immediate-release medications last about 3½–4½ hours, and most of the extended-release medications last 8–12 hours. First, check the entry in Chapter 10, 11, or 12 for the medication that your child is on. How long is it lasting? And when is the emotional lability most evident? If it seems that the emotional lability is displayed when medication is wearing off, then you can try three things:
  1. If your child is on immediate-release medications, switch to an extended-release medication.
  2. If your child is already on an extended-release medication and the emotional lability occurs only when medication is wearing off, then add a low dose of the immediate-release medication a half hour before it seems to wear off.
  3. Consider switching from an amphetamine to a methylphenidate or vice versa.

If you have tried these potential solutions without success, then add a second, non-stimulant medication (clonidine, guanfacine, atomoxetine). These medications are discussed in detail in Chapter 13. Give this second medication an hour before medication seems to be wearing off.

The secret to any time-related side effect is to understand the four important time periods for each child and for each medication:

1. Before medication is first given in the morning.
2. The period of effectiveness, after the medication has taken effect in the morning and before it begins to wear off.
3. The hour when medication is wearing off.
4. The remainder of the day (after medication has completely worn off and is no longer effective).

Before you next see your doctor, make sure you know during which of these four periods the emotional lability (or any other side effect, for that matter) is happening. You will be much closer to a solution if prepared with this information.

MOOD SUPPRESSION ("ZOMBIE EFFECT")

One day after lunch, I was looking through the list of patients I was scheduled to see for the afternoon. I recognized the name of a girl I had seen years ago when she was twelve years old. Michelle had been diagnosed with ADHD, primarily inattentive type, and treated with Ritalin LA. However, after a few visits, she had not returned. That was seven years ago.

She came into my office without her parents. She said that she thought she should go back on medication, but her parents didn't want her to, so she came by herself. She said, "I'm an adult now. I can make my own decisions."

I asked what had happened before, when she was diagnosed and then started on medication, but then did not return.

She paused for a while before responding. "Dr. Karniski," she started, "when you put me on that medication, I hated you. I hated the way that medication made me feel. I was able to concentrate better and my grades improved, but I just didn't like the way it made me feel."

"So, how did you feel?" I asked.

"Well, when I was studying, I was more serious, and I was able to concentrate better. But when I was with my friends, they told me that when I took that medicine, I wasn't as much fun to be around. Before I took the medicine, we were always laughing and telling jokes. After I took the medicine, I was more serious, and they didn't want to be around me anymore."

"I'm a freshman at the University of Florida now. And I know I am smart, but I am failing all my classes. I just can't seem to get organized."

So, I started her back on medication, and she returned in three weeks. She proudly told me that her grades had improved. "I am getting A's on all my tests now."

"So, what do your friends think?" I asked.

"That's the weird thing," she answered. "They think that I am a better friend when I am on my medication. They said that before I started taking medication, I was easily distracted, and I wouldn't listen to what they said. They said I interrupted all the time. But when I am taking my medication, I listen to them, and, well, I am just a better friend."

What happened here? Why did Michelle react differently to medication at twelve and nineteen years of age? Well, she didn't! She reacted the same way to medication at both ages. What changed was her friends. Her nineteen-year-old friends had different expectations from the friendship than her twelve-year-old friends.

What is the definition of impulsivity? Think about it for a moment before you respond. Impulsivity is to act without thinking of the consequences.

Now define spontaneity. Webster's dictionary defines spontaneous as "arising from a momentary impulse." And my thesaurus says that impulsivity and spontaneity are synonyms. But there is a big difference between these two words.

A spontaneous act is performed without much forethought. It is usually assumed to have a **positive** outcome, an unplanned activity leading to creative productiveness.

An impulsive act is performed without much forethought. It is usually assumed to have a **negative** outcome, an immature and irresponsible act leading to shame and guilt.

But both actions are initiated by the same pathways in the brain; it is often our social group that defines the difference between the two.

Stimulant medication decreases impulsive behavior; that is generally seen as a good thing. So, what do you think stimulant medication does to spontaneity? Impulsivity and spontaneity are virtually the same behaviors, so stimulant medication will reduce both.

David was another patient of mine, a bright, hyperactive, impulsive eight-year-old child with ADHD, and, according to his teacher, he had a very positive response to stimulant medication. His mother saw things differently.

When I saw him back in my office, two weeks after starting on medication, his mother was perplexed. "I think he is depressed," she said. When I asked her to elaborate, she said, "Well, when he comes home from school he goes to his room. He usually finishes his homework in twenty minutes, then he sits and reads till dinnertime."

"So why do you think he is depressed?" I asked.

She looked at me like I was mad. "But that's not David. He is usually running around the house, teasing the dog, accidentally knocking over lamps. I have never seen him sit and read for more than thirty seconds."

I turned to David, who was sitting next to his mother, playing a video game on her phone. "David, what books have you read recently. He looked up. "Oh, yesterday I finished reading Harry Potter. He's this kid who goes to this school to learn to be a wizard, and he plays Quidditch by flying around on a broomstick, and he fights off bad spirits, and he has a lot of friends. Have you read Harry Potter?"

"I have, and I think I loved it just as much as you do." He smiled and went back to his video game.

I turned back to his mother. "If David had been born to act like he does when he is on medication, if he had been born with a tendency to sit and enjoy reading for hours, would you have been concerned?"

"Well, no. Of course not."

"David is not depressed. This is the David that he would have been had he not been born with ADHD. Now that he is on medication, he is better able to express himself, and he is better able to communicate to you what he is thinking and feeling. So, medication is not depressing him but allowing him to be himself."

Stimulant medication reduces impulsivity. That is seen as a good thing. But stimulant medication may reduce spontaneity at the same time. Parents see this as an unwanted side effect of medication, but I offer it as freeing up the real child inside. Impulsivity is the nineteen-year-old Michelle who has friends who roll their eyes again and again when she interrupts. Spontaneity is the twelve-year-old Michelle who is popular with the other girls because she is so much fun.

Parents have a name for this side effect of stimulant medication. They call it the *zombie effect*. I can't tell you how often in my work with children with ADHD I have had parents say something like, "I know my son has ADHD, and that he would probably be helped by medication. But we don't want to turn him into a zombie."

One of the goals of using stimulant medication for the treatment of ADHD is to suppress impulsivity. Another equally important goal is to avoid reducing spontaneity. But if impulsivity and spontaneity are two sides of the same coin, how is that possible? It is all a matter of dose. It is the physician's job to find the medicine that is right for your child at the right dose, a dose that is high enough to bring out the natural intelligence hiding within each child and low enough that he retains his curiosity and creativity and the enhanced self-esteem that arrives when a skill is mastered, when a project is finished, when a friend says, "You are my best friend."

EMOTIONAL LABILITY (MEDICATION RELATED)

We now have talked about two different ways that stimulant medication can affect a child's mood. The first effect on mood is caused by an immediate-release medication given as two or three doses throughout the day. This results in constantly changing mood around the time that medication is wearing off. This is called emotional lability. The second way that stimulant medication can affect mood is the mood suppression just described. Medication reduces impulsivity, which can also be seen as a suppression of spontaneity. This is an expected effect of medication, but it is often seen as a "change in personality," or the zombie effect.

The third way stimulant medication can affect mood is an idiosyncratic side effect. That means that the side effect is not dose related or time related. It happens to some children and not others, regardless of the dose of medication or time of day. Even when medication is effective at treating the symptoms of ADHD, a child can become moody and irritable throughout the day while medication is working, then revert to his "usual" happy mood when medication wears off. This mood change can be a side effect of medication, but there is another possibility. This child may have ADHD with a comorbid condition, discussed in the next chapter. This is a situation when a non–stimulant (clonidine, guanfacine, atomoxetine, bupropion) should be considered, either in addition to a stimulant, or in place of the stimulant.

Does stimulant medication cause irritability? The answer is not a simple yes or no. An analysis of thirty-two different studies of ADHD medications involving 3,664 children with ADHD revealed some surprising findings. Amphetamine medications did cause irritability three times more often than a sugar pill (placebo), but methylphenidate medications resulted in a ***decline*** in irritability.

Occasionally when I see a new patient, I receive this complaint: "My son has been diagnosed with ADHD, and medication has really helped him, but he gets so irritated at the least little thing, at any time of day. We're worried about him."

I will often say, "Let me guess, Adderall?" and the parents nod their heads. This irritability effect of Adderall has a name. Gina Pera, who has written extensively about ADHD on her blog, calls this medication "Madderall."[20]

The solution to this problem is probably pretty obvious. If the child is on an amphetamine-based stimulant medication, especially Adderall, switch to a methylphenidate medication. If he is already on a methylphenidate medication, consider an increase or decrease in the dose. If neither of these strategies helps, then try adding a non-stimulant clonidine, guanfacine, atomoxetine).

HEADACHES AND STOMACHACHES

Stimulant medication can cause headaches and stomachaches, although these side effects occur relatively infrequently. When they do occur from stimulant medication, they are almost always a time-related side effect.

If a headache or stomachache is present when a child wakes up in the morning, before he takes his medication, it is very unlikely that stimulant medication is causing the pain, because a dose of medication given in the morning will be cleared from the body by the next morning. It is unlikely that medication is the culprit if the side effect is present only when no medication is in the body. Medication should be continued, and the cause of the headache or stomachache will likely be found from something unrelated to stimulant medication.

If headaches or stomachaches occur a few hours after a dose of medication is taken, and only then, and if they occur on a regular basis, then these pains occur when that medication would be expected to be at the highest daily concentration. Medication would then be the most likely culprit. A decrease in dose or a switch to a different stimulant would likely be the solution.

But for most children on stimulant medication, headaches and stomach-aches most frequently occur in the mid-afternoon, between 3:30 and 5. Two things are happening at that time. First, most extended-release medications wear off in the late afternoon, and a headache or stomachache could be part of the irritability that happens when some medications wear off.

The second possibility is that if your child did not eat much lunch because of the appetite suppression effect of stimulant medication, then he could be getting hungry in the late afternoon. Getting your child to eat something often eliminates the headaches and stomachaches.

If the pains persist, a small dose of immediate-release medication may help reduce any irritability, and the headaches or stomachaches should cease within 30–40 minutes. If that does not help, then a different stimulant should be tried.

However, as is always the case, changes in medication should be made by your physician only.

Any headache that persists longer than one day, any headache that wakes a child in the middle of the night, or any headache associated with vomiting, blurred vision, confusion, slurred speech, or imbalance should be brought to the attention of your physician immediately.

TICS

Stimulant medication does not cause tics, nor do stimulants make an existing tic disorder more severe or frequent. Therefore, tics are not a side effect of stimulant medication. This section is included because both parents and many physicians still believe that they are.

What Is a Tic?

A tic is not a six-legged insect (that's a tick). A tic is a rapid contraction of a small group of muscles, much like a twitch. Tics usually occur in the face and around the eyes or mouth. However, a tic can involve the neck and shoulders, and less often it can involve just about any other muscle in the body. A tic can even involve the muscles of the vocal cords, and can produce a symphony of sounds.

What Do Tics Look Like?

Tics most commonly occur in the face or neck and can appear as a wrinkling of the nose, a slight turn of the head, eye blinking, or facial grimacing. Grimaces can look like the child is "stretching" the face by opening the mouth and eyes. Tics can consist of a wrinkling of the brow, "scinching" of the nose, pursing the lips, or shrugging the shoulders. Sometimes tics can be more complex than just a simple twitch of a muscle. Sometimes a child will shoot his leg out, like he is kicking.

Sometimes tics can even affect the muscles of the throat or vocal cords, producing sounds, such as a sniffing, clearing of the throat, coughing, grunting, or "clicking" in the back of the throat. In more severe cases, tics can produce a whooping, yelping, or barking. When the tics are vocal and accompanied by other symptoms, they are given a different name (Tourette's syndrome).

How Often Do Tics Occur in Children?

Tics are common in childhood (5–25 percent of all children will have a tic at some time during childhood),[21] but because tics often come and go, only about 1–3 percent of children will have tics at any given time.[22] Finally, tics occur more frequently in children with ADHD, even before they are treated with stimulant medication.

Children with tics almost always have compulsive tendencies as well. As a matter of fact, a tic can be seen as an unconscious compulsive behavior. One adult with severe tics told me that his verbal tics made it difficult to work. He said that his facial tics and occasional vocalizations would start as an urge that he could suppress. However, in a few minutes the urge would gradually build so that he could think of nothing else. As soon as he made the facial grimace or sniffed, the urge would vanish. Soon, however, a new urge would emerge, and it would start all over again.

Does Stimulant Medication Cause Tics?

Contrary to popular belief among both parents and some physicians, stimulant medication does not cause tics.[23]

About 8 percent of children with ADHD who start on stimulant medication develop tics.[24] In a review of twenty-two separate studies involving more than twenty-three hundred children with ADHD, it was determined that when stimulant medication was started, new onset tics or worsening of tic symptoms were reported equally in children receiving stimulants and children receiving placebo (a sugar pill).[25]

For years, physicians have been told that stimulant medication should not be used in a child who has preexisting tics. However, more recent research indicates that there does not appear to be an increase in tic frequency or severity from stimulants. As a matter of fact, children who have both ADHD and tics before starting medication will often show a decline in tics when stimulant medication (especially methylphenidate) is started, and this remains true even after being on medication for a year.[26]

Can Children Control Their Tics?

Sometimes you can ask a child to stop the tics, and she can comply . . . for a short while. But as soon as she stops thinking about it, the tic will return. This can lead a parent to believe that the child is causing the tics and can stop them at will. This is not true. Children can consciously suppress a tic for a short time, but in most cases, a child is not even aware that she is exhibiting a tic until it is brought to her attention by a parent, teacher, or another child.

Should a Different Medication Be Used to Treat a Child with ADHD and Tics?

If tics develop in a child with ADHD who is taking a stimulant, then the first option is to try a different stimulant. Amphetamines may cause an increase in tics at higher doses, but in most cases neither amphetamines nor methylphenidates cause or increase the frequency of tics. If a child has tics on amphetamine, try switching to a methylphenidate medication. However, if tics continue to occur, it is time to consider a different medication.

Clonidine (Catapres, Catapres TTS, and Kapvay) and guanfacine (Tenex, Intuniv) are non-stimulant medications that are effective for the treatment of ADHD.[27] But they have an additional advantage. These medications are effective in reducing or eliminating tics, whether or not ADHD is present. Therefore, it might seem logical that any child who has tics and ADHD be treated with one of these non-stimulants.

A non-stimulant could be tried as a substitute for the stimulant, but generally the non-stimulants are less effective in the management of ADHD. I would consider a child with ADHD and tics as having two separate disorders. Use stimulant medication first to manage the ADHD symptoms. After establishing the optimum dose of a stimulant, if the tics are still problematic, start either clonidine or guanfacine. Then titrate the dose up or down until the optimum dose is found. As a matter of fact, some children require smaller doses of both medications if used in combination, as opposed to using either medication alone, exposing them to less likelihood of side effects from either medication.

No drug interactions are known between stimulants and non-stimulants, so children can be safely managed on both medications together.

CARDIAC

In 2005, the Canadian Public Health program suspended the marketing and sale of Adderall and Adderall XR over concerns of serious cardiovascular side effects of these medications. They cited case reports of twenty individuals who had been treated with Adderall or Adderall XR and had died suddenly. None of the cases were associated with overdose, misuse, or abuse. Fourteen of the cases were children, six adults. All of the cases occurred in the United States over a five-year period and were reported to the FDA.[28]

Even though these twenty patients were on stimulant medication for the treatment of ADHD, most of these patients had some additional concern that was more likely related to their death. One child was involved in strenuous exercise at the time of death, and another was dehydrated. A number of these deaths occurred in children and adults who had known physical abnormalities of the heart, or a family history of cardiac arrythmias. A few of the patients had toxic levels of Adderall (which would imply an accidental overdose or inappropriate dosing).[29]

At the time, the FDA did not have any research that indicated Adderall and Adderall XR were responsible for these deaths, so suspension of sales of these medications did not occur in the United States.

Six months after introducing the suspension of Adderall and Adderall XR, Canada rescinded this suspension and made these medications available again.

A review of thirty-eight different studies across five continents revealed that the rate of sudden death in the general pediatric population is 1–2 cases per 1.3–8.5/100,000 patient years, with an overall average of 1.7 cases per 100,000 years.[30] However, the rate of sudden death in children who were taking stimulants for ADHD was approximately the same or less.

The twenty deaths that initiated the action by Canada occurred over a five-year period, from 1998 to 2003. During that time, in the United States, approximately 300,000 individuals were taking immediate-release Adderall and 700,000 individuals were taking Adderall XR. Thus, twenty deaths occurred over a five-year period in approximately one million patients. The researchers conducting these studies concluded, "Thus, the rate of sudden death of children taking ADHD medications do not appear to exceed the base rate of sudden death in the general population."[31]

Any concern of potential lethal side effects from a medication must be taken very seriously. However, in this case, there is absolutely no evidence that would support any claim that stimulant medication therapy can cause sudden death in children or adults. On the other hand, consider the fact that trauma severe enough to require emergency room treatment is more likely in children with ADHD, but less likely in children with ADHD receiving stimulant medication.[32] How many children have been riding their bikes and were distracted? They looked left when a car was coming from the right and experienced a severe accident that could have been avoided if they had been on medication and had been more aware of their environment.

Nevertheless, concerns about the cardiac effects of these medication persisted. Finally, a pooling of data from ten different studies including more than four million individuals with ADHD found no correlation between ADHD medications and sudden death, arrythmia, stroke, heart attack, or death from any cause.[33]

Some minor cardiovascular side effects do occur more frequently in children who are taking stimulant medications. Eighteen studies involving almost six thousand children with ADHD revealed that amphetamines and atomoxetine (Strattera) caused an increase in heart rate and both systolic and diastolic blood pressure. Methylphenidate caused no increase in heart rate and an increase in diastolic blood pressure only.[34] However, these increases in heart rate (3–10 beats per minute) and blood pressure were small and probably not of any clinical significance.[35]

For a few years, some cardiologists recommended a cardiac evaluation of any child before starting to take stimulant medication. But after reviewing the research available at the time, the conclusion of some of the top researchers in the field was:

> No evidence currently indicates a need for routine cardiac evaluation (i.e., electrocardiography, echocardiography) before starting any stimulant treatment in otherwise healthy individuals.[36]

Chapter 9

COMORBIDITY

ADHD Does Not Dance Alone

By now, the behaviors associated with Attention Deficit Hyperactivity Disorder should be second nature to you. ADHD is a collection of behaviors, including difficulty focusing attention, distractibility, disorganization, and for most children, hyperactivity and impulsivity.

This chapter is one of the most important chapters in this book. Although all the previous chapters have been about the symptoms and behaviors of ADHD, and about how medication can reverse most of those behaviors and symptoms, this section describes behaviors that are often seen in children with ADHD but are *not* ADHD.

This chapter describes why the medication treatment of ADHD is often so unpredictable, and why two children, both with ADHD, can often respond to medication so differently. This chapter will help you avoid many of the potential complications of medication treatment.

Many years ago, I saw Lucas, a six-year-old boy. He had been moved to the gifted program recently because testing had confirmed that he was in the top 1 percent of children on an IQ test (a test of cognitive abilities). But he had been kicked out of three preschools because of his hyperactive and aggressive behaviors. He was inattentive, impulsive, and easily distracted. He had trouble concentrating for more than a few minutes. He would learn new concepts easily but would forget them by the next morning. Despite his intelligence, he was failing most of his work in the new classroom, not because he wasn't *able* to do the work, but because he wasn't *doing* any work. His teacher would remind him to get back on task and pay attention, but this reminder only caused him to get easily frustrated and angry. His frustration would lead to temper tantrums. He refused to follow classroom rules, was aggressive toward his friends, and often yelled at the teacher.

Lucas was diagnosed with ADHD and started on Concerta. Three weeks later, he then returned to see me.

I asked his mother, "Three weeks ago, we came to the conclusion that Lucas was having trouble at home and at school because of ADHD. We started him on a medication called Concerta. So, what have you noticed?"

"Well, doctor, that medication doesn't work."

I looked up from my notes, somewhat surprised. "Oh, I'm sorry to hear that. He is still having trouble in school? Trouble paying attention?"

"Oh no, he is doing great in school. His grades are all A's. His teacher said she knew that testing had shown that he was very bright, but she did not really realize how bright he was until she could see him stay focused on a subject for 10–15 minutes."

"That sounds excellent. So why do you think the medication isn't working?"

"Well, he still has temper tantrums."

Many children **with** ADHD have temper tantrums. Many children **without** ADHD have temper tantrums. Sometimes children with ADHD get so frustrated that they throw a temper tantrum. But sometimes children with ADHD have temper tantrums for the same reason that children without ADHD have temper tantrums, because they are young children who have not yet learned how to take control their emotions.

Lucas's tantrums were not caused by his ADHD. If they had been part of his ADHD, they most likely would have improved when he started on Concerta. I knew that Lucas had temper tantrums, and I should have distinguished between those behaviors that were part of his ADHD and those behaviors that were not. I should have told his mother that the tantrums may not improve with medication. His mother was concerned about his trouble paying attention in school, but she was more concerned about his tantrums. When they did not improve, she assumed that the medication was not working. By not preparing her for this possibility, I ran the risk that his mother would be disappointed by his "lack of response to medication" and discontinue medication without returning to see me again.

I no longer make that mistake. In my initial evaluations, I always ask about other, non-ADHD behaviors, and I am careful to identify for the parents which behaviors are likely to respond to medication and which are not. I tell the parents what to look for and to not discontinue medication, even if they feel that the medication is not helping.

About 30 percent of children with ADHD present with symptoms of ADHD only. They are considered "textbook" cases, and their response to medication is usually positive and dramatic. The other 70 percent of children will also have the "textbook" symptoms of ADHD, but in addition, other problematic behaviors will be evident. These other behaviors are called **comorbid behaviors**. A comorbid behavior is one that is often seen *with* ADHD but is not a behavior that occurs in all children with ADHD and is not part of the primary diagnosis of ADHD.

Most comorbid behaviors will often fit into one of the following categories. And children with ADHD may have more than one group of behaviors:[1]

ADHD Alone (without comorbid conditions)	30–35%
ADHD with Oppositional Defiant Behaviors	20–40%
ADHD with Mood Disorder Behaviors	4–30%
ADHD with Anxiety	12–34%
ADHD with Tics	5–11%
ADHD with Obsessive-Compulsive Disorder[2]	20–50%
ADHD with Sleep Disorders	23%
ADHD with Learning Disorders	56%

Notice that these numbers are highly variable from one study to the next. For example, one highly respected and frequently quoted study reported that 4 percent[3] of children with ADHD had a mood disorder; a second study, also highly respected, reported 30 percent.[4] Unfortunately, different studies used different criteria for the diagnosis. The message here is that when the diagnosis of ADHD is made, the job is only half done.

All of the above comorbidities can be separate disorders in their own right. They can occur with or without ADHD. A child can have an anxiety disorder or a mood disorder without ADHD. When the criteria are fully met, each disorder has a course of treatment separate from the ADHD treatment. A whole book could be written about that subject, but that is not the subject of this chapter.

However, many children with ADHD also have some of the behaviors present in some of these disorders but not enough to confirm a separate diagnosis. In those cases, it is important to identify for the parents those behaviors that are separate and may not be part of ADHD. In some cases, these behaviors will respond positively to stimulant medication, along with the ADHD behaviors, indicating that these behaviors were actually part of the ADHD. More often than not, the ADHD behaviors improve, predictably, but the comorbid behavior may worsen with stimulant medication. In some cases, a second medication may be added to the primary treatment of ADHD behaviors with stimulant medication. The medication treatment of ADHD with comorbid behaviors is discussed in the next section.

Understand that in many children with ADHD, the comorbid behaviors may be significant enough to interfere with learning and social relations but not severe enough to warrant a separate diagnosis. So, a child might be "on the anxious side" but not meet criteria for the diagnosis of an anxiety disorder.

One thing to remember when identifying comorbid behaviors: every one of these behaviors occurs in almost all children, at least some of the time. All of these behaviors are normal if they happen once in a while. But in children with ADHD, these behaviors can seem exaggerated, occurring more often and more intense. It is important to point out these behaviors to parents before starting medication, because these behaviors may react in a seemingly paradoxical way to stimulant medication.

ADHD WITH OPPOSITIONAL DEFIANT BEHAVIORS

Marcus (fictional): Marcus was excited about his first day at preschool. He had his backpack ready, filled with four of his Pokemon stuffed toys, and a Spiderman lunchbox, filled with his favorite foods.

"Marcus, did you finish your cereal?," I asked him.

"Yep, I ate it all up."

"And did you get your jacket?"

"I wanted to wear my Bruins jacket, but I can't find it."

"Wear your orange jacket instead. It's warmer anyway."

"No, I don't want to. I want to wear my Bruins jacket."

"Marcus, we have to leave now, or you will be late for your first day of school. And, anyway, I don't know what you did with that jacket. Wear the orange one."

"NO, NO, NO. I don't want to," he screamed. "I WANT TO WEAR THE BRUINS ONE," he screamed.

"Marcus, here is your other jacket. Put it on." We were running late, and my frustration should have been obvious, but Marcus didn't notice.

"No, I'm not going to wear that one." With that, he picked up his lunchbox and threw it at me. It hit my knee and hurt.

"Marcus," I screamed, "not good. That hurt. Now you lost all your iPad time in the car."

He ran out of the room, kicking over a wastebasket and running his hands along the counter as he ran, knocking his cereal bowl off the counter, with uneaten cereal and milk flying everywhere.

"I hate you. You're the worst mommy in the world. I hate you, and you should die. I want Daddy to take me to school."

This was not how I pictured his first day of school. I finally got him in the car, but he cried most of the way (and I did a little, too). But when we arrived, his teacher was there, and he saw two of his neighbor friends. After he hugged his teacher, he gave me a big smile and waved while I snapped a picture.

And that was the end of that. Or so I thought. A week later, I was picking him up in the afternoon, and his teacher brought him to the car. "How was his day?," I asked.

His teacher rolled her eyes. "We need to talk."

Children with oppositional and defiant (OD) behaviors are often described as "difficult." In addition to their ADHD behaviors, they are often irritable, aggressive, and do not respect authority. Because these behaviors are so socially unacceptable, they come to the attention of a child's parents and teachers fairly early, often in preschool. Barkley has referred to this as "deficient emotional self-regulation," and he sees it as a "central feature" of ADHD.[5] Although it is true that many children with ADHD exhibit these behaviors, not all do.

Oppositional Defiant Behaviors

ADHD behaviors accompanied by many of the following:

- Often loses temper
- Often argues with adults
- Often actively defies or refuses to comply with adult requests or rules
- Often deliberately annoys people
- Often blames others for his or her mistakes or misbehavior
- Often touchy or easily annoyed by others
- Often angry and resentful
- Aggressive
- Often vindictive

Every child exhibits these behaviors at one time or another. As children grow and learn, they meet new challenges, both in the classroom and out. Learning to navigate the rules that blanket social relationships can be more challenging than learning multiplication tables. Learning difficulties are frustrating because they almost always occur in a classroom, where your child's performance is compared to the performance of other children. Every child feels this "competition." Failure to learn academic material or social relationships can be frustrating. All children will express that frustration with a battery of some of these behaviors, some of the time, and that is not necessarily abnormal or part of a "disorder." But when these behaviors are present in an ADHD child before starting on medication, then they may represent a separate disorder.

ADHD WITH DYSPHORIC MOOD

Sophia (fictional): *I just got off the phone with Angela's mother. Angela would be unable to come to Sophia's tenth birthday party. When I told Sophia, she immediately broke into tears.*

"Sophia, I'm sorry that Angela won't be able to come to your party. She will be on a trip to see her grandparents."

"But she's my best friend," she sobbed.

I sat down next to her on the couch and gave her a big hug. "I know, honey. I'm sorry. So how many kids are coming?"

"Well, I think fifteen now."

"Angela, that's great. You invited the eighteen kids in your class. Almost everyone will be there."

"Yeah, but Olivia can't come either. I think they are going to the beach with her cousins who are visiting from Missouri. But I don't think most of the kids really want to come. Maybe their mothers are making them come."

"But I thought you told me that Sara and Kristen told you how excited they were about coming."

"Yeah, I guess so. And guess what? Martin said that he is coming, too. At first, he didn't think he could, but he said when he told his mom how much he wanted to come, she changed his dentist appointment."

"Well, see, you have a lot of good friends, and you'll have a great time."

"I guess so. But I still wish Angela could come." And she started crying again.

Dysphoric mood is a very general term that describes children with a mood that is often negative and constantly changing. Children with dysphoric mood often experience feelings of unease or dissatisfaction. This general term often refers to children who might have a major depressive disorder, or even bipolar disorder. But about 20 percent of children with ADHD have a cloud of negativity that seems to float around them.[6]

Children have disappointments every day. Some recover within minutes, but others brood about things for days. Most of the children do not have a major depression, they just seem to focus on the negative.

The following symptoms are more common in children with ADHD than in the general population. Some of those children are frustrated with their difficulties learning and social relationships, and those behaviors probably will improve with ADHD stimulant medication treatment. But some children with ADHD always seem to find the dark cloud. It is important to point out to parents that although some of these behaviors may improve with stimulant medication, some may not.

Dysphoric Mood Behaviors

ADHD behaviors accompanied by many of the following

- Emotional hypersensitivity and irritability
- Moods change at the drop of a hat
- Argues about every little thing
- Angry much of the time

- Negative attitude
- Little things become major issues
- Lack of spontaneity
- Sad or unhappy much of the time
- Often accompanies oppositional defiant disorder

You may notice that many of these behaviors overlap with oppositional defiant behaviors. Dysphoric mood shares some behaviors with oppositional defiant behaviors but without the severe anger and aggression.

ADHD WITH ANXIETY

Is anxiety a good thing or a bad thing? You probably responded that anxiety is a negative feeling. But anxiety is simply the body's way of motivating itself to get things done. If you have a book report due on Friday but have not yet read the book, you *should* be feeling anxious. As Friday gets closer, the anxiety builds. The best way to get rid of the anxiety is to read the book and write the report. And as soon as the report is finished, the anxiety vanishes.

Sometime it seems like children with ADHD have a *"deficiency of anxiety."* Children with ADHD have a tendency to put things off, to avoid deadlines. As Friday nears, they have the ability to ignore their anxiety, or maybe the anxiety is not produced at all. But, of course, that approach results in uncompleted projects, incomplete homework, and poor grades.

Children with ADHD are often described as risk takers. Because they lack anxiety, they are more willing to try things that could be unsafe or harmful, such as jumping off the bridge into a lake, or taking a hit on the joint offered by a friend.

So, a moderate amount of anxiety, at the right times, can be positive and productive.

However, a subgroup of children with ADHD will have anxiety at unpredictable times. They may not be anxious about the upcoming book report; more likely they worry that a monster is under the bed. An anxious child may be comfortable and enjoy playing with his best friend but uncomfortable in a group, even if his best friend is in the group.

Whereas many children with ADHD are bothered by their
a child with anxiety might have all A's but worry that mom
be upset by the B+ in history.

Anxiety Behaviors

ADHD behaviors accompanied by many of the following:

- Nervousness
- Fearfulness, especially in social situations
- Easily frightened
- Might be easily upset by noises in the house, especially at bedtime
- Afraid of separation from parent (getting the mail)
- Afraid of common things (fire alarms, a certain room, etc.)
- Upset by news reports (burglars, hurricanes, kidnapping)
- Resistant to trying new things
- Feel anxious without any reason

Anxiety can also make it difficult to pay attention, and it is sometimes
tricky to distinguish between the primary attention difficulties in a child
with ADHD and the attention difficulties that anxiety precipitates. No
blood test or CT scan will help your doctor make the distinction. But
the way to distinguish the two is relatively easy.

Before starting any medication, for three nights in a row, ask your
child to do her homework in the kitchen or family room (without the
TV on). While she is doing her homework, you can sit in the same
room or the next room and read (or pretend to read) a book. Don't
help your child with her homework and don't tell her to stay off her
phone or to pay attention or do her work; instead, just watch her out of
the corner of your eye. Pay attention to two things. First, how much of
the time is she actually working? Second, when she is actually engaged
with the work, how does she look? Ask yourself if she looks *carefree*
or *worried*. A child with ADHD will get up to get a drink of water,
go back to her room to get another pen, check her phone constantly,
laugh at something spontaneously, and seem, well, "carefree." On the
other hand, a child with anxiety will rub her lip while reading, complain
about how stupid algebra is, sigh frequently, make statements such as,

"I'll never get all this work done," and seem "worried." Your child may switch from one mode to the other, but ask yourself which mode she spends the most time in.

This method may not be an exact science and relies on parents' subjective interpretation of behavior, but I would guess that you can tell the difference in your own child. As your physician, I would not use the results of this experiment to make my diagnosis, but I would value this information to help determine which treatment to start.

If your child seems to spend more time in the "anxiety" mode, then I would not start a medication. Instead, I would have her start seeing a cognitive behavioral therapist. Counseling in children for anxiety has been found to be just as effective—or more effective—than many antianxiety medications.[7]

But if she seems to spend more time in the "carefree" ADHD mode, then I would start her on a stimulant—specifically a methylphenidate medication—at a lower-than-average dose. I would then increase the dose every 1–2 weeks, and I would ask these two questions: Is her attention improving on medication? Is her anxiety more problematic? If she has an anxiety disorder, her anxiety is likely to get worse. More often, the anxiety is due to the ADHD; and if that is true, her anxiety will lessen or disappear on stimulant medication.[8]

ADHD WITH COMPULSIVE BEHAVIORS

John was a patient of mine. He was a fourteen-year-old boy with ADHD and compulsive behaviors. He attends a school that specializes in teaching children with ADHD, and he has had a very positive response to stimulant medication. His self-confidence has improved along with his grades, but some of his compulsive behaviors are still problematic. On one follow-up visit, his mother asked if she could meet with me without John. I knew that John was a big baseball fan, so I asked him while he was waiting, "Could you write down the names of the top ten professional baseball players?"

When I returned to the waiting room twenty minutes later, John proudly handed me his list. He had written the names of sixty-four professional baseball players. And when I flipped it over, another fifty names were on the back side. Evidence of his compulsive tendencies can be seen in the fact that he wrote out the names of almost a hundred baseball players from memory, when I asked him to write only ten. But what is more striking is his handwriting. You can feel his compulsiveness (Figure 9.1).

His teachers stated that the ADHD medications had helped his attention tremendously, but they felt that his compulsiveness was still getting in the way of his learning. I asked his teacher to give me an example of how his compulsiveness was interfering with his learning. She said that one day he was asked to write a paragraph about his family. He wrote his name in the upper right corner of the paper, then erased it. He wrote his name again . . . and then erased it. After about five minutes

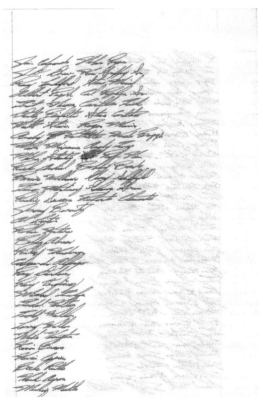

Figure 9.1 Handwriting sample of a 14-year-old boy with ADHD and obsessive-compulsive behaviors.

of this, he had erased a hole through the paper. He told his teacher that his name didn't look right, so he needed to try again.

Compulsive Behaviors

ADHD behaviors accompanied by many of the following:

- Tendency toward perfectionism
- Things have to be just a certain way
- Becomes upset if things in the room are out of order
- Has verbal routines (e.g., at bedtime you have to say a specific thing)
- Tactile sensitivity (socks, elastic, seams, or tags on the back of shirts bother them)
- Relatively higher probability of developing tics

Children with ADHD often seem to live in a state of chaos. When they change clothes, they just drop them on the floor. Their room looks like the aftermath of a Category 5 hurricane. They forget to bring home the right book for their homework. The next night, they bring home the book but forget to write down what pages to read.

On the other hand, some children have a subconscious tendency to impose a sense of order in their lives. The compulsive behaviors are comforting to them because they allow some control over the chaos. But when it is overdone, compulsiveness can be highly burdensome.

The teachers at our school once asked me to see Chloe, a nine-year-old girl from their classroom. They said that she was late to school most mornings, often by an hour or more. She frequently missed her first class. She told me that she had a fish tank with twelve tropical fish. She began telling me about each fish, his or her name, coloring, and so forth. When I asked her what this had to do with being late, she responded that she had to feed her fish each morning before going to school. But at the same time, her mother reached in her purse and pulled out a small notebook. Each page represented a day. Chloe had recorded what each fish had eaten and how much. Her mother said it often took an hour or more for her to feed the fish every morning and record their statistics. She had tried to put time limits on the feeding, but Chloe cried if she could not complete her task every morning.

We were able to get Chloe to do the fish feeding in the afternoon, and the addition of Intuniv, a non-stimulant ADHD medication, helped her feel more comfortable with the change in schedule. The teachers were thrilled that she was present at the beginning of class every morning, just like clockwork.

MEDICATION TREATMENT FOR ADHD
WITH COMORBID BEHAVIORS

Every comorbid behavior can be a normal behavior if it occurs occasionally, in isolation, and in response to the usual frustrations of childhood. But when comorbid behaviors occur many times a day, and when these behaviors occur in response to relatively mild problems, and when these behaviors interfere with a child's ability to learn, either in the classroom or in learning social interactions skills, then intervention is necessary.

When I see a child who meets criteria for the diagnosis of ADHD and that child also has significant comorbid behaviors, I would like to know which of three scenarios is most applicable to this child:

1. These behaviors are part of a normal response to frustration. Counseling is a better first choice than medication.
2. These comorbid behaviors can coexist along with the ADHD behaviors and can be triggered by the frustration of dealing with ADHD. In some children with ADHD, the comorbid behaviors will improve with stimulant medication. For other children, the comorbid behaviors may worsen with stimulant medication, requiring the addition of a second non-stimulant medication.
3. In some children, these behaviors are the predominant way a child handles frustration and may represent a separate diagnosis of oppositional defiant disorder, dysphoric mood, anxiety disorder, or obsessive-compulsive disorder. The primary disorder should be treated with a combination of counseling and a non-stimulant medication. Although children with ADHD often can be well managed by your pediatrician, if comorbid behaviors

are present, then a referral to a child psychiatrist for medication management might be appropriate.

For the first scenario, many books have been written and websites constructed to learn appropriate approaches to behavior management. The third scenario identifies the most common problems seen in child psychiatry, and a complete discussion of how to treat all of these comorbid diagnoses is way beyond the scope of this book.

This section will address the second scenario, a child who has ADHD as the primary diagnosis with some associated comorbid behaviors.

Physicians often prescribe medication to treat the comorbid behaviors. Two groups of medication are used frequently to treat anxiety, the **benzodiazepines** and the **selective serotonin reuptake inhibitors (SSRI)**. These medications are more likely to be used in adults, but doctors may prescribe these for some children as well. In many children, these medications can be effective in treating the comorbid behaviors in a child with ADHD, but one major problem with these medications should cause a physician to pause before prescribing.

Benzodiazepines are a group of medications that have been used for treating anxiety since 1955. Literally thousands of different benzodiazepines that have been produced but only fifteen approved by the FDA. These medications include Valium, Librium, Ativan, and Xanax.

The group of medications called the SSRIs also includes many different, medications, such as Prozac, Zoloft, Paxil, Lexapro, Celexa, and many others.

Both the benzodiazepines and the SSRIs are effective for treating anger, aggression, anxiety, dysphoric mood, and compulsive behaviors in children and adults. However, they have their own set of drawbacks. The benzodiazepines can be sedating. They have some potential for abuse and addiction. SSRIs can cause nausea, upset stomach, weight gain, and decreased libido. But the biggest concern in using both groups of medication in children with anxiety and ADHD is that **they very often cause the ADHD behaviors to worsen**.

So, a child has been appropriately diagnosed with ADHD. He is treated with stimulant medication and the ADHD behaviors improve, but the child is still oppositional or subdued or anxious or compulsive.

At this point, a benzodiazepine or an SSRI might be added to the stimulant medication. The comorbid behavior improves, but the ADHD behaviors may increase. The child becomes more hyperactive, impulsive, and inattentive. So, the dose of the stimulant is increased. Again, the ADHD behaviors improve, but the comorbid behavior returns. The dose of the benzodiazepine or SSRI is increased, and . . . Well, I think you see where I am going with this. Eventually a child is now on two medications at high doses for each, and the child is only marginally better. Instead, I would recommend that you discuss the following approach with your doctor:

Use behavioral questionnaires to measure both the ADHD behaviors and the comorbid behaviors. Each time a change in treatment is made (a different medication, a change in dose, starting counseling), you and the teacher would complete the questionnaire again so that you and your doctor can determine how each change affects the two different sets of behaviors.

If ADHD coexists with comorbid behaviors, first try to determine which of these behaviors is causing more disruption in the child's life and most interfering with his ability to learn and to get along with other children.

If the comorbid behaviors seem to be more disruptive to the child's learning and social relations, start with cognitive behavioral therapy[9] without medication. If therapy is not helpful, then try a methylphenidate medication.

If the ADHD behaviors are felt to be the most problematic, start with a methylphenidate-based medication (amphetamine medications such as Adderall and Vyvanse are more likely to cause irritability and worsen anxiety).[10]

Titrate the dose of the methylphenidate up or down until the optimal effect on attention is achieved.

If comorbid behaviors remain on an optimal dose of methylphenidate, and especially if it is more problematic, start a non-stimulant

ADHD medication (clonidine, guanfacine, atomoxetine). Try both a non-stimulant by itself and in combination with a stimulant.

For oppositional defiant behaviors and for tics, I would be more likely to start with the non-stimulant clonidine (Catapres, Kapvay) or guanfacine (Tenex, Intuniv); **for dysmorphic mood and compulsive behaviors**, I would be more likely to start atomoxetine (Strattera). Atomoxetine was initially used as an antidepressant and does help modulate mood, while, at the same time, it is helpful for the treatment of many of the ADHD symptoms. Clonidine (Catapres, Kapvay) is a little more sedating than guanfacine, so I would start with clonidine if there are associated sleep problems, or I would start with guanfacine (Tenex, Intuniv) if there are no sleep difficulties.

In most children, **ADHD behaviors will respond best to a stimulant, and comorbid behaviors will respond best to a non-stimulant.** These children will thus benefit from a combination of a stimulant and a non-stimulant.

If a stimulant and a non-stimulant will be used in combination, both medications should not be started at the same time because it will be difficult to tell which medication is doing what.

Children with ADHD and oppositional defiant behaviors are a special case. Sometimes the oppositional defiant behaviors are triggered by the impulsivity of ADHD and will respond to a stimulant, so a second medication will not be needed. If a child has ADHD and oppositional defiant behaviors who is also very active and impulsive and is under the age of six, many physicians are reluctant to start a stimulant and will instead start with clonidine (Catapres, Catpres TTS, Kapvay or guanfacine Tenex, Intuniv).

To summarize, children with ADHD often have comorbid behaviors as well. Before starting any medication treatment, it is difficult but important to distinguish between the ADHD behaviors and the comorbid behaviors. Then, identify how these two groups of behaviors respond to either a stimulant medication or a non-stimulant medication, or both.

Chapter 10

TWENTY BRAND-NAME METHYLPHENIDATE MEDICATIONS TO TREAT ADHD

This chapter will present a short profile of each of the twenty methylphenidate medications, including both its advantages and disadvantages. This knowledge should give you and your physician options to personalize medication treatment for your child and to maximize the benefits of medication while keeping side effects minimal to nonexistent.

All twenty of these medications contain the same active ingredient, methylphenidate. Some are immediate release and, therefore, last only a few hours. Some are extended-release preparations, lasting 7–20 hours. Some are liquid. Some are tablets that dissolve in the mouth so that they do not have to be swallowed. Some are chewable. Some come in a skin patch.

Some parents will have a tendency to read only the parts that describe the medication that their child is currently receiving. **I would encourage you to read through the entire next three chapters.** Your doctor will probably be well versed in the details of many of these medications but not all. This information gives you the opportunity to have an intelligent conversation with your doctor about whether an 8- or 10-hour medication might be better for your child. Or it might give you the knowledge to let your doctor know that your child has trouble swallowing a capsule. You can then discuss the benefits of a liquid preparation, or a chewable tablet, or an orally dissolving tablet.

Finally, detailed information of approximate costs of the medications will allow you to determine whether the minor or major difference from one medication is justified by the increased cost. Some medications will be covered by your insurance, whereas many others will not, so before discussing with your physician the different medications available, familiarize yourself with your specific insurance coverage. And understand that these costs are what is listed at the time of publication of this book. These costs can change on an almost daily basis, but the current listings can give you a basis of comparison. Check GoodRx.com to see if the prices have changed.

Understand that the following information is provided so that you can better understand the medications used to treat ADHD and ask the right questions of your physician. It is extremely important that you not make any changes in your child's medication without consulting with your physician first. Although the following information has been checked and rechecked, it changes frequently, and it cannot be guaranteed that all of the following information is 100 percent accurate.

Ritalin / Ritalin SR / Ritalin LA

Brand Name			Generic Name			
Ritalin Ritalin SR Ritalin LA			Methylphenidate Ritalin LA: 50% IR, 50% ER 50% dex, 50% levo			
Advantages			Disadvantages			
Because Ritalin is very short acting, it is a good medication to supplement a more long-acting medication (e.g., adding a second dose in the late afternoon or evening when a long-acting preparation might wear off).			Short acting Ritalin should almost never be used as the sole treatment of ADHD because irritability and other side effects can be caused by multiple, overlapping doses. A dose during the day at school may be needed.			
			Brand		Generic	
	Time	Preparations	w/o Ins	GoodRx	w/o Ins	GoodRx
Ritalin	4-5	Tablet 5-10-20mg	$117	$88	$96	$18
Ritalin SR	5-6	Tablet 10-20mg	Brand No Longer Available		$200	$24
Ritalin LA	7-8	Brand: 10-20-30-40-60mg Generic: 20-30-40mg Capsule	$440	$299	$230	$52

As far as medications go, Ritalin has a very mixed reputation. For the parents who have seen their child's self-esteem rise from the depths to sunlight, for those parents who have seen their child's grades improve overnight from failing to As and Bs, and for those parents who have seen a child's aggression and impulsivity melt away, Ritalin is a miracle drug. But this neurologic coin has another side. Many parents who have not had direct experiences with the medication will have spoken to a family member, or read a magazine article, or seen something online, so that almost no parent who has come to my office has never heard of Ritalin. Most parents are somewhat familiar with Ritalin, and many parents who have heard of Ritalin before have a negative opinion of it.

What has Ritalin done to garner this dubious reputation? It is not really Ritalin's fault. The only ingredient in Ritalin is methylphenidate, and methylphenidate is a very short-acting medication. Along with amphetamine, it is the most effective medication to treat ADHD, but from the time that it is swallowed until it ceases to be effective is usually about 3½–4 hours. But children have ADHD all day. Every day. To treat their ADHD by using two or three doses of short-acting methylphenidate exposes a child to potential emotional side effects. As each dose is absorbed, reaches a peak, and then wears off, a roller-coaster effect is created, which leads to emotional volatility throughout the day. This is described in more detail in Chapter 8 on side effects.

And treating a child's ADHD only during school hours makes no sense either. What about the third grader who takes an hour to complete fifteen minutes of homework? What about the twelve-year-old who has dance practice at 4? Or sees a tutor at 4:30? What about the teenager who is driving home after school and then to a job stocking shelves? Having to take medication three times a day might not only produce the emotional side effects described, but also could lead to a lack of compliance with the medication as prescribed. The teenager driving to his afternoon job at the grocery store forgets to take his afternoon dose of medication and because he is running late, doesn't go home to get his dose. So, he works without his medication, forgets to stock a whole cart of hamburger buns, and then is fired. If he had been using a longer-acting medication, he might have avoided his termination.

For years, we physicians begged Novartis, the pharmaceutical company that had been producing Ritalin, to come up with a more long-term solution. At the end of the 1990s, Novartis released Ritalin SR. The company combined the raw methylphenidate with cellulose (which is a completely natural ingredient that is the "fiber" in most plants). The cellulose slows the absorption of methylphenidate, producing a longer-acting medication. Unfortunately, Ritalin SR only extended the effective life of methylphenidate by an hour or two and was discontinued in 2014, but it is still available as a generic.

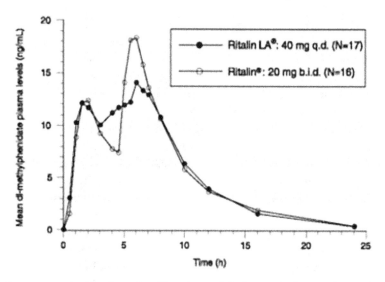

Figure 10.1   Blood levels produced by 2 doses of Ritalin vs. a single dose of Ritalin LA.

Ritalin LA (long acting) was released by Novartis in 2005. Ritalin LA comes in a capsule with a mixture of two different beads. Half the beads are simply methylphenidate, released exactly like regular Ritalin. They are absorbed quickly, take effect in 20–30 minutes, and last 3½–4 hours. However, the other half of the beads consist of coated methylphenidate beads using the SODAS® (spheroidal oral drug absorption system) technology. The methylphenidate in these beads is more slowly absorbed and lasts longer (7–8 hours). The combination of these two beads produces a curve with two peaks (corresponding to the immediate-release beads and the extended-release beads), but it is a much smoother curve than two doses of Ritalin (see Figure 10.1),[1] avoiding the "ups and downs" of regular methylphenidate and, thus, significantly reducing emotional lability.[2]

Brand-name Ritalin LA is expensive (more than $400 for sixty brand-name pills or approximately $300 with a GoodRx coupon). A generic is available for much less. The brand name is not prescribed very often anymore because there are so many other better, extended-release options. However, if Ritalin LA is one of the few long-acting medications that your insurance company covers, it is a good medication with which to initiate treatment. The drawback is that the beneficial effects last about 7–8 hours. If it is taken early (7 a.m.), it will start wearing off around 3, necessitating an additional dose of the short-acting methylphenidate to last through homework, soccer, tutoring, and after-school jobs.

Concerta

Brand Name	Generic Name
Concerta	Methylphenidate 22% IR, 78% ER 50% dex, 50% levo
Advantages	**Disadvantages**
Longest acting of the oral meds (with exception of Jornay), "smoother" effect throughout the day. An excellent choice to initiate first-time treatment of ADHD. Generic often covered by insurance, and the generic from Patriot is exactly the same as the brand, but significantly cheaper. It is necessary to specify "generic from Patriot" (see below).	Moderately expensive.

	Time	Preparations	Brand		Generic	
			w/o Ins	GoodRx	w/o Ins	GoodRx
Concerta	10-11	18-27-36-54 mg capsule	$504	$383	$295	$45

Ritalin LA was good as a long-acting medication for ADHD, but in 2000, Concerta was released by Janssen Pharmaceuticals. It was a game changer. Three years after its release, Concerta accounted for 26 percent of all medications prescribed for ADHD.[3]

Concerta is a long-acting preparation of methylphenidate, and although it only lasts a few hours longer than Ritalin LA, those few hours make all the difference. Ritalin LA lasts about eight hours, but Concerta lasts about 10–11 hours. That means that a dose of Ritalin LA given at 7 a.m. will wear off around 2 or 3 p.m., whereas Concerta will last until 4 or 5 p.m. No longer would you have to worry about your child getting medication at school. Concerta instead will be wearing off around dinnertime, allowing appetite to return. And Concerta wears off gradually, so that emotional lability is much less likely or even absent. Concerta is ideal for this situation because a second dose is usually not needed.

Concerta extends the medication time duration in a way like no other medication. In order to achieve this extended-release effect, Concerta uses a unique technology called osmotic-controlled release oral delivery system (OROS):

Concerta starts with a plastic pill (which does not dissolve; it will pass through the GI tract and emerge in the stool).

The outside surface of the pill is coated with 22 percent of the total short-acting methylphenidate (4 mg for the 18mg pill).

The one-way membrane that forms the pill allows water to seep from the GI tract into the pill (but water cannot exit back into the GI tract).

Inside the pill are three different compartments.

The bottom compartment, the push compartment, contains a substance that expands when it gets wet, like a sponge.

The other two compartments contain methylphenidate in differing concentrations.

A microscopic hole has been drilled with a laser at the end of the pill opposite the push compartment. The size of the hole determines how fast the medication will be released to the body.

So here is what happens when the pill is swallowed:

The outside coating of methylphenidate is absorbed within the first twenty minutes and begins to take effect in 30–40 minutes.

Water from the stomach begins to seep into the push compartment, and it begins to expand.

The expanding push compartment pushes the methylphenidate in compartment 1 out the laser-drilled hole. The microscopic hole is precisely designed to allow the methylphenidate out at a predetermined rate.

The push compartment continues to expand until all of the methylphenidate in compartment 1 and most of the methylphenidate in compartment 2 has emerged from the hole.

This elaborate mechanism produces a steady level of methylphenidate in the bloodstream (and thus the brain) that simulates the administration of three doses of the short–acting methylphenidate.

Even though a number of other options for long-acting methylphenidate are available, Concerta is still one of the best oral, pill-based strategies for treating ADHD.

Janssen Pharmaceuticals developed and marketed the original brand-name Concerta. However, when its brand-name exclusivity expired, Janssen knew that generic versions of Concerta could now be sold by generic pharmaceutical companies at a much lower price than the brand name. To counter this loss of revenue, Janssen developed a licensing agreement with Actavis Pharmaceuticals, a subsidiary of Janssen, that allowed Actavis to market a generic of Concerta. However, this "generic" would be produced in the same lab, using exactly the same pharmaceutical techniques, and even labeling the pill with the same markings. This "generic" is, in reality, brand-name Concerta.

In the recent past, when a physician wrote a prescription for Concerta, that physician could specify that the prescription be filled with the authorized generic from Actavis, and their patients would get brand-name Concerta at the significantly lower generic prices. And many physicians did just that.

However, the authorized generic is no longer available through Actavis but is now available through Patriot Pharmaceuticals, another subsidiary of Janssen Pharmaceuticals, the company that produces brand-name Concerta. Your physician then has three choices when writing a prescription for Concerta:

1. Your doctor can simply write the prescription for Concerta without specifying anything, and that is what is usually done. The pharmacist may fill the prescription with brand-name Concerta (at $400 without insurance). However, if the insurance company does not cover the brand name, the pharmacy might fill the prescription with one of ten different generics. These long-acting methylphenidate generics usually use some form of coated beads, some of which are immediate release and some of which are extended release), usually producing a medication that lasts around 7–8 hours, not nearly as long as with the brand-name Concerta.

2. Or the physician can specify Concerta, brand-name only, and the pharmacist must fill the prescription with the Concerta brand name. But Concerta brand name is expensive and often not covered by insurance.

3. Or the physician can specify that the prescription must be filled with the **authorized generic from Patriot**. Patriot is the only "generic" of Concerta that uses the same OROS technology as Concerta. The two are the same in every way, except that the brand-name Concerta costs around $400 without insurance, whereas the generic of Concerta from Patriot costs around $200 without insurance.

If your physician wants to be sure that you obtain the brand-name medication at generic prices, he can specify the National Drug Code (NDC) for each prescription. The NDC number is a unique number assigned to each strength of a medication. Your physician can find the NDC for any medication through the FDA website: https://www.accessdata.fda.gov/scripts/cder/ndc/index.cfm.

The unique NDC codes for the Patriot Concerta generic are:[4]

- 18mg: 10147-0685
- 27mg: 10147-0688
- 36mg: 10147-0686
- 54mg: 10147-0687

If your insurance company covers brand-name Concerta, then you have nothing to worry about. But I have seen insurance companies that once covered the brand name revert to covering the generic only. To prevent the substitution of a "generic" that is not identical to Concerta, the physician should write the name of the medication on the prescription as "*Concerta (generic by Patriot only, NDC = 10147-0685)*"[5] (with an understanding that the NDC code is different for each different dosage).

Metadate CD

Brand Name			Generic Name		
Metadate CD			Methylphenidate Metadate CD: 30% IR, 70% ER 50% dex, 50% levo		
Advantages			**Disadvantages**		
Multiple dosages allowing for easier titration. Capsule can be opened and sprinkled on applesauce or pudding. Good for a younger child. Less expensive than Concerta.			Brand name is no longer available, but an **identical** generic, made by a subsidiary of the company that produced Metadate CD. Shorter lasting than Concerta, but may be a good choice for a younger child.		
	Time	Preparations	Brand		Generic	
			w/o Ins	GoodRx	w/o Ins	GoodRx
Metadate CD	8-9	10-20-30-40-50-60mg capsule	Brand Name Not Available		$171	$38
Metadate ER	6-7	10-20 mg	Brand Name Not Available		$220	$24

Metadate CD is an extended-release methylphenidate medication that lasts about 8–9 hours after an oral dose. Metadate CD uses the same medication release mechanism as does Ritalin LA, a mixture of two types of coated beads, one that is immediate release and the other that is extended release. The immediate-release beads function just like plain methylphenidate or Ritalin, taking about 20–30 minutes to take affect and lasting about 3–4 hours. The extended-release beads are coated to delay the onset for about 3–4 hours and last another four hours. The combination of the two beads results in a medication that begins to take effect in 20–30 minutes and lasts for 8–9 hours after an oral dose. In this way, Metadate CD is very similar to Ritalin LA. The only difference is that the bead mixture in Ritalin LA is 50 percent immediate release and 50 percent extended release, whereas Metadate CD is 30 percent immediate release and 70 percent extended release. Because Metadate CD has relatively more extended-release beads, it has a slightly longer effect (8–9 hours) than Ritalin LA (7–8 hours).

One advantage of Metadate is that unlike some other extended-release medications such as Concerta, this capsule can be opened and sprinkled on a spoonful of pudding or ice cream or applesauce. However, the small beads must be swallowed without chewing (if they are chewed, all of the medication will be released too early and would cause the child to get more medication than intended).

Brand name Metadate CD was discontinued by its manufacturer in April 2017. However, multiple generics are available, and if a physician writes a prescription for Metadate CD, it will be filled with a generic. UCB, the company that originally produced Metadate CD, sold Metadate CD to Lannett Pharmaceutical Co. as an authorized generic. Although Lannett sells the medication as a generic, it is actually identical to brand-name Metadate CD.

Metadate CD is no longer available as brand name, so ask your physician to write the prescription as follows:

Metadate CD 10mg (generic from Lannett only NDC = 00527-4579-37)

For most pharmacies, the above prescription without the NDC is usually effective, and most physicians are not used to using the NDC code. However, with so many different methylphenidate generics,[6] to be sure of getting Metadate CD brand (now generic) it is best to specify the NDC code. The NDC code is different for each strength:

- 10mg: 00527-4579-37
- 20mg: 00527-4580-37
- 30mg: 00527-4581-37
- 40mg: 00527-4582-37
- 50mg: 00527-4583-37
- 60mg: 00527-4584-37

Adhansia XR / Aptensio XR

Brand Name	Generic Name
Adhansia XR Aptensio XR	Methylphenidate AdhansiaXR: 20% IR, 80% ER Aptensio XR: 40% IR, 60% ER 50% dex, 50% levo
Advantages	**Disadvantages**
These two medications use the same technology as Ritalin LA and Metadate CD (but with different ratios of Immediate Release to Extended Release). These two medications are almost identical to Ritalin LA or Metadate CD, but with Aptensio XR lasting 8 – 9 hour and Adhansia XE lasting 14-16 hours.	The high cost (without insurance) is not justified by the subtle differences.

	Time	Preparations	Brand		Generic	
			w/o Ins	GoodRx	w/o Ins	GoodRx
Adhansia XR 20% IR 80% ER	14-16	25-35-45-55-70-85mg capsules	$392	$346	Generic Not Available	
Aptensio XR 40% IR 60% ER	8-9	10-15-20-30-40-50-60mg capsule	$304	$251	Generic Not Available	

Adhansia XR and Aptensio XR are two newer extended-release methylphenidate medications, very similar to Ritalin LA and Metadate CD, although they last a little longer.

All four medications have methylphenidate as the active ingredient. All four medications use the same technology as these medications, a combination of uncoated beads of medication (releases immediately over one-half hour) and coated beads (released over about 8–10 hours).

If all four of these medications use the same technology (coated beads) and all four medications have methylphenidate as their main ingredient, then what makes them unique? And why does the FDA not consider them to be generics of Ritalin LA? The *only* substantial difference in these four medications is that they are produced with a different ratio of immediate release-beads to extended-release beads. Adhansia XR lasts longer than the other three medications because it contains 80 percent extended release versus 70 percent for Metadate CD, 60 percent for Aptensio XR, and 50 percent for Ritalin LA. On the other hand, the higher the percentage of extended release means a lower percentage of immediate release, which can cause Adhansia XR to take longer to take effect in the morning. Adhansia XR would be expected to last the longest because it has 80 percent extended-release beads.

It is great to have options that can be tailored to each child, but are the extra few hours gained from Adhansia XR worth the very significant increase in cost? Without insurance, you would pay $254 a month more for Adhansia XR than Metadate CD, or more than $3,000 per year. If insurance covers Adhansia XR, it would be a good option for your older child, who goes to sleep later, but if Adhansia XR is not covered by your insurance, you should question the benefits of Adhansia XR. Finally, you should consider that Concerta contains the same active ingredient (methylphenidate) and lasts nearly as long as Adhansia XR.

Remember what was said earlier about evergreening? Evergreening is the practice of making subtle changes to the active-ingredient molecule or in the delivery system in order to get FDA approval as a brand name, rather than a generic. Why? Because they can charge more. Adhansia XR and Aptensio XR are unique medications with some minor advantages, but overall, this is a perfect example of evergreening.

On the other hand, this is one case where the attempt by the pharmaceutical companies to make more money gives you and your physician more options for treating your child's ADHD.

One small advantage of Metadate CD, Adhansia XR, and Aptensio XR is that unlike Concerta, these capsules can be opened and sprinkled on a spoonful of applesauce or pudding or ice cream. However, the small beads must be swallowed without chewing (if they are chewed, all of the medication will be released too early and would cause the child to get more medication than intended).

The bottom line is that Adhansia XR lasts a little longer than other bead-delivery forms of methylphenidate, and Aptensio XR takes effect a little quicker in the morning. But they are both expensive, not usually covered by insurance, and probably not worth the significant increase in cost. In most cases, Concerta would usually be a better choice.

Note: Aptensio XR has been available in Canada as Biphentin since 2006. Same medication, different name.

Methylin

Brand Name			Generic Name			
Methylin			Methylphenidate 50% IR, 50% ER 50% dex, 50% levo			
Advantages			**Disadvantages**			
No real advantage. Brand name no longer available.			The tablets are simply short-acting methylphenidate. The ER dose does not last much longer than the shorter acting tablets. The chewable tabs and the liquid are short-acting and multiple doses would be needed, causing variability throughout the day.			
	Time	Preparations	Brand		Generic	
			w/o Ins	GoodRx	w/o Ins	GoodRx
Tablets	4-5	5-10-20mg	$116	$50	$96	$18
Chewable	4-5	2.5-5-10mg	Brand No Longer Available		$252	$61
Liquid	4-5	5mg/5ml 10mg/5ml 150-225-300-450-600-675 ml bottles	Brand No Longer Available		$218	$31

Methylin was a version of methylphenidate that came in four different forms: an immediate-release tablet, a chewable tablet, an extended-release tablet, and a liquid. However, the brand name for each of these four preparations has been discontinued, although pharmacists will still fill a prescription for "Methylin" with a generic. And that is just as well, because other brand name and generics of each of those four preparations are better choices of each of the four preparations. This information is included for completeness only.

Methylin tablets have been discontinued, but they were actually the same as plain old Ritalin, raw methylphenidate in a tablet form. Many different generics have essentially the same characteristics.

Methylin chewable tablets have also been discontinued, but for children who cannot swallow a pill, QuilliChew ER (see below) is a better option anyway, because QuilliChew ER lasts about eight hours whereas Methylin chewable tablets only lasted about 4–5 hours.

Methylin liquid was a good medication because it was easy to fine-tune the dose of medication without being restrained by pills that, for example, come in 5mg, 10mg, or 15mg preparations. However, Methylin liquid is also short acting. Quillivant XR is another liquid form of methylphenidate, but due to a unique manufacturing process, it lasts eight hours while still having the advantage of a liquid that will allow fine-tuning of the dose and make it easy to swallow. Quillivant XR is, therefore, a better medication, although it is much more expensive if not covered by insurance.

Methylin ER has also been discontinued. It was initially a generic of Ritalin SR, which has also been discontinued. Neither preparation adds much therapeutic benefit, because Ritalin SR and Methylin ER only lasted about 5–6 hours.

Daytrana

Brand Name			Generic Name		
Daytrana			Methylphenidate 50% IR, 50% ER 50% dex, 50% levo		
Advantages			**Disadvantages**		
Flexible duration. Patch can be removed at different times depending on daily demands. **Flexible fine-tuned dosage**, by cutting patch. **Crash-resistant**. Because it wears off gradually. The irritability that can occur when a stimulant wears off at the end of the day is greatly reduced. **Compliance**. (Parent knows that a child had the patch on all day, because if removed, it cannot be reapplied.)			Expensive, not often covered by insurance. Mild skin irritation is common, but treatable. Rarely an allergic reaction may prevent use. Leukoderma, a discoloration of the skin, is rare, but when it occurs, it is permanent.		
	Time	**Preparations**	**Brand**		**Generic**	
			w/o Ins	**GoodRx**	**w/o Ins**	**GoodRx**
Skin Patch	5- 20	10-15-20-30 mg Skin Patch	$504	$441	Generic Not Available	

Of all the medications used to treat ADHD, Daytrana is probably the most unique medication available. If it were not for two problems, Daytrana could be the single best form of methylphenidate to use in both children and adults with ADHD.

Daytrana is not a pill but a skin patch. It is another method of delivering methylphenidate to the body, and it is the only stimulant medication available as a skin patch (Catapres TTS is the only other medication treatment for ADHD that is currently available in a skin patch, but Catapres is not a stimulant, does not contain methylphenidate or amphetamine, and is not as effective at treating the ADHD symptoms. Noven Pharmaceuticals is currently developing a skin patch for delivery of dextro-amphetamine for children with ADHD. Clinical trials are ongoing, and early results are very promising, but at the time of this printing, this medication has not yet been approved by the FDA.)

Many other medications deliver medication into the body through a skin patch (estrogen and testosterone are frequently prescribed in a patch form), as well as other medications that need a constant level of medication in the bloodstream throughout the day (scopolamine for motion sickness, opioids for chronic pain, and nicotine for smoking cessation). However, most of these patches are designed with a reservoir in the middle of the patch surround by adhesive that keeps the patch attached to the skin.

Instead, Daytrana is produced by mixing methylphenidate with an adhesive, and this mixture is applied to a plastic sheet. This sheet is then cut into smaller squares. The size of the square dictates how much medication will be available in the patch for treatment.

The main reason that Daytrana excels as a stimulant treatment for ADHD can be summed in one word: *flexibility*.[7] This skin patch preparation of methylphenidate excels compared to other ADHD medications for four reasons. Daytrana is the only ADHD stimulant medication that allows the physician and patient to determine how long the medication will last, and it is the only medication other than the liquid preparations (Quillivant XR and Methylin liquid) that allows the physician and patient to fine-tune the dose. It wears off more gradually than any other methylphenidate medication, which usually prevents the emotional "crash" that can occur as other medications wear off at the end of the day. Finally, it is the only ADHD medication that gives the parent a way to monitor whether the child is taking the medication:

1. Flexible Medication Duration Time

With any other oral medication, once you have swallowed the medication, the specific characteristics of the medication and your body determine how long that medication will remain effective by how rapidly it is absorbed through the stomach and intestines and how rapidly it is metabolized in the body, broken down, and eliminated by the liver or kidneys. It is as if the duration of Ritalin and every other oral ADHD medication is preprogramed, and once it is swallowed, you can't do anything to change that.

When the research was done to demonstrate to the FDA that Daytrana lasts throughout the day, the patch was routinely removed after nine hours. This "wear time" would allow Daytrana to be compared to other long-acting preparations of methylphenidate (Ritalin LA, Metadate CD, Concerta, etc.), which typically are effective for 8–12 hours.

Daytrana is designed to deliver a steady dose of medication throughout the day. In order to keep the dose per hour relatively stable, much more medication is affixed to the patch than can be released in a nine-hour period. But here is where the patch gets "sticky." Daytrana comes in four dosages (10mg, 15mg, 20mg, 30mg). A 10 mg patch actually contains 27.5 mg of methylphenidate, a 15mg patch contains 41.3 mg, and so on. A 10mg patch will release about 1.1 mg per hour and in nine hours will release 9 x 1.1mg or 10 mg in a nine-hour period. However, that means that at the end of nine hours, only 36 percent of methylphenidate has been released, and 17.5 mg still remains on the patch, most of which can still be absorbed if the patch remains affixed to the skin past nine hours. When the FDA approved Daytrana as a treatment for ADHD, it added the directive that the patch be removed after it had been worn for nine hours, because that is the only scenario studied prior to FDA approval. However, leaving the patch affixed to the skin for more or less than nine hours has no drawback and gives you more flexibility in determining how long the medication will last.

If the patch is applied when Danny wakes up at 7 a.m. on a school day, it is slow to take effect, but is generally effective from 1½ hours after applying the patch. The positive therapeutic effect of the medication wears off about 1–2 hours after removing the patch. That would mean that in the FDA nine-hour wear-time scenario, the patch would be removed at 4 p.m. and it would cease being effective around 5–6 p.m. This might be ideal for a child in school.

But what if Danny is very sensitive to the appetite suppression side effect of methylphenidate? If a patch lasts until 6 p.m., and Danny's family eats dinner at 5:30, the methylphenidate may still be in his system suppressing his appetite. Removing the patch after less than nine hours will cause the blood levels of methylphenidate to diminish earlier and allow him to eat better.

But what about the weekend? Danny gets up at 7 a.m. during the week, but he sleeps in till 10:30 on the weekend. If he took a long-acting oral medication such as Ritalin LA, Concerta, Adderall XR, or Vyvanse at 11 a.m., then these medications would wear off around 7 to 8 p.m. Here is where the patch excels. In this case, the patch might be applied at 11 a.m. and then removed at 4 p.m. so that he would feel hungry at dinner and ready for bed at 8:30 p.m. Through trial-and-error, you can find the application times and removal times that work best for your child.[8]

This flexibility is even more important for college students with ADHD. On Wednesdays, your daughter at college might have an 8:30 class but nothing throughout the rest of the day. She might go to the library and study till noon and then go back to the dorm for lunch. So, she might remove the patch after lunch for a wear time of only five hours. However, on Thursdays, she might have two classes in the morning and a lab at 7 p.m. And she has a test Friday morning, so she might stay up until 1 a.m. studying. On Fridays she would put the patch on at 7:30 a.m. and remove it at midnight, for a wear time of 16½ hours. By strategic planning, the patch might be applied and removed at different times to adapt to each child's different daily schedules.

You might be interrupting here to inform me that because of your daughter's lack of organization, you cannot imagine her planning each different day. But you would be pleasantly surprised at how little planning this requires and how well the ADHD college student adapts to this daily variability, and even prefers it.

2. Flexible Fine-Tuned Dosage

One of my patients was a seven-year-old boy with ADHD. A 10mg Daytrana patch had no effect. His attention and schoolwork showed no improvement. A 15mg patch was then prescribed, and the mother told me that the teacher could not believe how alert and attentive he was. His learning and grades had improved dramatically. However, he was very quiet and did not engage with the other children. His mother felt that the dose was too high. What was I to do? There is a 10mg patch and a

15mg patch but nothing in between. Many physicians might consider switching to a different oral medication at this point.

But there is another option. The patches are easily cut. Remember that the patch is initially produced on a large sheet and then cut to different sizes. The size of the patch dictates how much medication will be delivered. So, one strategy for this seven-year-old boy would be to cut off a small strip of the patch to deliver a slightly lower dose. Cutting one-fourth inch off a 15mg patch would deliver about 13 mg in nine hours instead of the 15 mg delivered by the uncut patch.

This strategy was effective for this child for a few years. As he got older and as he grew, the patch seemed to be losing its effectiveness. At this point, I told her to stop cutting the patch. He now received the full dose from the 15mg patch, and his attention improved again, this time without the mood suppression. This approach allows you and your doctor to fine-tune the dose for each individual child. It lets the child's individual metabolism determine the right dose for each individual child, to achieve the best response with the least side effects.

This approach is described as an option to be discussed with your physician. Never cut the patch without consulting with your physician first.

But Daytrana still has two more advantages.

3. Crash-Resistant

In the chapter on side effects, it was evident that multiple doses of a short-acting stimulant medication resulted in emotional lability and irritability. Methylphenidate is a fast-acting medication. It begins to take effect within a half hour after swallowing a pill and it wears off 3½–4 hours later. This rapid onset and offset means that at least two and often three doses per day of this medication are required. Further, this rapid onset and offset can produce irritability and variability in mood throughout the day that is highly problematic and one of the biggest drawbacks of the many short-acting medications used to treat ADHD (see Chapter 8 on side effects).

Because Daytrana releases the methylphenidate steadily and gradually throughout the day, and because it wears off very gradually, this emotional lability, or the "crash" at the end of the day, rarely occurs.

4. Compliance

One drawback of the patch is that a child can remove the patch without your knowledge and go to school without his medication. But a child who is taking a pill can put the pill in his mouth, let it sit in his cheek for a few minutes, then go to the bathroom, and spit it out. You would never know that he did not take his medication that day. You cannot prevent your child from removing a patch, but you can check at the end of every day to make sure the patch is still attached to the skin. If the patch had been removed earlier, it cannot be reapplied because it will not stick to the skin again.

If a child resists taking a pill in the morning or applying a patch, it is important to understand why he does not want to take the medication in the first place. Is it because he doesn't like the taste? Or because he has trouble swallowing it? Or because he is experiencing side effects that he has not revealed to you?

Daytrana Side Effects

Because Daytrana is methylphenidate, it has the potential to produce all the same side effects that the other methylphenidate preparations can produce (appetite suppression, insomnia, irritability, etc.), although Daytrana might be less likely to do so because of the flexibility in duration and dosage that Daytrana provides. But three potential side effects are unique to Daytrana, and all three are produced by the direct effect of the patch on the skin.

About half the children who use Daytrana develop irritation and redness at the site of application. (This is usually referred to as **irritant contact dermatitis**.) This redness is usually just under the patch, lasts for 12–24 hours, and usually disappears without treatment by the next day.[9] That is why it is recommended to change the site of application every day. This type of skin irritation is usually relatively mild, and it is not usually necessary to discontinue medication.[10]

Although this common side effect does not usually require any treatment, sometimes the skin redness will be accompanied by a mild to moderate itching or burning. A moisture cream applied after removing the patch can help alleviate these symptoms. Calmoseptine,[11] an over-the-counter cream, creates a moisture barrier with cooling menthol, zinc oxide, and calamine. Also, olive oil works well for this. Over-the-counter steroids (1 percent) can be applied to the site *before* applying the patch in the morning,[12] but it is necessary to wait about 15–20 minutes for the steroid cream to dry, or the patch will not adhere well to the skin. Over-the-counter steroids will rapidly reduce the burning and itching if applied after the patch is removed at the end of the day.[13] It is important to point out that none of these treatments has been well studied.

Two other skin reactions to the Daytrana patch are very rare. Some patients may have an allergic reaction to the patch. An allergic reaction usually happens within the first hour after the patch is applied and then may gradually increase as the day goes on. The redness and irritation from an allergic reaction usually covers more skin area beyond the skin covered by the patch. If this happens, there does not seem to be a work-around, and Daytrana will need to be discontinued and an alternative medication started.

A very small number of patients have developed **leukoderma**, or a permanent loss of skin pigmentation, leaving white patches on the skin. This may be bothersome for Caucasian children but more troublesome for children of color, because the discoloration may be more apparent and permanent.

The FDA reviewed the cases of leukoderma that had been referred to them and it concluded:

> We reviewed cases of chemical leukoderma associated with the Daytrana patch reported to the *FDA Adverse Event Reporting System (FAERS) database* and described in the medical literature. FAERS includes only reports submitted to FDA so there are likely additional cases about which we are unaware. FDA identified 51 FAERS cases from April 2006 to December 2014 and one published case that was not recorded in FAERS. The time to onset of leukoderma after starting Daytrana ranged from 2 months to 4 years. All of the patients described a decrease in or loss of skin color. In most cases, the loss of skin color was limited to the areas around where the patch was rotated. However, a small number of patients also reported skin color changes on parts of the body where the patch was never applied. In all cases, the decreased skin color was permanent.[14]

So, to summarize, after removing the patch, if the skin is red, treat, but don't discontinue using the patch. If the skin is whiter than the surrounding area, stop using the patch, and talk to your doctor.

Sometimes the protective liner can be hard to remove from the patch. This can sometimes occur if the patch is left in a warm area (such as a car on a sunny day). If you feel that the patch is hard to remove, try storing the unused patches in the refrigerator (not the freezer).[15]

Noven Pharmaceuticals produces Daytrana. It recommends the following:

1. Carefully cut open the pouch containing the patch, and make sure it is not damaged. The patch should separate easily from the protective liner. Do not use patches that have been damaged in any way. Throw away the patch if the protective liner is hard to remove.
2. Hold the patch with the protective liner facing you—the word "Daytrana" will appear backwards because you are looking at the bottom of the patch.
3. Gently bend the patch along the faint line, and slowly peel half the liner to expose the sticky surface underneath. Try to avoid touching the sticky part with your fingers. If you do touch it, wash your hands immediately after application.
4. Place the sticky side of the patch firmly on the hip and smooth it down. Make sure the skin is clean, dry, and cool. Alternate the hip on which the patch is worn each day to reduce potential irritation. Try not to use the same application site on either hip for several days.
5. Gently fold back the other half, and slowly peel off the remaining protective liner.
6. Press the entire patch firmly into place and hold for about thirty seconds. This ensures good adhesion of the patch to the skin. Go over the edges with your fingers to make sure that it's well-placed and secure.

The patch can take 1–2 hours before it begins to effectively manage the symptoms of ADHD. This can cause difficulty getting ready for school in the morning. One solution is to go into your child's bedroom and try to place the patch on his hip an hour or two before he wakes up, although this can be tricky. This will allow the medication to begin working earlier and ease the process of getting dressed, eating breakfast, and getting ready for school. Another solution is to add a dose of regular short-acting methylphenidate as soon as your child gets out of bed and then put on the patch just before your child leaves the house for school.

A generic of Daytrana is not yet available. As a result, Daytrana is an expensive medication if not covered by insurance, costing about $500 for thirty patches.

Noven Pharmaceuticals is currently working on a similar skin patch for amphetamine, but it has not yet been approved by the FDA.

Focalin / Focalin XR

Brand Name			Generic Name			
Focalin Focalin XR			dextro-methylphenidate 50% IR, 50% ER 100% dex, 0% levo			
Advantages			Disadvantages			
Less side effects than other methylphenidate meds because levo-methylphenidate is not included as it is in most other methylphenidate medications.			Covered by some insurance plans, but many others do not cover. Focalin is relatively inexpensive, but Focalin XR is much more expensive. Significant reduction in cost through a GoodRx coupon. Novartis does have a program for reducing the cost of Focalin XR to a $10 co-pay (FocalinXR.com).			
	Time	Preparations	Brand		Generic	
			w/o Ins	GoodRx	w/o Ins	GoodRx
Focalin	4	2.5-5-10mg Tablet	$119	$85	$93	$18
Focalin XR	8-9	5-10-15-20-25-30-35mg Capsule	$517	$387	$263	$53

In the previous chapter, I discussed the presence of mirror-image molecules in both methylphenidate and amphetamine. All the methylphenidate medications are a mixture of 50 percent dextro-methylphenidate and 50 percent levo-methylphenidate, with two exceptions: Focalin (and Focalin XR) and Azstarys.

Dextro-methylphenidate is responsible for most or all of the positive, therapeutic effects of methylphenidate, whereas levo-methylphenidate is next to useless and might actually increase the probability of side effects. So, the thinking goes, what if we removed the levo-methylphenidate and treated ADHD children with dextro-methylphenidate alone? You would expect the same benefit as with the 50 percent–50 percent combination, but by removing the molecule that does not produce benefit, you might reduce the side effects as well. This was the thinking behind Focalin.

And there do appear to be fewer side effects with Focalin, although the difference is not large. I have found that the irritability often seen with methylphenidate is reduced with Focalin and Focalin XR compared to most other forms of methylphenidate. Focalin XR does not last as long as other preparations of methylphenidate (Concerta, Daytrana), but it is often a good place to start.

Focalin XR is the extended-release preparation of dextro-methylphenidate. Focalin is also available in a short-acting form that can be used at the end of the day, to extend the effects into the early evening, if needed for homework, sports, or tutoring.

Focalin XR uses the SODAS® (spheroidal oral drug absorption system) technology, exactly like Ritalin LA, Metadate CD, Adhansia XR, and Aptensio XR, with the exception that Focalin XR is only dextro-methylphenidate. Focalin XR comes in a capsule with a mixture of immediate release beads lasting 3½–4 hours and extended-release beads that are more slowly absorbed and last longer (7–8 hours). The pharmaceutical company that produces Focalin XR claims that the therapeutic effects can be seen for 11–12 hours, but research (and my experience) indicate that the true therapeutic affects begin to wear off at eight hours, and little benefit is seen after nine hours. One study compared Focalin XR to Concerta and found that Focalin XR began to take effect more quickly (25–30 minutes for Focalin XR and 30–60 minutes for Concerta). However, Concerta lasted longer (10–12 hours) than Focalin XR (8–9 hours).[16] The combination of these two beads produces a smoother curve than two doses of Focalin, avoiding the "ups and downs" of regular methylphenidate and, thus, significantly reduces the emotional lability.

A dose of Focalin and Focalin XR is equally effective as one-half the dose of Ritalin and Ritalin LA, respectively. That is what you would expect to see, because half of the medication, the ineffective stereoiso-mer, has been removed.

One of my patients was a very bright sixteen-year-old girl with ADHD. I started her on Concerta, which certainly helped improve her ability to focus and concentrate. However, she became irritable as it wore off in the late afternoon. Her parents said that she does not seem irritable to them and they really don't notice that much difference. But they then told me that on the previous Sunday afternoon, she was studying for a test on the family room couch. All of a sudden, she began kicking her legs up in the air and pounding her fists on the couch. "I hate the way this medication makes me feel." She told me that when this happens, usually in the late afternoon, she feels mad but doesn't know what she is mad about. I switched her to Focalin XR, and it worked just as well as Concerta, but the late-afternoon irritability completely disappeared.

Quillivant XR

Brand Name			Generic Name			
Quillivant XR			Methylphenidate 20% IR, 80% ER 50% dex, 50% levo			
Advantages			Disadvantages			
The only Extended-Release **liquid** preparation of methylphenidate. It is easier to swallow, and easier to fine-tune a dose by using a marked dropper or medication cup. This can result in maximum effect and minimum side effects. Lasts longer than many other XR release medications.			Expensive and not usually covered by insurance. Do not mix with other liquids or food.			
	Time	Preparations	Brand		Generic	
			w/o Ins	GoodRx	w/o Ins	GoodRx
Quillivant XR	8-12	25mg/5ml 60-120-150-180ml Liquid	$353	$318	Generic Not Available	

Quillivant XR is the only extended-release *liquid* preparation of methylphenidate approved for the treatment of ADHD. There had been liquid preparations of methylphenidate before Quillivant XR, but they were simply methylphenidate suspended in a syrup (e.g., Methylin liquid). Such liquid preparations were a big advantage for young children who could not swallow a pill, but the methylphenidate only lasted four hours, requiring multiple doses during the day. It can be very difficult for children in school to get a dose around noon, because schools are reluctant to dose liquid medications.

Quillivant XR uses the LiquiXR technology. Methylphenidate is bound to microscopic resin particles, which come in three forms. The uncoated resin particles release the medication into the stomach almost immediately and allow for effective medication treatment within the first half hour. The two remaining resin particles are coated, some with a small amount of coating, others with a larger coating. As the coating dissolves, the two different coated particles release the methylphenidate gradually over 8–12 hours.

Quillivant ER Liquid has two advantages over pill preparations of methylphenidate:

1. Quilivant XR is easier to swallow than a pill, although some younger children may still have difficulty swallowing from a spoon.
2. Quillivant XR is one of the best methylphenidate medications for children who are very sensitive to dose. In the section above on Daytrana, we discussed how for some children a 10mg dose of Metadate CD or Ritalin LA might have no effect, but the next dose up, 15 mg, might be too much medication, reducing appetite or making it difficult for the child to fall asleep. By using a dropper or a marked medication cup, the dose of liquid Quillivant XR can be customized specifically for each child.

Quillivant should not be mixed with water, milk, or other liquids. If a child does not drink every drop of the water or milk, you cannot be sure that he or she is getting the prescribed dose.

The biggest disadvantage to Quillivant XR is that it is expensive, about $300 for a month's prescription. It does not come in a generic yet, and is not usually covered by insurance.

QuilliChew ER

Brand Name			Generic Name			
QuilliChew ER			Methylphenidate 20% IR, 80% ER 50% dex, 50% levo			
Advantages			**Disadvantages**			
Excellent choice for a child who cannot swallow a pill. The only Extended-Release chewable preparation of methylphenidate. Lasts longer than many other XR release medications (8-12 hrs.)			Expensive and not usually covered by insurance.			
	Time	Preparations	Brand		Generic	
			w/o Ins	GoodRx	w/o Ins	GoodRx
QuilliChew ER	8-12	20-30-40mg Chewable tablet	$487	$349	Generic Not Available	

QuilliChew ER is the only methylphenidate preparation in an extended-release chewable tablet. Methylin Chewable is also methylphenidate in a chewable tablet, but it consists of short-acting medication only, lasting 3½–4 hours. A chewable pill is a better solution for children who cannot swallow a pill and might also have trouble with the liquid Quillivant XR.

QuilliChew ER has another advantage. Like Quillivant XR liquid, QuilliChew is a combination of 20 percent immediate release and 80 percent extended release. Because of the greater proportion of extended-release particles, both Quilllivant ER and QuilliChew last longer (10–12 hours) than many other extended-release medications.

QuilliChew ER only comes in three dosages, 20mg, 30mg, and 40mg pills. The pills are scored, so that intermediate dosages are possible. For example, you can get 25 mg by giving one-half of a 20mg pill (10 mg) and one-half of a 30mg pill (15 mg), but this requires two prescriptions a month for a medication that is expensive and not usually covered by insurance.

Cotempla XR-ODT

Brand Name	Generic Name
Cotempla XR-ODT	Methylphenidate 30% IR, 70% ER 50% dex, 50% levo
Advantages	**Disadvantages**
Cotempla is an Extended-Release form of methylphenidate, lasting 8-9 hours. In addition, it comes as a grape flavored Orally Dissolving Tablet for children who have trouble swallowing a pill.	Expensive and not usually covered by insurance.

	Time	Preparations	Brand		Generic	
			w/o Ins	GoodRx	w/o Ins	GoodRx
Cotempla	8-9	8.6-17.3-25.9mg Capsule	$474	$442	Generic Not Available	

Cotempla XR–ODT has two unique characteristics. First, Cotempla is another extended-release methylphenidate, lasting about 8–9 hours. In order to extend the release of methylphenidate over 8–9 hours, it uses a unique microparticle delivery technology, similar to the technology that Quillivant XR Liquid uses. Some 30 percent of the particles are immediate release and 70 percent are extended release. The combination of these particles allows Cotempla XR ODT to last 8–9 hours.

The second unique characteristic is that Cotempla is a grape-flavored orally dissolving tablet. Many young children, when given a pill, hold the pill in their mouths but refuse to swallow it. Cotempla dissolves in a few minutes and can be followed with a glass of water so that the child does not spit out the orally dissolved solution. This is the only methylphenidate preparation available as an orally dissolving tablet.

Notice that Cotempla is available in three unusual dosages, 8.6mg, 17.3mg, and 25.9mg. Why is that?

When methylphenidate is outside the body, it is hooked to a salt, hydrochloride. The hydrochloride salt does little, except that it keeps the charge on the molecule neutral. Before methylphenidate can have an effect in the brain, the hydrochloride is removed. The hydrochloride does not change the effectiveness or side-effect profile of a medication.

When Cotempla XR-ODT is absorbed into the brain, methyl-phenidate is not hooked to hydrochloride. As a result, 10 mg of meth-ylphenidate hydrochloride is equivalent to 8.6 mg of methylphenidate (MPH). And that is why Cotempla has such odd dosing options.

10 mg of MPH-HCl is equal to 8.6 mg of Cotempla XR-ODT.
20 mg of MPH-HCl is equal to 17.3 mg of Cotempla XR-ODT.
30 mg of MPH-HCl is equal to 25.9 mg of Cotempla XR-ODT.

So, if a child is receiving 10 mg of Metadate CD or 10 mg of Ritalin LA, and needs to switch to Cotempla, he should start on 8.6mg Cotempla XR-ODT.

Jornay PM

Brand Name			Generic Name			
Jornay PM			Methylphenidate 30% IR, 70% ER 50% dex, 50% levo			
Advantages			**Disadvantages**			
A dose given at 6:30pm does not begin taking affect until 6:30am, 12 hours later. It then lasts another 12 hours. An excellent medication if you are having difficulty getting your child ready for school in the morning.			Timing of the dose is critical. Give too early the night before and it would take effect earlier, affecting breakfast appetite. Give too late and it may not take effect early in the morning, but last much longer in the evening affecting sleep. Difficult to balance timing effects with changes in daily schedule, such as sleeping in on the weekends. Expensive and not usually covered by insurance.			
	Time	Prepar-ations	Brand		Generic	
			w/o Ins	GoodRx	w/o Ins	GoodRx
Jornay PM	12hr to onset then works for 12hr	20-40-60 80-100mg Capsule	$485	$310	Generic Not Available	

One unique characteristic of most ADHD medications is that a reduction in the ADHD behaviors is usually evident the first day after starting medication, and within an hour of the first dose. However, that hour can be wicked. You are under a time limit to get your child dressed, feed him breakfast, brush his teeth, and get ready to get in the car or out of the house to catch the bus. Oh, and you have to remember to remind him to bring his homework that he spent two hours on last night, and, oh, yes, don't forget his lunch, his jacket, and that candy sculpture that he wants to bring to school for show and tell.

If your child wakes up at 6:30, and you must leave for school at 7:30, then you have an hour to accomplish all these tasks. One solution is to make sure to give him his medication as soon as he wakes up so that it will kick in as soon as possible, usually in a half hour.

Next, have him eat before he gets dressed and before his medication kicks in. But that only gives you a half hour of workable time. And once his medication begins to take effect, it may decrease his appetite.

Or you could give him a newer medication, Jornay PM. Jornay PM is a very long-acting methylphenidate medication designed to help with exactly this situation. Jornay PM does not start to take effect until twelve hours after it is swallowed, so it is given the night before. A dose given at 6:30 p.m. will start to take effect about 6:30 a.m. the next morning, about the time your child wakes up.[17] This is a big advantage, because you don't have to wait the half hour that other medications would require to take effect. On the other hand, because the medication is already effective when he wakes up, his appetite may be decreased as well.

Jornay PM has one other potential benefit. The irritability that often occurs in the afternoon as other medications wears off is less likely with Jornay PM, although this had not been well studied.

Jornay is similar to the coated beads that other medications (Ritalin LA, Metadate CD) use, but it has an extra-thick coating on the outside to delay the release of the medication until twelve hours after taking it.

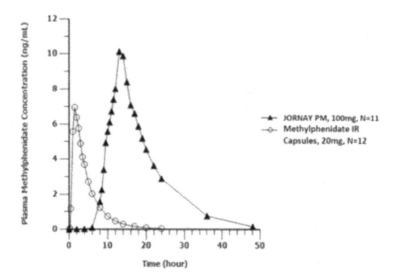

Figure 10.2   Blood levels produced by a single dose of Ritalin vs. a single dose of Jornay.

Jornay PM has one potential problem. Look at this graph (Figure 10.2). The twelve-hour delay in onset is clearly evident. But the medication reaches its peak around 14–15 hours, which would be around 8:30 a.m.–9:30 a.m. (for a dose given at 6:30 the night before). From that point on, the medication gradually becomes less effective.

The blood and brain levels, therefore, are decreasing after that time. For most children, a higher dose in the afternoon is needed to achieve what the lower levels did in the morning. That might result in strong benefits in the morning but much less benefit in the afternoon, where a higher blood level is usually preferable. Finally, notice that some methylphenidate remains in the body twenty-four hours after a dose. That may result in more difficulty falling asleep.

For some families, Jornay PM will be an excellent choice. However, it may take some time to determine the exact right time to take the medication. Give it too early, and it kicks in too early in the morning. This might wake up your child too early and then not last long enough at the end of the day. And an earlier onset may mean more trouble with breakfast appetite. Give it too late, and it won't kick in until later in the morning, defeating the whole purpose for using this medication. If it is given too late the night before, it will last longer the next day and may have adverse effects on appetite at dinner and may cause more difficulty falling asleep. Time of dose should be adjusted if the child plans to sleep in the next morning, such as on a weekend. Finally, if your child forgets to take the medication the night before, you should have an "emergency prescription," such as Concerta or Metadate, to take in the morning in its place. I suspect that some families will find this medication to be perfect for them; many others might feel that it is too much trouble.

Azstarys

Brand Name	Generic Name
Azstarys	dextro-methylphenidate 70% ser-dex-methylphenidate 30% dex-methylphenidate
Advantages	**Disadvantages**
Like Focalin, this medication contains only the active stereoisomer dextro-methylphenidate. By eliminating the inactive levo-methylphenidate, side effects may be reduced. This medication is a pro-drug (which cannot enter the brain if it is snorted or injected) therefore it cannot be abused. However, abuse of methylphenidate by children with ADHD is rare.	This medication was only very recently approved by the FDA (March 2021), so little is known about this medication in clinical use. Difficult to switch from another medication to Jornay because of the dosage preparations. Expensive and are not often covered by insurance.

	Time	Preparations	Brand		Generic	
			w/o Ins	GoodRx	w/o Ins	GoodRx
Azstarys	11-12 hours	26.1mg/5.2mg 39.2mg/7.8mg 52.3mg/10.4mg Capsule	$467	$388	Generic Not Available	

Azstarys was approved by the FDA for the treatment of ADHD in March 2021. Because it was so recently approved, few physicians have had experience in prescribing this medication.[18]

Azstarys is another extended-release form of methylphenidate. Azstarys is different from the other methylphenidate medications listed above in two ways. First, the active ingredient is dextro-methylphenidate only. Dextro-methylphenidate is the right-handed version of methylphenidate, which is the only ingredient in Focalin (to understand what dextro-methylphenidate is, please see the section on mirror-image molecules in Chapter 7). Dextro-methylphenidate is responsible for most or all of the benefit in all of the methylphenidate medications listed above, while its mirror-image (levo-methylphenidate) is virtually useless. As stated above in the discussion on Focalin, a medication based on dextro-methylphenidate alone might have fewer side effects, because you are eliminating the half of the molecules that contribute to the side effects without benefiting the patient.

Second, Azstarys is unique in that it is a prodrug. A prodrug is created when the active ingredient (in this case, dextro-methylphenidate) is combined with another chemical entity (in this case, the amino acid serine) so that the new combined medication, ser-dextro-methylphenidate, is not active and cannot even get into the brain. Once the pill is swallowed, the body metabolizes the medication so that the serine amino acid is removed, leaving the active ingredient to do its work.

This new methylphenidate prodrug has two main advantages. Because the prodrug must be metabolized by the body before it can be absorbed into the brain to do its business, the onset is usually a little delayed, but in the end the drug will last longer. The pharmaceutical company that makes Azstarys claims that its studies indicate that this medication lasts up to thirteen hours. Unfortunately, I cannot comment on the clinical use of this medication. Because of its recent release, we do not have any clinical experience with it yet, and studies by scientists independent of the pharmaceutical company that makes the medication have not been performed.

Another advantage of the combined chemical entity is that if someone wanted to abuse the drug by crushing the pill and snorting it, that person would not get high because the methylphenidate, combined with serine, cannot pass into the brain. This virtually eliminates the possibility of abuse.

However, much of this is beside the point. Methylphenidate is not often abused because it produces only a minimal high in people without ADHD. Children with ADHD treated with methylphenidate do not feel a high at all, because medication simply allows the brain chemistry to function the same way it does in all other children without ADHD.

If a prodrug is being prescribed for an eight-year-old, it is unlikely that an eight-year-old will consider snorting the medication. So, then, why use the expensive brand-name drug when a medication such as Concerta costs much less and will do exactly the same thing as the pro-drug? The pro-drug concept is a good idea, but in reality, prodrugs are another example of evergreening. Prodrugs have benefits (they prevent abuse and they usually last a little longer, but at the expense of taking longer to take effect in the morning). At the same time, prodrugs are also used by pharmaceutical companies to claim that they have a new drug that the FDA will approve as a brand-name drug for which they can charge much more.

Chapter 11

SIXTEEN BRAND-NAME AMPHETAMINE MEDICATIONS TO TREAT ADHD

The previous chapter was a review of each of the methylphenidate medications available to treat ADHD. But remember that when Bradley gave medication to the boys in the Bradley Home in 1937, he gave them Benzedrine. Benzedrine was the brand name for amphetamine, a drug that had been sold since 1932 by the pharmaceutical company Smith, Kline & French (now GlaxoSmithKline). At that time, it was an inhaler and was a treatment for asthma and other forms of congestion.

Bradley performed his groundbreaking studies on children who had been institutionalized for severe developmental and behavioral disorders. About twenty years passed before the medical community recognized that this medication could also be valuable for a milder but similar problem, minimal brain dysfunction, which we now know as ADHD.

The methylphenidate medications in Chapter 10 differed by how they delivered the medication to the patient (tablet, capsule, liquid, orally dissolving tablet, skin patch). Or they differed by how long they were effective for the symptoms of ADHD. By altering the ratio of immediate-release to extended-release methylphenidate coated beads, or by using different methods for delaying the release of methylphenidate, the pharmaceutical companies have produced medications that differed primarily by how long they last. But pharmaceutical companies have done something completely different with the amphetamine medications.

All of the medications in this section contain amphetamine as the active ingredient. Much like the methylphenidate medications, the amphetamine medications also have different delivery mechanisms. A liquid form (Dexedrine Liquid, Procentra, Dynavel XR, Adzenys ER), a chewable pill (Vyvanse chewable), and orally dissolving tablets (Adzenys XR-ODT, Evekeo ODT) are available for children who have trouble swallowing a pill. And like the methylphenidate medications, some of the medications are short acting only, whereas others are long acting.

Earlier, we learned that most medications have a specific molecular structure that is present in mirror-image forms, called "stereoisomers" (see Chapter 6). All of the methylphenidate medications (with the exception of Focalin and Azstarys) are a combination of 50 percent of the right-sided molecule (dextro-methylphenidate) and 50 percent of the left-sided molecule (levo-methylphenidate). And for all of these medications, the levo-methylphenidate is just there. It does virtually nothing.

But here is where the amphetamine medications differ significantly from the methylphenidate medications.

The amphetamine that Bradley used was simply . . . amphetamine. It was a combination of 50 percent dextro-amphetamine and 50 percent levo-amphetamine. But the earliest amphetamine used on a regular basis for children with ADHD in the 1970s was Dexedrine (duration time about four hours) and then later Dexedrine Spansule (duration time 7–8 hours). Both medications consisted only of the right-sided molecule, dextro-amphetamine. And that seems appropriate, as dextro-amphetamine is responsible for most of the benefit in treating ADHD, while levo-amphetamine adds almost nothing. But in 1996, Adderall was introduced as a combination of the right- and left-sided molecules. In essence, it started with dextro-amphetamine (as in Dexedrine) and then **added levo-amphetamine**. That was a surprising decision.

Dextro-amphetamine is responsible for most or all of the therapeutic benefits of the amphetamine medications, while levo-amphetamine has nothing to offer the ADHD patient, except possibly more side effects.

Why would a pharmaceutical company do that? No rationale has ever been given for adding an ineffective form of medication, other than the ability to sell the new medication at brand-name prices. Nevertheless, Adderall quickly became one of the most frequently prescribed medications for the treatment of ADHD. Other pharmaceutical companies entered the ADHD medication market by altering the ratio of the two different stereoisomers. But since dextro–amphetamine is responsible for most or all of the benefit, and levo–amphetamine is responsible for little benefit and more side effects (see Chapter 7), the only difference for many of the amphetamine medications is that those with a higher percentage of levo–amphetamine will have more side-effects and will require a higher dose (because there is less of the effective dextro-amphetamine). However, in the process, a number of very useful medications were created.

Dexedrine tab / Dextrostat tab / Zenzedi

Brand Name	Generic Name
Dexedrine tab	dextro-amphetamine
Dextrostat tab	100% IR, 0% ER
Zenzedi	100% dex, 0% levo
Advantages	Disadvantages
Dextro-amphetamine is an Immediate Release (IR) medication, short-acting medication. There were three different brand names of dextro-amphetamine, but Dexedrine and Dextrostat brand names are no longer available. The IR form can be used with an Extended-Release form in the morning, before the ER has kicked in or at the end of the day to extend the effect after the ER has worn off.	Because dextro-amphetamine is a short-acting medication (3.5-4 hr.) it should not be used as the primary medication to treat ADHD, but instead can be used to supplement an IR form. There is no advantage to the brand name Zenzedi, except that it comes in multiple dosages not available in the generic. The generic is substantially cheaper and equally effective.

	Time	Preparations	Brand		Generic	
			w/o Ins	GoodRx	w/o Ins	GoodRx
Dexedrine	3.5-4.0 hr	5-10 mg tablet	Brand Name Not Available		$163	$25
Dextrostat	3.5-4.0 hr	5-10 mg tablet	Brand Name Not Available		$183	$26
Zenzedi	3.5-4.0 hr	Brand: 2.5-5-7.5-10-15-20-30mg Generic: 5-10-15-20-30 tablet	$551	$26	$183	$23
Dexedrine Liquid	3.5-4.0 hr	5mg/5ml 75-150-225-300-450ml Liquid	$550	$26	$253	$72

In 1937, the same year that Bradley conducted his experiments, the pharmaceutical company Smith, Kline & French took Benzedrine (which was the combination of dextro-amphetamine and levo-amphetamine). It then removed the inactive levo-amphetamine, leaving only dextro-amphetamine, and called it Dexedrine. It was approved by the FDA in 1940 as a treatment for obesity and nasal congestion. Later, in the 1970s, after physicians took note of Bradley's work, Dexedrine was approved for the treatment of ADHD.

Shortly after this, Shire Pharmaceuticals (which eventually would develop Adderall in the 1990s) signed on with its own version of dextro-amphetamine, which it called Dextrostat. Dexedrine and Dextrostat were identical forms of dextro-amphetamine. More recently, Zenzedi was introduced, and it also is identical to Dexedrine and Dextrostat.

For twenty years, Dexedrine and Ritalin ruled the market for ADHD medication treatments. But the problem with Dexedrine, Dextrostat, and Zenzedi is that they are all short-acting, immediate-release medications, lasting only about 3½–4 hours, requiring multiple doses per day. This would produce the same roller-coaster effect as described with Ritalin in Chapter 8 on side effects. Therefore, the use of only immediate-release amphetamine in multiple doses throughout the day is not recommended.

Two scenarios would justify using these short-acting immediate-release amphetamines. First, some long-acting extended-release amphetamines (Vyvanse) can take up to an hour to take effect in the morning. While you are waiting for the medication to begin to take effect, you are scrambling to get ready to leave for school, and distractibility and impulsivity will not help. In this case, an immediate-release amphetamine that takes effect in a half hour can be given as soon as your child gets out of bed, and the extended-release amphetamine can be given as you are leaving the house in the morning.

The second scenario occurs when an extended-release amphetamine is given in the morning but wears off in the late afternoon. A dose of the immediate-release medications could then be given as your child sits down for dinner, which will take effect a half hour later, allowing your child to eat with a good appetite and the medication to then take effect as homework is started after dinner.

    Zenzedi has one small advantage over Dexedrine, Dextrostat, and the other short-acting generics. Zenzedi comes in multiple dosage options (2.5 mg, 5 mg, 7.5 mg, 10 mg, 15 mg, 20 mg and 30 mg), which should make it easier to fine-tune the dosage.

    Dexedrine also comes in a liquid, which is easier for some children to swallow and even easier to fine-tune the dose. However, Dexedrine Liquid is available only as short-acting liquid, while two other liquid preparations of amphetamine (Dynavel XR Liquid and Adzenys ER) are available in an extended-release form lasting 8–10 hours.

    Dextro-amphetamine did come in a liquid, as Immediate Release Dexedrine Liquid, but is no longer available. However, Zenzedi is virtually identical to the original Dexedrine Liquid.

    Currently, the only short-acting, immediate-release dextro-amphetamine available as a brand name is Zenzedi; the immediate-release brand-name versions of Dexedrine and DextroStat are no longer available. However, more than twenty different pharmaceutical companies have produced inexpensive generics of the immediate-release dextro-amphetamine.

    It is not clear why anyone would prescribe such an expensive brand-name medication when much cheaper generics are available that are just as effective as the brand name. If your insurance covers Zenzedi or if the GoodRx app is used, the cost is almost the same for the brand name as for the generic ($26 vs. $23); in that case, prescribing the brand name would be appropriate.

    Zenzedi does offer a copay savings card, which ensures that you pay no more than $75 per prescription (Zenzedi.com).

Evekeo

Brand Name			Generic Name		
Evekeo			Amphetamine 100% IR, 0% ER 50% dex, 50% levo		
Advantages			Disadvantages		
Evekeo tablet is a combination of d-AMP and l-AMP, so it is different from Dexedrine, Dextrostat, Zenzedi and their generics, but because L-AMP is not as effective as d-AMP and can produce more cardiovascular side effects, it offers no real advantage. Evekeo ODT is an Orally Dissolving tablet and is much easier to swallow than other medications.			Evekeo is a short-acting amphetamine that is expensive and does not provide any real advantage over the generics of Dexedrine, Dextrostat or Zenzedi. May have more appetite and cardiovascular side effects.		
	Time	Preparations	Brand		Generic
			w/o Ins	GoodRx	w/o Ins	GoodRx
Evekeo	3.5-4.0 hr	5-10 mg Tablet	$500	$413	$403	$56
Evekeo ODT	3.5-4.0 hr	5-10-15-20 mg Orally Dissolving Tablet	$485	$399	Generic Not Available	

Evekeo is another brand–name, short–acting amphetamine. It is different from Dexedrine, Dextrostat, and Zenzedi because it is the combination of dextro–amphetamine and levo–amphetamine. But because levo–amphetamine offers little benefit for the treatment of ADHD, there seems to be little rationale for using Evekeo.

On the other hand, Evekeo is also available as an orally dissolving tablet (ODT) and Evekeo ODT does provide an alternative for children (and adults) who have difficulty swallowing a tablet. An orally dissolving tablet is placed in the mouth, and within minutes it dissolves and is followed by a drink of water, milk, or juice. However, Evekeo ODT is an immediate-release medication, lasting only 3½–4 hours. An extended-release orally dissolving tablet is available as Adzenys XR-ODT, which is a much better alternative. It requires only one dose per day, versus the 2–3 per day that would be needed with the short–acting Evekeo.

Procentra

Brand Name			Generic Name			
Procentra			dextro-amphetamine 100% IR, 0% ER 100% dex, 0% levo			
Advantages			**Disadvantages**			
One of four liquid preparations of amphetamines, thus easier for children to swallow and dose can be more easily fine-tuned.			Short-acting. Moderately expensive, does not come in a generic and is not usually covered by insurance.			
	Time	Preparations	Brand		Generic	
			w/o Ins	GoodRx	w/o Ins	GoodRx
Procentra Liquid	3.5-4	5mg/5ml 75-150-225-300-450mg Liquid	$293	$79	Generic Not Available	

Procentra is one of four *liquid* preparations of amphetamine approved for the treatment of ADHD. Dexedrine is available as a liquid, but like Procentra, it is short acting (3½–4 hours). Dynavel XR and Adzenys ER are also amphetamine liquids, and they are long-acting liquids. A liquid preparation of amphetamine might be easier than a capsule for some children to take. However, because Procentra employs immediate-release dextro-amphetamine only, it will require multiple doses per day, potentially producing the roller-coaster effect described in Chapter 8 on side effects.

Procentra has two advantages over other *pill* preparations of amphetamine:

1. Because it is a liquid, Procentra dose can be more easily customized specifically for children who are very sensitive to dose. By using a dropper or a marked medication cup, the dose of Procentra can be customized specifically for each child.
2. Procentra is bubble-gum flavored and easier to swallow than a pill.

Nevertheless, Procentra XR is still immediate release only. The biggest disadvantages to Procentra XR are that it is moderately expensive, does not come in a generic, and is not usually covered by insurance.

Dexedrine Spansule

Brand Name			Generic Name		
Dexedrine Spansule			d-amphetamine 50% IR, 50% ER 100% dex, 0% levo		
Advantages			Disadvantages		
Extremely expensive medication without insurance, but usually covered by insurance. Generics are usually equally effective and much less expensive than brand name.			Extremely expensive if not covered by insurance. Lasts 7-8 hours, but may need another short-acting dose in the afternoon. Other medications last longer.		
	Time	Preparations	Brand		Generic	
			w/o Ins	GoodRx	w/o Ins	GoodRx
Dexedrine Spansule	7-8	5-10-15 mg Capsule	$797	$700	$133	$37

Dexedrine Spansule was released in the 1970s as the first long-acting extended-release form of dextro-amphetamine and is still available today. It uses a coated bead technology similar to the way Ritalin LA and Metadate CD are formulated for methylphenidate. The Spansule did for dextro-amphetamine what Ritalin LA did for methylphenidate. Immediate-release Dexedrine takes about a half hour to take effect and lasts for 3½–4 hours, necessitating multiple doses per day, often leading to the emotional swings described in Chapter 8 on side effects. Dexedrine Spansules last about 7–8 hours and in younger children, often require only a single dose per day, avoiding the need for a dose at school and 2–3 doses throughout the day. On the other hand, older children need their medication to last into the evening. A dose taken at 7 a.m. wears off around 2–3 p.m., often requiring a dose of short-acting Dexedrine in the late afternoon or early evening when homework is more likely to be done. There are extended-release amphetamine medications that last longer (Adzenys XR-ODT, Adzenys ER liquid, Adderall XR, Dynavel XR, and Vyvanse).

The brand-name Dexedrine Spansule is often not covered by insurance and is expensive ($850 per month), so generally it is not a good option. If you use GoodRx.com, the generic is available for $40 or less.

Adderall / Adderall XR

Brand Name			Generic Name			
Adderall **Adderall XR**			Amphetamine (mixed salts) 50% IR, 50% ER 75% dex, 25% levo			
Advantages			**Disadvantages**			
Effective for treating ADHD, but it holds no advantage over other medications like Dexedrine, Dextrostat and Zenzedi. The brand name is expensive, the generics are very inexpensive and Adderall is usually covered by insurance.			More likely than methylphenidate medications to caused irritability as it wears off in the afternoon, and more likely to cause appetite reduction.			
	Time	Preparations	Brand		Generic	
			w/o Ins	GoodRx	w/o Ins	GoodRx
Adderall	3.5-4	5-7.5-10-12.5-15-20-30mg Tablet	$273	$249	$50	$11
Adderall XR	7-8	5-10-15-20-25-30mg Capsule	$279	$228	$185	$22

To understand Adderall, we have to start with an older medication, Obetrol. Remember that Obetrol was an early form of amphetamine, used to treat obesity in the 1940s, 1950s, and 1960s. Initially, Obetrol contained meth-amphetamine, which is now better known as "speed," and this may have explained its initial popularity. Even though the meth-amphetamine was removed from Obetrol, in 1973 the FDA withdrew its approval because of nationwide concerns that amphetamines had significant abuse potential.

However, although the name Obetrol has faded from history, its legacy has persisted. Shire Pharmaceuticals acquired the rights to Obetrol in 1994. Initially, Obetrol was a mixture of the two stereoisomers (mirror images: dextro-amphetamine and levo-amphetamine) in a 50 percent–50 percent ratio. Shire changed the ratios so that a single pill contained 75 percent dextro-amphetamine and 25 percent levo-amphetamine and then went back to the FDA. Because of this change in the ratio of the stereoisomers, this new formulation could be approved as a new brand-name medication.

But this time, Shire did not ask that Obetrol be approved for the treatment of obesity. Instead, Shire asked the FDA to approve it as a treatment for ADHD, which the FDA did in 1996.

Shire Pharmaceuticals made one more change to this new formulation: it changed the name of Obetrol to Adderall (short for "ADD for all").

Dexedrine consists only of dextro-amphetamine., whereas Adderall is a combination of 75 percent dextro-amphetamine and 25 percent levo-amphetamine. However, the inclusion of levo-amphetamine in any ratio has never been shown to be superior in any way to simple dextro-amphetamine alone.

Further, in Adderall, the two isomers of amphetamine (dextro and levo) are also combined to different salts. However, the different salts add absolutely nothing. Once the medication is absorbed, the salt is stripped away from the amphetamine molecule and discarded. Nevertheless, Adderall is often referred to as mixed amphetamine salts (MAS).

So, Adderall is really Dexedrine (dextro-amphetamine) combined with levo-amphetamine and with different salts. But what benefit do you get from such a concoction?

As it turns out, zero.

Some studies have shown that levo-amphetamine is a little better than dextro-amphetamine at reducing hyperactivity and aggressiveness, but it has little significant effect in the brain in enhancing attention in children with ADHD.[1] Another study showed that dextro-amphetamine was "consistently superior to levo-amphetamine." Further, researchers found that dextro-amphetamine began to take effect during the first few days, whereas levo-amphetamine would take up to three weeks before any benefit could be seen, and then the benefit was minimal.[2]

But there is more. Levo-amphetamine is also more likely to cause side effects (appetite reduction and mild increase in blood pressure and heart rate), and the mixture of salts affixed to the amphetamine molecule has absolutely no therapeutic benefit.

Because dextro-amphetamine is much more effective than levo-amphetamine,[3] one-third of Adderall is virtually useless. And the mixed amphetamine salts are nothing more than window dressing. So why go to all the trouble to produce mixed amphetamine salts in this new ratio of stereoisomers when it has no advantage over plain old Dexedrine (dextro-amphetamine)? By now, you should be able to answer this question. These machinations made Adderall unique, in a chemical way, allowing the FDA to grant its production as a brand-name medication.

John S. Markowitz, a scientist who has researched amphetamines extensively, stated, "The reasoning behind the inclusion of disparate amounts of dextro- and levo-amphetamine, and the range of salt forms incorporated, appears to have been one more of pharmaceutical convenience than scientific rationale."[4]

When I asked this same question of a representative from Shire Pharmaceuticals, he spoke extensively about the subtle differences of the left- and right-handed versions of amphetamine, but in the end, he admitted, "It was a business decision." What he meant was that because Obetrol had already been formulated and had been approved by the FDA, it could be presented as another treatment for ADHD without having to go through all the effort to come up with a new medication.

My clinical experience with Adderall is that Adderall and Dexedrine are equally effective for the treatment of ADHD, but I do see a difference in side effects. Adderall is more likely to cause irritability when it wears off than the methylphenidate preparations. It got to the point that when I saw a new patient, I occasionally received this complaint, "My son has been diagnosed with ADHD and medication has really helped him, but he gets so angry when he gets home from school. We're worried about him."

I will often say, "Let me guess, Adderall?," and the parents nod their heads. This irritability effect of Adderall has a name. Gina Pera, who has written extensively about ADHD on her blog, calls this medication "Madderall."[5]

Adderall XR is the extended-release version of Adderall. It employs a similar coated bead technology used in Ritalin LA, Focalin XR, and Metadate CD to last about eight hours. It was approved by the FDA in 2001.

Adderall and Adderall XR are very effective medications to treat ADHD, but they offer no real benefit over the much less expensive

Dexedrine and Dexedrine Spansules and their generics.[6] Adderall is usually covered by insurance, but without insurance, it is an expensive drug that shows no advantage over the much less expensive Dexedrine Spansule with the added burden of more side effects. Nevertheless, in 2016, it was the forty-fifth most prescribed medication in the United States, with more than seventeen million prescriptions per year.[7]

Adzenys ER Liquid / Adzenyz XR ODT

Brand Name	Generic Name
Adzenys ER Liquid **Adzenys XR ODT**	Amphetamine (mixed salts) 50% IR, 50% ER 75% dex, 25% levo
Advantages	**Disadvantages**
These two medications, one a liquid, the other an Orally Dissolving Tablet (ODT) are identical to Adderall XR, but they do provide an alternative to traditional tablets, that might be difficult to take for some children. Liquid preparation that is much easier to swallow. Because it is liquid, it is easier to fine-tune the dose and to give intermediate dosages.	Expensive, not usually covered by insurance. Except for the alternative delivery mechanism, they provide no real treatment advantage over the much less expensive generic Adderall XR.

	Time	Preparations	Brand		Generic	
			w/o Ins	GoodRx	w/o Ins	GoodRx
Adzenys ER Liquid	8-9	1.25mg/ml 90-120-150-270-450 Liquid	$720	$670	Generic Not Available	
Adzenys XR-ODT	8-9	3.1-6.3-9.4-12.5-15.7-18.8mg ODT	$525	$429	Generic Not Available	

Equivalent Doses of ADZENYS ER-ODT, Adzenys ER and ADDERALL XR						
Adzenys ODT Adzenys ER Liquid	3.1 mg (2.5 mL)	6.3 mg (5 mL)	9.4 mg (7.5 mL)	12.5 mg (10 mL)	15.7 mg (12.5 mL)	18.8 mg (15 mL)
Adderall XR	5 mg	10 mg	15 mg	20 mg	25 mg	30 mg

Adzenys ER Liquid and Adzenys XR-ODT are all about making it easier for some children to swallow their medication. Both provide an alternative to traditional tablets that are easier for most children to take.

Adzenys ER is one of two extended-release *liquid* preparations of amphetamine approved for the treatment of ADHD (the other is Dynavel XR). Procentra and Zenzedi liquids are also liquid preparations of amphetamine, but both are short acting (3½–4 hours). Adzenys ER is a mixture of the dextro- and levo-amphetamine salts, in the same ratio as in Adderall XR. For all practical purposes, Adzenys ER *is* Adderall XR in a liquid form. It has an orange flavor. Adzenys ER Liquid is an expensive medication, not usually covered by insurance. Because it is almost identical to Adderall XR, it does not provide any real therapeutic advantage, except that it is easier for many children to swallow. Further, it is just as likely as Adderall to cause irritability.

As with all liquid preparations, it is better to administer the liquid in a dropper or with a marked medication cup to ensure the proper dose. It should not be mixed with other liquids (milk, water) or solid food, as you cannot ensure that all the medication will be consumed. However, if your child resists taking the medication in its raw liquid form, you could take a half spoonful of applesauce or pudding, leaving enough space to empty the dropper onto the spoon. This can get a little tricky.

There is some indication that Adzenys ER may be discontinued by the manufacturer in the near future.

Adzenys XR-ODT is an extended-release form of amphetamine that is prepared in an orange flavored, orally dissolving tablet (ODT). It also is bioequivalent to Adderall XR.

It comes in a blister pack, and the pills should not be removed from the blister pack until just before taking the pill.

If a child is on Adderall and is switched to Adzenys XR-ODT, you cannot use a mg to mg conversion. Because of the way that the amphetamine molecule is prepared, it is necessary to use the above conversion chart instead.

Dynavel XR

Brand Name			Generic Name		
Dynavel XR			Amphetamine 50% IR, 50% ER 76% dex, 24% levo		
Advantages			**Disadvantages**		
Liquid preparation that is much easier to swallow than a pill. Because it is liquid, it is easier to fine-tune the dose and to give intermediate dosages.			Very expensive and not usually covered by insurance.		
	Time	Preparations	Brand		Generic
			w/o Ins	GoodRx	w/o Ins	GoodRx
Dynavel XR Liquid	8-9	2.5mg/ml 60-90-120-150-180ml Liquid	$1370	$340	Generic Not Available	

Dynavel XR is one of two extended-release *liquid* preparations of amphetamine approved for the treatment of ADHD (the other is Adzenys ER. Procentra and Zenzedi are also liquid preparations of amphetamine, but they are both short-acting [3½–4 hours]). It is produced by Tris Pharma, the same pharmaceutical company that produces Quillivant XR, and uses the same LiquiXR technology.

Dynavel has two advantages over other pill preparations of amphetamine:

1. Dynavel XR is easier to swallow than a pill, and
2. Dynavel XR is one of the better amphetamine medications for children who are very sensitive to dose. By using a dropper or a marked medication cup, the dose of Dynavel XR can be customized specifically for each child.

The biggest disadvantage to Dynavel XR is that it is expensive, about $1,370 for a month's prescription without insurance, $340 with a GoodRx coupon. It does not come in a generic yet, and is not usually covered by insurance.

Mydayis

Brand Name			Generic Name			
Mydayis			Amphetamine (mixed salts) 33% IR, 67% ER 75% dex, 25% levo			
Advantages			Disadvantages			
Lasts longer than any other amphetamine-based ADHD medication.			Significantly more appetite and sleep problems.			
	Time	Preparations	Brand		Generic	
			w/o Ins	GoodRx	w/o Ins	GoodRx
Mydayis	15-16 hrs.	12.5-25-37.5-50mg Capsule	$372	$325	Generic Not Available	

Throughout this book, I have emphasized the importance of maintaining a steady blood level of the stimulant medications to prevent the need for multiple dosing throughout the day. Multiple dosing increases the likelihood that a child will miss a dose during the day. In addition, multiple doses result in a roller-coaster effect of the medications, moving in and out of the therapeutic index range, leading to emotional volatility.

Many of the medications listed here have delivery mechanisms that delay and slow the release of amphetamine. Mydayis may have taken this to an extreme.

Mydayis is a capsule that contains coated beads, much like Ritalin LA, Metadate CD, and Adderall XR. Those three medications have two different types of beads: an immediate release that releases its medication right away and lasts for about four hours, and extended-release beads that then kick in and last another 4–5 hours. Mydayis takes this one step further by adding a third bead that has an additional, second coating so that it releases additional medication over the next eight hours, bringing the time of total effectiveness up to sixteen hours.

The active ingredient in Mydayis is exactly the same as Adderall XR (mixed amphetamine salts), and the ratio of dextro-amphetamine to levo-amphetamine is 75 percent to 25 percent, again, just like Adderall XR. Levo-amphetamine adds little benefit. In addition, the different salts add nothing to the therapeutic benefit of the medication. The only difference is that Adderall XR lasts about nine hours, whereas Mydayis is designed to last 15–16 hours. If Adderall XR is taken at 7 a.m., it will wear off around 4 p.m., whereas Mydayis, if taken at 7 a.m., should last until 10–11 p.m. That is a huge benefit for the older child who might not start homework until late in the evening.

However, a medication that lasts until 11 p.m. predictably will have more side effects than any other preparation of amphetamine-based medication, and Mydayis does not disappoint. In studies done by the pharmaceutical company, children who took Mydayis were 30 percent more likely to experience reduced appetite, and more than 30 percent had trouble falling asleep.[8] These studies were done in children thirteen years of age and older. One would expect the rate to be even higher for younger children.

Mydayis is approved for children thirteen years of age and older. Doctors have the right to prescribe a medication "off label" (for a purpose or at a dose not approved by the FDA), so it can be prescribed for younger children. If Mydayis is used in younger children, remember that if it wears off at 11 p.m., then that younger child may not be able to fall asleep until midnight or even later. So, a medication lasting 15–16 hours might be a better option for a sixteen-year-old, but it is likely to cause significant problems with sleep in a ten-year-old.

Many children with ADHD have significant sleep difficulties, and this has been thoroughly discussed in Chapter 8 on side effects. Interestingly, some children might actually sleep better on Mydayis (as long as they can *get* to sleep), because it has been shown that some existing sleep difficulties will decrease or even disappear when stimulant medication is started.

Finally, when considering whether Mydayis is right for your child, consider whether it is covered by insurance and consider the cost. Mydayis might be right for your child as long as it does not last too long and cause significant sleep and appetite difficulties and as long as it is covered by insurance. Otherwise, consider another long-acting amphetamine (such as Dexedrine Spansules, Adderall XR, or Vyvanse) or consider a long-acting methylphenidate medication (such as Concerta, Daytrana, or Focalin XR).

Mydayis comes as a capsule that can be opened and sprinkled on applesauce or pudding to make it easier to swallow.

Vyvanse / Vyvanse Chewable

Brand Name	Generic Name
Vyvanse Vyvanse Chewable	lisdexamfetamine 0% IR, 100% ER 100% dex, 0% levo
Advantages	**Disadvantages**
Vyvanse lasts about 10-12 hours, so that multiple daily dosing is not necessary. The abuse of amphetamine medications can be curtailed with Vyvanse because if snorted, it will not be absorbed into the brain. However, the risk of abuse of stimulant medications in children with ADHD is low. It is usually covered by insurance.	Vyvanse is nothing more than dextro-amphetamine, the same ingredient in multiple amphetamine medications. It is expensive and if it is not prescribed for its abuse reduction, it does not have much advantage over much less expensive medications. It takes longer to take effect in the morning.

	Time	Preparations	Brand		Generic	
			w/o Ins	GoodRx	w/o Ins	GoodRx
Vyvanse	10-12	10-20-30-40-50-60-70 Capsule	$380	$354	Generic Not Available	
Vyvanse Chewable	10-12	10-20-30-40-50-60mg	$380	$338	Generic Not Available	

Vyvanse (lis-dextro-amphetamine) is an extended-release version of dextro-amphetamine that uses a novel technology to extend its effect for 10–12 hours. In addition, it is a medication that prevents some forms of inappropriate use or diversion to other students. Here's how all of this is accomplished.

Adderall XR was developed by Shire Pharmaceuticals (now part of Takeda), and for about fifteen years it enjoyed patent protections and exclusivity (meaning that no generic of Adderall XR could be produced by another pharmaceutical company). It was one of the most frequently prescribed medications for the treatment of ADHD, but that was all about to change. Adderall XR was losing its patent protection, so that after January 2009, generic medications would be allowed to compete for Adderall XR's market share.

Right after the beginning of the new millennium, Shire began working on a new concept for ADHD medications. A pro-drug is a medication that is inactive when ingested, but the body's metabolic processes convert it into a medication with active properties.

Since the 1970s, it has been recognized that amphetamines can be abused. They are not usually abused by adolescents with ADHD, because when they take an amphetamine, they feel . . . well, normal. However, the more medication they take, the more it supresses their spontaneity, and most adolescents don't like that feeling. So, they tend to resist taking their medication. This hardly sounds like a drug that would be abused.

However, it is not uncommon for adolescents or college-age students with ADHD to give or sell their medication to a friend or acquaintance who may *not* have ADHD. That friend will then use the amphetamine medication to help stay awake while studying late at night. This is called "diversion." But some of those friends or acquaintances have learned that if you take an Adderall pill and crush it into a powder, you can snort Adderall, which delivers the medication to the brain quickly, allowing them to experience a high. Children with ADHD do not experience this high (at least at prescribed doses), because the medication allows their brain to function more like other children function off medication.

However, if Vyvanse (lis-dextro-amphetamine) is snorted . . . nothing happens. If Vyvanse is taken orally, it gets into the brain and works the way it was designed to treat ADHD, but when it is snorted, it does not get into the brain at all and has no effect.

Amino acids are a group of about twenty small molecules that are the building blocks of proteins. Shire took dextro-amphetamine and joined it to one of these amino acids, lysine. Snorting Vyvanse won't produce a high because the lysine attached to the dextro-amphetamine prevents its absorption into the brain.

On the other hand, if lis-dextro-amphetamine is swallowed, it is absorbed into the bloodstream, then into the red blood cells. Once inside the red blood cell, lysine is separated from dextro-amphetamine, and the remaining molecule is released from the red blood cell back into the bloodstream.

So, what's left? Once lysine is separated from the molecule, the original dextro-amphetamine remains. This molecule easily crosses into the brain and acts on the neurons just as all the other amphetamine medications do. The dextro-amphetamine that gets into the brain from Vyvanse is exactly the same as the dextro-amphetamine that Bradley used in 1940 to produce the first positive effects of this medication in children.

This medication, dextro-amphetamine linked to the lysine amino-acid, is Vyvanse. By altering the chemical structure of dextro-amphetamine, even temporarily, three things are accomplished:

1. A new treatment for ADHD is created that dramatically limits the possibility of it being abused nasally, even though abuse at the low doses used for treating ADHD is extremely unlikely.

2. Dextro-amphetamine lasts for about 3½–4 hours, but the whole process of having a medication absorbed by red blood cells, metabolized, and then released as dextro-amphetamine takes time. Shire Pharmaceuticals can then produce a medication that lasts up to 9–10 hours without using the coated beads that most other extended-release medications employ.

3. Shire knew that it would be relatively easy to prove to the FDA that Vyvanse is safe and effective, because when Vyvanse gets to the brain, it becomes the same medication that is present in many other medications (Dexedrine, Dexedrine Spansule, Dextrostat, Zenzedi, Procentra, Evekeo, etc.). Yes, Shire was losing exclusivity for Adderall XR but was able to replace the lost revenue from Adderall XR with new revenue from Vyvanse. Vyvanse was approved by the FDA in 2007. By the time Adderall XR lost its patent protection and exclusivity in 2009, Vyvanse was already marketed as a better alternative to all these other medications.

I have a confession to make. Shortly after Vyvanse was approved, I was asked by Shire to attend a three-day conference where a new medication for the treatment of ADHD would be introduced. I felt obligated to attend so that I could learn about this new medication that would be a big help for my patients. The fact that the conference was being held at the Atlantis Hotel in the Bahamas was further encouragement. Oh, and the fact that all travel, hotel, and food expenses would be paid by Shire didn't hurt. Neither did it hurt that we were given a $1,000 stipend for other expenses.

More than six hundred developmental pediatricians, psychiatrists, and neurologists attended. The first day there, we went on a snorkeling expedition. That night we attended a beachfront dinner with a live band and an open bar. The next day was all conferences. Many of the most respected researchers in the ADHD field presented the results of their studies on this new medication. I actually learned a lot from these presentations.

The third day was different. That morning I checked in and was told that I needed to go to a smaller conference room on the fourth floor. I found myself in a small room with about thirty other physicians and one representative from Shire Pharmaceuticals. He started the meeting by asking if we were enjoying our stay in the Bahamas; general agreement was that everyone was learning much and having a great time.

Then I sensed that the mood in the room changed a little. He said, "Yesterday we learned about Vyvanse, a novel medication that was recently approved by the FDA for the treatment of ADHD. We learned about the pharmacokinetics of this medication and the result of a number of very successful trials. And we learned about how Vyvanse can prevent diversion and abuse. But today, all of the attendees to this conference have been divided into smaller groups like this one, and each group has been tasked to address a different issue."

"Your job," he continued, "is to help us describe the medical situations for which Vyvanse should be prescribed as the medication of *first choice*" for ADHD. Our group quickly and enthusiastically entered into a discussion of the advantages of Vyvanse. Obviously, we might want to prescribe Vyvanse first if we suspected that an adolescent or college student might have a history of substance abuse or a history that would suggest propensities to give or sell his medication to a friend or roommate. But the pharmaceutical representative began pushing us to extend the recommendation for Vyvanse to more common situations, such as a typical student with ADHD who might need medication for a longer period throughout the day. Vyvanse's extended duration would help here.

I had not participated much during this discussion, and by this time, I was getting uncomfortable. I began to see what was happening here. I felt that I had to speak up.

"If I have a child with typical ADHD without associated comorbid difficulties, I am going to start with a methylphenidate medication first, because there are fewer side effects. If for some reason the child does not respond to the methylphenidate medication, I might consider switching to an extended-release amphetamine such as Dexedrine Spansules. Only if I suspect the possibility of abuse or diversion would I then switch to Vyvanse. But other than this, I don't see a situation where I would start first with Vyvanse." I remember that the pharmaceutical rep quickly switched the subject and began soliciting other answers from other attendees.

I was never invited to one of these conferences again.

For years, Adderall was marketed as a better medication than Dexedrine (dextro-amphetamine), because it is a mixture of mixed amphetamine salts, with both dextro-amphetamine and levo-amphetamine. Now Vyvanse is marketed as a better medication because it is just dextro-amphetamine. But why pay for expensive Vyvanse when Dexedrine is just as effective as Vyvanse at one-tenth the cost? Yes, Vyvanse does last an hour or two longer at the end of the day, because the metabolism taking place in the red blood cells takes time. But this long duration comes at the cost of taking an hour or even longer before it begins to take effect in the morning.

Vyvanse is a highly effective medication for treating ADHD, but after a diagnosis of ADHD is made, there is very little reason to consider it the first-choice treatment. Some adolescents respond better to amphetamine medications than to the methylphenidate medications, but we have no way to predict this in advance. For a child who is newly diagnosed with ADHD and who has never been treated with medication, I usually start with a methylphenidate medication such as Concerta or Daytrana, and only switch to an amphetamine medication such as Vyvanse or Adderall XR if that child either did not show a positive response to methylphenidate or experienced side effects that prevented its use.

Vyvanse is expensive, but it is often covered by insurance. No generic is available.

Note: Because lis-dex-amphetamine, linked to the amino acid lysine, is a bigger molecule than dextro-amphetamine alone, more Vyvanse must be given (by weight) to achieve the same benefit that would be realized from dextro-amphetamine alone. Therefore, 70 mg of Vyvanse equates to 20.8 mg of dextro-amphetamine alone.[9]

Amphetamine Transdermal System

Brand Name	Generic Name
Amphetamine Transdermal System	Dextro-amphetamine 0% IR, 100% ER 100% dex, 0% levo
Advantages	**Disadvantages**
A skin patch for stimulant medication has 4 advantages: **Flexible Duration** Patch can be removed at different times depending on daily demands. **Flexible fine-tuned dosage**, by cutting patch **Crash-resistant** Because it wears off gradually. The irritability that can occur when a stimulant wears off at the end of the day is greatly reduced. **Compliance** (parent knows that a child had the patch on all day, because if removed, it cannot be reapplied.)	Skin irritation

	Time	Preparations	Brand		Generic	
			w/o Ins	GoodRx	w/o Ins	GoodRx
Amphetamine Transdermal System	4-24	4.5-9-13.5-18mg Skin Patch	?	?	Generic Not Available	

Noven Pharmaceuticals is currently developing a skin patch for the delivery of dextro-amphetamine for children with ADHD. Clinical trials are ongoing, and early results are very promising. Once these clinical trials are complete, Noven will apply to the FDA for final approval. No brand name has yet been announced.

Noven is the same company that produces Daytrana, the only other skin patch for a stimulant medication approved by the FDA, which has been used for approximately the past fifteen years. Daytrana uses methylphenidate, but the new patch will use dextro-amphetamine. Another skin patch is also available for clonidine (Catapres TTS), which is a non-stimulant also used for the treatment of ADHD. Catapres TTS is not as effective as the stimulant medications.

A skin patch has two significant advantages: First, it is the only delivery system for an ADHD medication that gives the physician and patient complete flexibility in how long a medication lasts. Current trials indicate that the amphetamine skin patch takes about two hours to take effect and lasts at least nine hours (which is how long the patch was worn in these trials). However, the patch can be removed earlier or later than that time, allowing for a flexible duration of effectiveness determined by how long the patch remains in contact with the skin.

Second, the dosage can be fine-tuned by cutting the patch. (See the section on Daytrana for a detailed explanation of the advantages of cutting the patch to fine-tune the dose and of removing the patch at different times to customize the effect of medication throughout the day.)

Because of the flexibility, Daytrana is an excellent medication for treating ADHD. However, significant skin irritation is an added side effect. Unfortunately, not much more information will be available about this new medication until it is approved by the FDA and physicians start using it. A decision about brand name has not yet been made.

Just a note about all amphetamine medications: Taking any amphetamine medication with fatty foods delays the time that it takes to reach the peak concentration in the blood by 1–2 hours. That doesn't mean that your child cannot take it with food, but understand that it might delay the onset and peak times. Further, acidifying agents/foods may lower absorption of amphetamine (requiring a slightly higher dose), while alkalinizing agents/foods may increase absorption (requiring a slightly lower dose). This effect is not seen with methylphenidate medications. However, in practice, the effect of food intake does not usually alter the effectiveness by any significant degree.

Chapter 12

TEN NON-STIMULANT
MEDICATIONS TO TREAT ADHD

Brand Name	Generic Name	Neurotransmitter Affected
Catapres	Clonidine	Norepinephrine
Catapres TTS		
Kapvay		
Tenex	Guanfacine	
Intuniv		
Qelbree	Viloxazine	
Strattera	Atomoxetine	Dopamine & Norepinephrine
Wellbutrin	Bupropion	
Wellbutrin SR		
Wellbutrin XL		
The Stimulants	Methylphenidate	
	Amphetamine	

Stimulant medications are highly effective for the treatment of ADHD, but these medications can cause irritating side effects (decreased appetite, insomnia, irritability, mood changes, etc.). Wouldn't it be great if we could find a medication that worked as well as the stimulants without the annoying side effects?

Five **non-stimulant** medications have been approved for the treatment of ADHD (clonidine, guanfacine, atomoxetine, bupropion, and viloxazine) and these five generic medications have been produced in ten different brand-name medications. Remember that ADHD is associated with a decrease in activity of two neurotransmitters in the brain, dopamine and norepinephrine. Stimulant medications increase the activity of these two neurotransmitters.

On the other hand, all non-stimulants work primarily by increasing only the norepinephrine activity in certain areas of the brain[1] (especially the frontal cortex,[2] just behind the eyes). Clonidine, guanfacine, and viloxazine have little effect on dopamine. The two other non-stimulants (atomoxetine and bupropion) also have their primary effect on norepinephrine but with some smaller effect on dopamine as well. However, none of these five medications has the same effect on dopamine as do the stimulants.

Because these medications have their primary effect on norepinephrine, you might expect the non-stimulants to be less effective as the stimulants in treating ADHD. And this is, indeed, the case. These medications help reduce the hyperactivity and impulsivity of ADHD as well as the stimulants, but they have much less beneficial effect on a child's ability to maintain focus and attention.

Strattera (atomoxetine) and Wellbutrin (bupropion) also have their primary effect on norepinephrine, but they also have a mild to moderate effect on increasing activity of dopamine as well. That is why Strattera and Wellbutrin perform better than clonidine and guanfacine for attention and distractibility.[3]

All of the non-stimulants have one big advantage over stimulants: they do not cause the irritating side effects often seen with stimulant medications[4] (appetite suppression, insomnia, irritability, and mood suppression). As a matter of fact, the non-stimulants **treat and reduce** many of the side effects that stimulants produce.

Because non-stimulants increase the activity of norepinephrine and because increased norepinephrine activity has a positive effect on mood, it is not surprising that non-stimulants have a tendency to stabilize mood as well.

Many children with ADHD have trouble controlling their emotions. They are easily excitable, overreact to disappointment, anger more easily, and can be very irritable. When a child with ADHD, who also has emotional hypersensitivity, starts on stimulant medication, he usually shows the same positive effects on hyperactivity, impulsivity, distractibility, and attention. And sometimes, unpredictably, emotional hypersensitivity decreases, or disappears entirely. But many other children with ADHD and emotional hypersensitivity become even more hypersensitive and irritable when started on a stimulant.

And that's where non-stimulants come in. They can be used in place of a stimulant or combined with a stimulant to improve the symptoms of ADHD without causing the side effects of a stimulant alone.

If a non-stimulant is used alone, it usually reduces hyperactivity and distractibility equally as well as a stimulant. And it may help with the attention and distractibility problems but less successfully than stimulants. However, it is likely that the non-stimulant will result in improved emotional stability.[5]

Other children with ADHD exhibit no emotional volatility before starting medication. Once a stimulant is introduced, the expected improvements in attention and distractibility are seen, but the children become moody and irritable, especially as the stimulant is wearing off in the late afternoon or early evening. A non-stimulant will often reduce emotional hypersensitivity and irritability, especially as medication wears off. And if tics existed prior to starting medication or emerged with stimulant medication, guanfacine and clonidine are likely to reduce or eliminate the tics as well.

Because pediatricians pay close attention to growth and because stimulants decrease appetite, physicians (especially pediatricians) are often reluctant to use a stimulant in a child under six years of age. As a result, physicians have developed a tendency to use a non-stimulant (especially Intuniv) for children under six with ADHD.

Preschools and kindergarten are all about children learning to live well with other people (following rules, sharing, taking turns, listening, etc.). In addition, some preschools and all kindergartens teach academic skills (letter recognition, number recognition, early reading, and number skills). Hyperactivity and impulsivity are the most disruptive symptoms in a preschool-age child with ADHD because these behaviors most interfere with a child's ability to learn to get along with other children. Preschool children with ADHD almost always have trouble focusing and attending as well, if you look hard enough, but these symptoms are usually less concerning at this age. The non-stimulants clonidine and guanfacine are usually effective in reducing hyperactivity and impulsivity but usually have less impact on distractibility and attention. Because these medications do not produce difficulty falling asleep or cause decreased appetite like stimulants, physicians are more likely to use these medications for a newly diagnosed child with ADHD under six years. However, once a child with ADHD gets older and is required to pay attention and focus, it is often necessary to add or switch to a stimulant. Very few children with ADHD can be treated with a non-stimulant alone throughout childhood.

A child with ADHD, at any age, should almost always be tried on a stimulant first. But for children who develop significant insomnia, irritability, or other side effects from a stimulant, the addition or substitution of a non-stimulant can make all the difference.

Catapres / Catapres TTS / Kapvay

Brand Name			Generic Name		
Catapres Catapres TTS Kapvay			clonidine		
Advantages			**Disadvantages**		
Clonidine is only moderately effective for ADHD symptoms. but it is a good alternative for very young children. It has the advantage that when used with a stimulant, clonidine will minimize most of the stimulant side effects (insomnia, tics, irritability). One patch lasts 7 days. It is often covered by insurance.			Sedation and low blood pressure are the two most common side effects. Sedation is usually mild and if a stimulant is added, the sedation will disappear. Low blood pressure can cause light headedness or fainting, but this is not usually a problem at the low doses used to treat ADHD.		

	Time	Preparations	Brand		Generic	
			w/o Ins	GoodRx	w/o Ins	GoodRx
Catapres Tab	4-6	0.1-0.2-0.3mg Tablet	$206	$164	$17	$4
Catapres TTS Patch	7 days	0.1-0.2-0.3mg per patch	$382	$293	$120	$24
Kapvay	12	0.1-0.2mg Tablet	$284	$249	$133	$18

Clonidine is not a stimulant like methylphenidate and amphetamine but is in a group of medications called alpha-2 agonists. It was one of the first non-stimulant medications approved for the treatment of ADHD.

In the 1960s, clonidine was used to treat nasal congestion. However, it had two side effects. Patients on clonidine were somewhat sedated, and their blood pressure dropped. This was about the time physicians had identified the dangers of high blood pressure and were beginning to be more aggressive in its treatment. Clonidine was restudied, then received approval from the FDA for the treatment of hypertension.

Tourette's syndrome is a medical condition characterized by obsessive-compulsive behaviors and vocal tics. In 1979, it was reported that children with tics due to Tourette's syndrome improved on clonidine.[6] Tourette's syndrome is often accompanied by ADHD in children, and physicians noted that children on clonidine had significantly fewer tics, but they became less hyperactive as well. Research studies showed that all of the symptoms of ADHD improved, although not as dramatically as with stimulants (methylphenidate and amphetamine).[7] In 2008, clonidine was approved for the treatment of ADHD.

Early in my career, I saw a five-year-old boy who was hyperactive, impulsive, and having trouble focusing and attending in school. That was difficult enough, but this child was also disrespectful to adults, easy to anger, and aggressive toward other children. The least little thing would precipitate a twenty-minute tantrum of screaming, spitting, and kicking. I diagnosed ADHD and a second disorder, oppositional defiant disorder (ODD).

I started him on Ritalin LA. His hyperactivity disappeared. He was more attentive in school, although he still had some difficulty attending to something that did not interest him. Unfortunately, he was still aggressive, angry, and oppositional, and it seemed that these behaviors had actually increased since starting Ritalin LA. Further, since starting to take Ritalin LA, he would take an hour and a half to fall asleep. I discontinued the Ritalin LA and started an amphetamine-based stimulant (Dexedrine Spansule). Like the Ritalin LA, Dexedrine significantly improved his ability to focus and concentrate, but his moodiness, anger, and aggressiveness were even worse than with Ritalin LA, and he even had more difficulty falling asleep.

I was aware of research studies that indicated that clonidine might be therapeutic in situations like this. I discontinued the Dexedrine Spansule and started clonidine.

He and his mother returned in two weeks. She said that since starting the clonidine, his personality had changed. Before, he was angry, irritable, and aggressive. Since he started taking clonidine, he was almost always smiling, happy, and agreeable. He seemed to enjoy pleasing his parents and his teacher. His teacher said it was like magic. In addition to these gains in behavior and school, it was only taking fifteen minutes to fall asleep at night. Unfortunately, on clonidine alone his hyperactivity had returned (although milder than before medication), and he was having more trouble attending for long periods of time, although these symptoms were better than without any medication.

Because the symptoms of ADHD had disappeared with Ritalin LA and then returned with clonidine, I continued the clonidine and started Ritalin LA again, at a lower dose than before. His hyperactivity again vanished. He was attentive and focused in school, and the teacher said he was like a model student. At home, he was happy and agreeable. The combination of these two medications treated two different sets of symptoms. Ritalin LA increased his ability to focus, attend, and concentrate while reducing his hyperactivity and impulsivity. At the same time, Ritalin LA was responsible for increasing his anger and aggressiveness. Clonidine minimized the negative effects of Ritalin LA, helped stabilize his volatile moods, and helped him get to sleep and sleep more soundly.

Many parents hesitate before agreeing to medical treatment of their child's ADHD. I understand why a parent of a young child would balk even more at the suggestion of using two medications in combination to treat ADHD. You would expect two medications to have twice the side effects of one medication.

But here is where things get surprisingly unexpected. The stimulants have a number of relatively mild side effects (difficulty falling asleep, deceased appetite, moodiness, and irritability). And clonidine has side effects as well (low blood pressure, dry mouth, and sedation are the most common). ***But almost every side effect that can result from a stimulant will be diminished or eliminated with a non-stimulant. And the side effects that clonidine causes are diminished when a stimulant is added.***

Physicians try to avoid using multiple medications because the more medication a patient is on, the more likely are side effects. Further, the *interaction* of two or more medications together can produce additional side effects. But with a non-stimulant and a stimulant together, side effects are almost always reduced or eliminated. A child who is on a stimulant may have trouble falling asleep but usually will fall asleep more easily and quickly with clonidine or guanfacine. Tics occur often in children with ADHD, and clonidine and guanfacine are an effective treatment for tics. Stimulants almost always cause some appetite suppression, and although clonidine and guanfacine do not increase appetite, they do stimulate the production of growth hormone. The irritability that occurs when a stimulant medication wears off is usually eliminated with clonidine.[8] Stimulants can cause a mild increase in heart rate and sometimes an increase in blood pressure, whereas clonidine and guanfacine decrease heart rate and lower blood pressure. Finally, clonidine causes sedation during the day, but if a child is on a stimulant with clonidine, the daytime sedation will be absent.

Clonidine and guanfacine start working within a half hour after taking it, and the positive effects last about 4–5 hours.[9] Some physicians will give clonidine at night to help with sleep problems that are much more common with ADHD. They have noted that when the child wakes up the next morning, clonidine may still be helping, with a positive effect on mood. That is true, but the beneficial effects are not optimal and will not continue throughout the day on just an evening dose of regular clonidine. Another dose of clonidine is then needed in the morning. And if a dose is given in the morning, it may not last until late afternoon or early evening, so a second dose will almost always be needed.

Kapvay is the extended-release form of clonidine. Kapvay lasts about twelve hours, so a child would need only a single dose of Kapvay in the morning, and then could take a dose of the immediate-release clonidine when he gets home from school. On the other hand, a dose of Kapvay, at night only, will continue to have some positive effects into the late morning. However, the optimal effects of Kapvay are best realized when given both in the morning and evening.

Generic clonidine is inexpensive ($20 for a month supply) and is usually covered by insurance, whereas brand-name Kapvay is more expensive. Kapvay is less likely to be covered by insurance. Clonidine is also available as a skin patch (Catapres TTS). Generally, a skin patch is an excellent choice for the treatment of ADHD. A skin patch allows for complete flexibility in dosing. Unlike the methylphenidate skin patch (Daytrana), which lasts an entire day, the positive effects of the Catapres skin patch can last up to seven days. In addition, some skin patches can be cut to fine-tune the dose as well (see the section on Daytrana for a more detailed explanation of these benefits). The pharmaceutical company that produces the skin patch usually will advise against cutting a skin patch, because it may lead to variability in dosing. Some skin patches have a reservoir of medication in the middle of the patch. Cutting this kind of patch would open the reservoir and could lead to a sudden release of medication, and possibly to a child getting more medication than expected. However, Catapres TTS is produced as a large number of micro-reservoirs, so that cutting the patch will not increase the dose.

One patch can last up to seven days. It can take a few weeks to determine how often to put on a new patch; some children may be able to do well if the patch is left on longer than seven days, but that is not recommended because of skin irritation if left on past that time.

Catapres TTS skin patch is an excellent option for children with ADHD who experience multiple side effects to a stimulant. The generic patch is often covered by insurance, but the brand name is usually not covered and is expensive.

Because of the similarities between guanfacine and clonidine, please read the section on clonidine above, before reading the following.

Tenex / Intuniv

Brand Name			Generic Name			
Tenex Intuniv			guanfacine			
Advantages			**Disadvantages**			
Tenex and Intuniv are only moderately effective for ADHD symptoms. but it is a good alternative for very young children. It has the advantage that when used with a stimulant, guanfacine will minimize most of the stimulant side effects (insomnia, tics, irritability).			Sedation and low blood pressure are the two most common side effects. Sedation is usually mild and if a stimulant is added, the sedation will disappear. Low blood pressure can cause light headedness or fainting, but this is not usually a problem at the low doses used to treat ADHD.			
	Time	Preparations	Brand		Generic	
			w/o Ins	GoodRx	w/o Ins	GoodRx
Tenex	5-6	1-2mg	Brand Name Not Available		$54	$12
Intuniv (guanfacine ER)	10-12	1-2-3-4mg	$360	$294	$255	$13

Tenex is the brand name for another non-stimulant, guanfacine, that has been approved for the treatment of ADHD. Guanfacine has a chemical structure similar to clonidine and was also initially used as a treatment for high blood pressure. When the benefits of clonidine for ADHD were realized, studies of guanfacine confirmed suspicions that it would work for ADHD as well. Studies showed that it did have a positive effect on reducing the hyperactivity and impulsivity of ADHD,[10] but just like clonidine, the attention problems and impulsivity of ADHD showed minimal benefit from guanfacine when compared to stimulants. Everything discussed above for clonidine applies equally to guanfacine, with one exception. Guanfacine is a little less sedating than clonidine, so I often use clonidine if a child has sleep problems and guanfacine if not.

Children with ADHD are more likely to have tics, and guanfacine is an effective treatment for them. The irritability that occurs when stimulant medication wears off is usually minimized or eliminated with guanfacine. Stimulants almost always cause some appetite suppression, and although guanfacine does not increase appetite, it does stimulate the production of growth hormone.[11] Stimulants can cause a mild increase in heart rate and, rarely, an increase in blood pressure. Guanfacine decreases heart rate and lowers blood pressure. Finally, guanfacine results in less sedation than clonidine, and if a child is on a stimulant with guanfacine, daytime sedation is almost always absent.

Intuniv is the brand name for extended-release guanfacine. It has all the benefits of Tenex (immediate-release guanfacine),[12] but a single dose usually lasts nine hours, so a dose is not needed at school. Therefore, Intuniv can be started in the morning, and the beneficial effects will last most of the day.[13] A second dose is often added in the early evening to help with any coexisting sleep problems (although clonidine is more likely to help with sleep).

Both clonidine and guanfacine are approved for children ages 6–17. However, when many physicians are confronted with a four-year-old who meets criteria for a diagnosis of ADHD they are often reluctant to use a stimulant because of the effect on appetite. Instead, it has become common practice initially to use Intuniv without a stimulant for pure ADHD in younger children. This probably works because if a child is diagnosed with ADHD as a four-year-old, the most troublesome symptoms are usually hyperactivity, impulsivity, anger, and aggression. Intuniv is an excellent treatment for those symptoms.[14] Intuniv generally is not nearly as effective as stimulants for attention difficulties, but this is usually of less concern in a four-year-old. So, the younger the child with ADHD, the more likely he or she is to be started on Intuniv first, adding a stimulant later or switching to a stimulant as the child grows older and is confronted with more difficulty focusing and attending.

I have a different practice for young children with ADHD. Even though preschool children are less likely to be asked to attend for long periods of time, they still need to attend. And stimulants are still the best medications to help with the attention difficulties in ADHD. So, my feeling is why not start with the most effective medication[15] (the stimulants methylphenidate or amphetamine) and if side effects occur, only then switch to Intuniv or add Intuniv to the stimulant treatment.[16]

Strattera

Brand Name			Generic Name			
Strattera			atomoxetine			
Advantages			Disadvantages			
Treats most of the symptoms of ADHD (hyperactivity, impulsivity) but less effective for treatment of inattention of distractibility. Does not cause the side effects of the stimulants (insomnia, decreased appetite, irritability). Usually covered by insurance.			Not as effective as stimulants for treatment of ADHD. Can take 2-3 weeks or longer before optimal benefits realized.			
	Time	Preparations	Brand		Generic	
			w/o Ins	GoodRx	w/o Ins	GoodRx
Strattera	9-10	10-18-25-40-60-80-100mg Capsule	$520	$430	$376	$31

About twenty years ago, I was attending a dinner after a major medical conference on ADHD. Strattera had just been approved for the treatment of ADHD in 2002. One of the researchers who performed the safety and efficacy studies for Strattera was present, and he was asked how Strattera was "discovered." He stated that they had been searching for a non-stimulant treatment for ADHD and asked some of the pharmaceutical companies if they had any potential prospects. One pharmaceutical company had been developing atomoxetine in the 1980s as a potential new treatment for depression. However, about the same time, Prozac was developed, and this pharmaceutical company did not feel that atomoxetine could compare favorably to Prozac. As a result, atomoxetine was shelved and no further development was pursued.

However, because atomoxetine was a norepinephrine reuptake inhibitor, and because this researcher was well aware of the role of nor-epinephrine in the treatment of ADHD, he felt that atomoxetine might be a good alternative to stimulant medications.

In initial studies, the positive effects in treating ADHD were encouraging. They pursued further studies of the safety and effectiveness in children with ADHD and received FDA approval for Strattera (atomoxetine) as a treatment for ADHD in 2002. In 2017, researchers looked back at their experience with Strattera (atomoxetine) and found that in forty-two studies of 8,398 children and adolescents, atomoxetine was consistently effective at treating the primary symptoms of ADHD.[17] Effect size was 1.37, which is considered highly effective and comparable to the stimulant medications. However, another review of eleven studies of more than two thousand children with ADHD found that atomoxetine was effective for the treatment of ADHD, but that Concerta[18] and Adderall[19] were superior to Strattera.

Remember that ADHD is associated with decreased activity of the neurotransmitters norepinephrine and dopamine in three prominent brain areas. It was initially felt that atomoxetine functioned as a norepinephrine reuptake inhibitor, increasing the activity of the neurotransmitter norepinephrine in the brain. Further research demonstrated positive effects on dopamine as well. As a result, Strattera is an effective non-stimulant option for the treatment of ADHD, because it functions in a similar way to the stimulant medications but without the stimulant side effects.

Although Strattera does not produce the common side effects seen with stimulant medications (insomnia, irritability, mood suppression), it does have its own side-effect profile. The most common side effects to Strattera are a decrease in appetite, abdominal pain, vomiting, upset stomach, and sedation.[20] Strattera can also increase heart rate and blood pressure (in contrast to clonidine and guanfacine, which lower blood pressure and heart rate), although no evidence indicates that Strattera causes serious cardiac side effects.

When I first started prescribing Strattera, I did not feel that it was very effective in my patients, and I was considering discontinuing its use. However, a major drawback of Strattera is that it can often take 2–3 weeks to take effect, and the full effects might not be seen until 4–6 weeks. This can be a major disadvantage. You have to wait six weeks to see the optimal effect of Strattera, and if you don't see much benefit, you might increase the dose, requiring another wait of six weeks. Although I would still start treatment of ADHD with a stimulant, especially methylphenidate, I do consider Strattera to be a good option to stimulants if side effects prevent their effective use, especially mood side effects and irritability.

Qelbree

Brand Name		Generic Name			
Qelbree		viloxazine			
Advantages		**Disadvantages**			
Treats most of the symptoms of ADHD (hyperactivity, impulsivity) but less effective for treatment of inattention of distractibility. Does not cause the side effects of the stimulants (insomnia, decreased appetite, irritability). Usually covered by insurance.		Not as effective as stimulants for treatment of ADHD. Can take 2-3 weeks or longer before optimal benefits realized.			
	Time	**Preparations**	**Brand**		**Generic**
			w/o Ins	GoodRx	w/o Ins	GoodRx
Qelbree	8 hrs.	100-150-200 mg Capsule	$360	$320	Generic Not Available

Qelbree (viloxazine) is an extended-release norepinephrine reuptake inhibitor, just like Strattera (atomoxetine). It has been used as an antidepressant in Europe for more than twenty years, with the brand names Vivalan or Emovit, but it has not been approved for that purpose in the United States. Qelbree (viloxazine) was very recently approved by the FDA for the treatment of ADHD (April 2021). Only a few research studies have been published for viloxazine and ADHD, and although they do demonstrate that viloxazine is effective for the treatment of ADHD, many of these studies were funded by the pharmaceutical company.

Qelbree was made available in pharmacies in May 2021, but it is still too early to determine how it is doing in clinical practice. Researchers have not yet had much chance to study Qelbree independent of the pharmaceutical company. As a result, clinicians have had very little experience with this medication.

Remember that ADHD is associated with a decrease in activity of the two neurotransmitters norepinephrine and dopamine in three prominent areas of the brain. On the other hand, decreased activity of the neurotransmitter serotonin is associated with depression. Many of the most commonly prescribed antidepressants work by increasing the activity of serotonin. Because Qelbree also increases the activity of serotonin, because of its success as an antidepressant in Europe, and because it is effective for the treatment of ADHD, one can speculate that Qelbree might be especially helpful for children with ADHD with associated irritability or mood difficulties, but no research has been done to document this relationship.

Qelbree holds promise as a new non-stimulant for the treatment of ADHD, but it is too early to make any definitive statements about its use in clinical practice.

Wellbutrin / Wellbutrin SR / Wellbutrin XL

Brand Name			Generic Name			
Wellbutrin Wellbutrin SR Wellbutrin XL			bupropion			
Advantages			Disadvantages			
Primarily used as an anti-depressant, but is a non-stimulant that is effective for ADHD. Used uncommonly and primarily when stimulants cause mood, anxiety and obsessive compulsive behaviors. Brand name is expensive but generic is very inexpensive.			Can take 3-4 days to begin to see benefit and 4-6 weeks before optimal effects achieved. Can cause seizures at high dosage, but not at usual dosage.			
	Time	Preparations	Brand		Generic	
			w/o Ins	GoodRx	w/o Ins	GoodRx
Wellbutrin		75-100mg Tablet	Brand Name Not Available		$38	$9
Wellbutrin SR		100-150-200mg Tablet	$288	$230	$34	$9
Wellbutrin XL		150-300 Tablet	$1829	$1688	$65	$13

A few years ago, I saw a twelve-year-old boy who had been having a very difficult time. Since preschool, he had trouble sitting still, attending, and was hyperactive and impulsive. He had been seen by three doctors, all of whom diagnosed ADHD. He had been treated with six different stimulant medications, and all of them caused his ADHD symptoms to improve, but he developed major side effects including depression, anxiety, and severe picking of his skin, causing it to bleed.

While on Vyvanse, he because so depressed that he told his parents, "I just want to be with Jesus." His parents said "he has lost his zest for life and learning." Lexapro, an antidepressant, had been tried with a stimulant, but his ADHD symptoms just got worse.

Almost all children who have developed these kinds of side effects to the stimulant medications had some evidence of these symptoms before starting medication. However, the parents were adamant that that was not the case with their son. They said that when he was not on medication he was "sweet, easy-going, and a joy." I checked with his teachers, and they confirmed this. They said that when he was on his medication, he was angry and defiant. Off medication, he was happy and silly and inattentive and distractable.

What was I to do? It looked like everything I would recommend in a case like this had already been tried, without success. After going back to my textbooks and scouring the internet and the National Library of Medicine, I stumbled on bupropion. I found a few studies that suggested that bupropion might be useful in a situation like this. But bupropion was not approved by the FDA for the treatment of ADHD.

So, I explained to the parents that bupropion was a possible solution. I explained that bupropion had been shown to be effective for the treatment of ADHD but was usually less successful than the stimulants. I explained the side effects and risks, and after further discussion and debate, the parents agreed.

After one week on Wellbutrin his teachers reported that he was a model student in the classroom. He was attentive, and his distractibility had completely vanished. And at home, the dreaded mood side effects did not emerge. His mother reported that "it has been a lovely weekend." She reported that this was the best Mother's Day present she had ever received. She stated that her son was "spontaneous, fun, and obedient, and even spontaneously said, 'I love you' last night."

Wellbutrin (bupropion) is an older antidepressant medication. It is also sold under the brand name Zyban to help patients stop smoking. In 2018, it was the twenty-seventh most commonly prescribed medication in the United States accounting for more than twenty-four million prescriptions.

Wellbutrin is not approved by the FDA for the treatment of ADHD. That does not mean that it is ineffective or had too many side effects. It just means that no pharmaceutical company has applied to the FDA for that purpose. Physicians can prescribe medications for purposes other than for what they received approval; this is called "off-label" prescribing.

However, numerous research studies have found Wellbutrin to be effective in treating ADHD.[21] Effect size was 0.6, comparable to the other non-stimulants, but less effective than stimulants with an effect size of 0.8 to 1.2.[22]

The most common side effects to Wellbutrin are similar to the stimulants.[23] Wellbutrin can cause difficulty falling asleep, although that difficulty is generally less than with stimulants. Some children have trouble falling asleep because they are anxious. He may be worried about monsters in the closet, or she may be worried about the fight she had with her best friend. Children who have significant anxiety in addition to their ADHD may actually fall asleep easier with bupropion; whereas stimulant medication (methylphenidate and amphetamine) can increase anxiety, bupropion is an excellent *treatment* for anxiety. Bupropion does not usually cause sedation. If anxiety is causing a child to have trouble falling asleep, then bupropion may actually help that child to fall asleep easier, by treating the anxiety, in addition to treating the ADHD.

Bupropion has been found to be safe with few side effects when used with moderate dosages. However, extremely high single doses (>400 mg) of bupropion may cause seizures even in patients who have never had a seizure before.[24] But at recommended doses, bupropion is not known to cause seizures.

Bupropion does not work as quickly as the stimulants. It can take 3–4 days before any benefit is realized and 4–6 weeks before the full effect is achieved.

Since I saw this twelve-year-old boy, I have tried bupropion in 8–10 other patients with a similar presentation of major side effects to stimulants that did not exist prior to starting medication, and I have had the same surprising but highly therapeutic result. This is not a medication I would use often, but in some cases, bupropion can be a lifesaver.

AFTERWORD

Suddenly I realized that this work is complete. I have tried to present many complex medical issues in a way that is easily understandable and then to back up everything with a careful review of the scientific research. After forty years of working with children with ADHD and their families, I realized that everything they have taught me is reflected in this book. I hope that I have been true to their legacy. This book belongs to them.

I am sure that this book will have many critics. I am sure that I will be accused of offering medication as an easy solution to a complex problem. Some will accuse me of being overzealous in my enthusiasm for medication. And that's fine.

No, it is not fine. The problem is that this story is still about your child. I have sat with almost five thousand children and their parents. I have listened to your concerns and your frustrations. I hear your heart-breaking stories. I hear your unease about what your children are experiencing in school and on the playground and in your homes. I hear your apprehension about what the future holds for them. I understand that teachers are frustrated that what was known yesterday is forgotten today. I understand that your child comes home from school in tears because he is beginning to doubt his intelligence, his competence, and his very being. You wonder whether your child will get into college, and then you wonder if your child can survive the frightening independence of living away from home, no longer under the protection of their parents and teachers. You hold hope for the future, but are uncertain about what to expect, while your child blames himself when he wants to excel but can't remember to write down a homework assignment.

And here is my dilemma. I have seen medication treatment awaken the creative intelligence that hides behind inattentiveness and distraction. I have seen medication treatment transform self-doubt into self-confidence. I have seen medication convert feelings of failure to the pride of success and accomplishment.

Would these changes have occurred without medication? Maybe. Maybe next year's teacher will understand your child so that she will be able to teach to your child's individuality. Maybe a coach will be the spark to motivate your child. Maybe other children will suddenly appreciate your child's unique talents. Some children with ADHD mature, without medication, but most do not. I would like to be able to tell you to just wait it out, but unfortunately, for most children, ADHD plagues their adulthood the same way that it haunts their childhood, but with even greater consequences. Fortunately we have a solution.

This book is not meant to magically turn you into a developmental pediatrician. But I hope it has given you the knowledge and the confidence to have an intelligent conversation with your doctor about the options that medication offers. ADHD medication is safe and it is effective. It is not for everyone, but it might be just right for your child.

MEDICATION LIST

STIMULANT MEDICATIONS for ADHD

BRAND NAME	GENERIC NAME	Hours Effective	PREPARATIONS	COMMENTS
			Methylphenidate – Immediate Release	
Ritalin	methylphenidate	3½-4	5-10-20mg Tablet	Short-acting, requires multiple doses per day resulting in roller-coaster effect of medication, producing irritability and other mood changes, requiring a dose at school. Should only be used to supplement an ER preparation, in the morning before the XR takes effect or at the end of the day to extend the effect as Extended Release is wearing off. Inexpensive compared to most other medications.
Methylin Tablets	methylphenidate	3½-4	5-10-20mg Tablet	
Methylin Chewable	methylphenidate	3½-4	2.5-5-10mg Tablet	
Methylin Liquid	methylphenidate	3½-4	5mg/5ml 10mg/5ml 150-225-300-450-600-675ml bottles	One of two liquid preparations of methylphenidate. Liquid easier to swallow than a pill and far easier to fine-tune dose. Much shorter lasting than Quillivant XR liquid.
Focalin	dextro-methylphenidate	3½-4	2.5-5-10mg Tablet	Less side effects than other MPH meds, especially emotional lability, because levo-methylphenidate is not included as it is in most other methylphenidate medications. Covered by some insurance plans, but many others do not cover. Focalin is relatively inexpensive, but Focalin XR is much more expensive.

Methylphenidate – Extended Release				
Ritalin SR / Methylin ER / Metadate ER	methylphenidate	5-6	10-20mg Tablet	Brand Name has been discontinued for all three, available in generic only. They are the shortest-acting of the Extended Release methylphenidate options. A second dose of short-acting med would be necessary.
Ritalin LA	methylphenidate	7-8	Brand: 10-20-30-40-60mg Generic: 20-30-40mg Capsule	Long-acting, but does not last as long as other preparations. Still may require dose in late afternoon or early evening. 10 and 60mg available in Brand Name only.
Focalin XR	dextro-methylphenidate	8-9	5-10-15-20-25-30-35mg Capsule	Less side effects than other MPH meds, especially emotional lability, because levo-methylphenidate is not included as it is in most other methylphenidate medications. Covered by some insurance plans, but many others do not cover. Focalin is relatively inexpensive, but Focalin XR is much more expensive.
Metadate CD	methylphenidate	8-9	10-20-30-40-50-60mg Capsule	Capsules can be opened and partially sprinkled on food to titrate dosage (better for younger children). Comes in 10-20-30-40-50-60mg, easier to titrate dose.
Aptensio XR	methylphenidate	9-10	10-15-20-30-40-50-60mg Capsule	Uses the same technology as Ritalin LA and Metadate CD (but with different ratios of Immediate Release to Extended Release) so that it lasts longer. May have more side-effects on appetite and sleep.

(Continued)

Methylphenidate – Extended Release

BRAND NAME	GENERIC NAME	Hours Effective	PREPARATIONS	COMMENTS
Concerta (generic by Patriot)	methylphenidate	10-12	18-27-36-54 mg Capsule	One of the longest acting of the oral meds (with exception of Jornay or Daytrana), "smoother" effect throughout the day; gradual wear-off, less irritability. A good choice for first-time treatment of ADHD. Generic often covered by insurance, and the generic from Patriot is exactly the same as the brand, but significantly cheaper. It is necessary to specify "generic from Patriot" (see text). Capsules cannot be cut or chewed. Difficult to titrate dose in younger children.
Quillivant XR	methylphenidate	10-12	25mg/5ml 60-120-150-180ml Liquid	One of two liquid preparations of methylphenidate, but much longer lasting than Methylin liquid (3½-4hrs.). Easier to swallow than a pill and far easier to fine-tune dose.
QuilliChew ER	methylphenidate	10-12	20-30-40mg Chewable Tablet	One of two chewable methylphenidate for children who cannot swallow pills. Long-acting (10-12 hrs.) vs. Methylin which is short-acting (3½-4 hrs.)
Adhansia XR	methylphenidate	10-12	25-35-45-55-70-85mg Capsule	Uses the same technology as Ritalin LA and Metadate CD (but with different ratios of Immediate Release to Extended Release) so that it lasts longer. May have more side effects on appetite and sleep.

			Methylphenidate – Extended Release	
Cotempla XR-ODT	methylphenidate	10-12	8.6-17.3-25.9mg Orally Dissolving Tablet	Orally dissolving pill for children difficulty swallowing. Expensive, not usually covered by insurance.
Azstarys	Ser-dextro-methylphenidate	10-12	26.1mg/5.2mg 39.2mg/7.8mg 52.3mg/10.4mg Capsule	The only pro-drug for methylphenidate. May limit abuse. Just approved by FDA 4/2021, so minimal clinical experience.
Jornay PM	methylphenidate	36	20-40-60 80-100mg Capsule	Given at night, takes effect in the morning so that medication is effective while children getting ready for school. Intriguing, but new med, no experience. May take longer to titrate appropriate timing of dose. Effect on sleep??
Daytrana Transdermal Skin Patch	methylphenidate	4-24	10-15-20-30 mg Skin Patch	Skin Patch, much smoother onset and offset. **Flexible dose** by removing at different times depending on daily demands. **Crash-resistant** because it wears off gradually. Irritability that occurs when a stimulant wears off at the end of the day is greatly reduced. **Compliance** (parent knows that a child had the patch on all day, because if removed, it cannot be reapplied.) Expensive and may not be covered by insurance. Takes 1.5-2 hrs. to take effect, frequent skin irritation.

(Continued)

			Methylphenidate - Liquid	
BRAND NAME	GENERIC NAME	Hours Effective	PREPARATIONS	COMMENTS
Methylin Liquid	methylphenidate	3½–4	5mg/5ml 10mg/5ml 150-225-300-450-600-675 ml bottles	One of two liquid preparations of methylphenidate. Liquid easier to swallow than a pill and far easier to fine-tune dose. Much shorter lasting than Quillivant XR liquid.
Quillivant XR	methylphenidate	10–12	25mg/5ml 60-120-150-180ml Liquid	One of two liquid preparations of methylphenidate. Liquid easier to swallow than a pill and far easier to fine-tune dose. Much longer lasting than Methylin liquid.
Methylphenidate – Chewable & Orally Dissolving				
Methylin Chewable	methylphenidate	3½–4	2.5-5-10mg Chewable Tablet	One of two chewable methylphenidate for children who cannot swallow pills. Short-acting (3½–4 hrs.) vs. Quillichew ER which is long-acting (10-12 hrs).
QuilliChew ER	methylphenidate	10–12	20-30-40mg Chewable Tablet	One of two chewable methylphenidate for children who cannot swallow pills. Long-acting (10-12 hrs.) vs. Methylin which is short-acting (3½–4 hrs.)
Cotempla XR-ODT	methylphenidate	10–12	8.6-17.3-25.9mg Orally Dissolving Tablet	Orally dissolving pill for children difficulty swallowing.

Methylphenidate – Skin Patch			
Daytrana Transdermal Skin Patch	methylphenidate	4-24	10-15-20-30mg Skin Patch	Skin Patch, much smoother onset and offset. **Flexible dose** by removing at different times depending on daily demands. **Flexible duration** by cutting patch. **Crash-resistant** because it wears off gradually. Irritability that occurs when a stimulant wears off at the end of the day is greatly reduced. **Compliance** (parent knows that a child had the patch on all day, because if removed, it cannot be reapplied.) Expensive and may not be covered by insurance. Takes 1.5-2 hrs. to take effect, frequent skin irritation.

(Continued)

BRAND NAME	GENERIC NAME	Hours Effective	PREPARATIONS	COMMENTS
			Amphetamine – Immediate Release	
Dexedrine, Dextrostat	D-amphetamine 100%	3 ½–4	5-10mg Tablet	Short acting, requires multiple doses per day resulting in roller-coaster effect of medication, producing irritability and other mood changes, requiring a dose at school. Should only be used to supplement an ER preparation, in the morning before the XR takes effect or at the end of the day to extend the effect as Extended Release is wearing off. Inexpensive compared to most other medications.
Zenzedi	D-amphetamine 100%	3 ½–4	2.5-5-7.5-10-15-20-30mg Tablet	Exactly same as Dexedrine, Dextrostat, but more dosages options.
Adderall	D-amphetamine 75% L-amphetamine 25%	4	5-7.5-10-12.5-15-20-30mg Tablet	Effective for treating ADHD, but it holds no advantage over other medications like Dexedrine, Dextrostat and Zenzedi. The brand name is expensive, the generics are very inexpensive but Adderall is usually covered by insurance. More likely than methylphenidate medications to caused irritability as it wears off in the afternoon, and more likely to cause appetite reduction
Evekeo	D-amphetamine 50% L-amphetamine 50%	4	5-10mg Tablet	Essentially a generic of Adderall at three times the cost with a different ratio of stereo-isomers. Insufficient research to justify change in stereo-isomer ratio.

			Amphetamine – Immediate Release	
Evekeo ODT	D-amphetamine 50% L-amphetamine 50%	3 ½-4	5-10-15-20mg Orally Dissolving Tablet	One of two ODT amphetamines. Short acting, requires multiple doses per day resulting in roller-coaster effect of medication, producing irritability and other mood changes. Requires a dose at school.
Dexedrine Liquid	D-amphetamine 100%	3 ½-4	5mg/5ml 75-150-225-300-450ml Liquid	Dexedrine and Procentra are 2 of 4 liquid amphetamine preparations, but much shorter lasting than other amphetamine liquids. Liquid easier to swallow than a pill and far easier to fine-tune dose. These short-acting medications should be used to supplement a long-acting amphetamine only, and not as the sole treatment option
Procentra Liquid	D-amphetamine 100%	3 ½-4	5mg/5ml 75-150-225-300-450mg Liquid	
			Amphetamine – Extended Release	
Dexedrine Spansule	D-amphetamine 100%	7-8	5-10-15mg	The first Extended Release preparation of amphetamine but not as long-acting as other preparations. Very expensive. Much better options available.
Adzenys XR-ODT	D-amphetamine 75% L-amphetamine 25%	8-9	3.1-6.3-9.4-12.5-15.7-18.8mg Orally Dissolving Tablet	One of 2 ODT amphetamines and the only long-acting ODT amphetamine.
Adderall XR	D-amphetamine 75% L-amphetamine 25%	8-9	5-10-15-20-25-30mg Capsule	Longer acting capsules can be opened and sprinkled on food. Because of multiple strengths, dose is more easily customized. May cause more irritability and more compulsive behaviors.

(*Continued*)

Amphetamine – Extended Release

BRAND NAME	GENERIC NAME	Hours Effective	PREPARATIONS	COMMENTS
Adzenys ER Liquid	D-amphetamine 75% L-amphetamine 25%	9-10	1.25mg/ml 90-120-150-270-450ml Liquid	These two medications are long acting liquid amphetamines, easier to swallow than a pill and far easier to fine-tune dose. Adzenys is virtually identical to Adderall. Dynavel is almost identical to Adderall with a slightly different ratio of stero-isomers, although the difference is not clinically significant and cannot be justified by research.
Dynavel XR Liquid	D-amphetamine 76% L-amphetamine 24%	10-12	2.5mg/ml 60-90-120-150-180ml Liquid	
Vyvanse	Lis-dex-amfetamine	10-12	10-20-30-40-50-60-70mg Capsule	Longer lasting than most, very difficult to abuse. After metabolism, it is the same medication as Dexedrine Spansule. Can take up to 90 minutes to take effect, but then lasts longer at the end of the day.
Vyvanse Chewable	Lis-dex-amfetamine	10-12	10-20-30-40-50-60mg Chewable Tablet	Only chewable amphetamine. Longer acting than ODT, very difficult to abuse. After metabolism, it is the same medication as Dexedrine Spansule, and can take up to 90 minutes to take effect, but then lasts longer at the end of the day.
Mydayis	D-amphetamine 75% L-amphetamine 25%	15-16	12.5-25-37.5-50mg Capsule	Essentially a generic of Adderall XR with less dosage options, but because of the higher proportion of Extended Release, it lasts much longer. More likely to have appetite and sleep problems.

Amphetamine Transdermal System (No Brand Name Yet)	D-amphetamine 50%	4-24	4.5-9-13.5-18mg Skin Patch	Will be the only amphetamine skin patch, but not yet approved by FDA. Made by same pharmaceutical company as Daytrana, so probably will act in similar way. Skin patch can customize how long it lasts by when it is removed. Dose can be fine-tuned by cutting patch. Less likely to cause irritability when it wears off. Skin irritation is common.
Amphetamine - Liquid				
Dexedrine Liquid	D-amphetamine 100%	3½-4	5mg/5ml 75-150-225-300-450ml Liquid	Two of four liquid preparations of amphetamine. Liquid easier to swallow than a pill and far easier to fine-tune dose. Much shorter lasting than other amphetamine liquids. Inconvenient to transport, a little more likely to give accidental overdose.
Procentra Liquid	D-amphetamine 100%	3½-4	5mg/5ml 75-150-225-300-450mg Liquid	
Dynavel XR Liquid	D-amphetamine 76% L-amphetamine 24%	8-10	2.5mg/ml 60-90-120-150-180ml Liquid	Two of four liquid preparations of amphetamine. Liquid easier to swallow than a pill and far easier to fine-tune dose. Long acting. Inconvenient to transport, a little more likely to give accidental overdose.
Adzenys ER Liquid	D-amphetamine 75% L-amphetamine 25%	8-10	1.25mg/ml 90-120-150-270-450ml Liquid	

(Continued)

BRAND NAME	GENERIC NAME	Hours Effective	PREPARATIONS	COMMENTS
Amphetamine – Chewable & Orally Dissolving				
Evekeo ODT	D-amphetamine 50% L-amphetamine 50%	3½-4	5-10-15-20mg Orally Dissolving Tablet	One of two ODT amphetamines for children with difficulty swallowing pills. Short acting, requires multiple doses per day resulting in roller-coaster effect of medication, producing irritability and other mood changes, and a dose at school
Adzenys XR-ODT	D-amphetamine 75% L-amphetamine 25%	8-9	3.1-6.3-9.4-12.5-15.7-18.8mg Orally Dissolving Tablet	One of two ODT amphetamines for children with difficulty swallowing pills and the only long-acting ODT amphetamine.
Vyvanse Chewable	Lis-dex-amfetamine	10-12	10-20-30-40-50-60mg Chewable Tablet	Only chewable amphetamine. Longer acting than ODT, very difficult to abuse. After metabolism, it is the same medication as Dexedrine Spansule, and although it lasts a little longer, much more expensive.
Amphetamine – Transdermal Skin Patch				
Not Yet Determined (Not Yet FDA Approved)	D-amphetamine 50%	4-24	4.5-9-13.5-18mg Skin Patch	Made by same pharmaceutical company as Daytrana, so probably will act in similar way. No experience yet, as not yet approved by FDA (although likely will be).

Non-STIMULANT MEDICATIONS for ADHD

Tenex	guanfacine	4-6	1-2 mg Tablet	Tenex is short-acting, Intuniv is long-acting guanfacine. Brand Name of Tenex no longer available.
Intuniv	guanfacine	10-12	1-2-3-4mg Tablet	Good medication for ADHD with comorbidities (ODD, anxiety, mood lability, obsessive-compulsive or tics). Reduces hyperactivity and impulsivity with less beneficial effect on attention and executive function. Less sedating than the clonidine preparations.
Catapres	clonidine	4 - 6	0.1-0.2-0.3mg Tablet	Catapres is short-acting, Kapvay is long-acting clonidine. Good medication for ADHD with comorbidities (ODD, anxiety, mood lability, obsessive-compulsive or tics). Reduces hyperactivity and impulsivity with less beneficial effect on attention and executive function. More sedating than the guanfacine preparations.
Kapvay	clonidine	12	0.1-0.2 Tablet	
Catapres-TTS	clonidine	7 days	0.1-0.2-0.3mg Skin Patch	Skin patch, one patch lasts 7 days. More exact titration of dose and duration. Good medication for children with ADHD and comorbidities. Expensive
Strattera	atomoxetine	9-10	10-18-25-40-60-80-100mg Capsule	Treats most of the symptoms of ADHD (hyperactivity, impulsivity) but less effective for inattention and distractibility. Does not cause the side effects of the stimulants (insomnia, decreased appetite, irritability). Good for children with ADHD and mood dysphoria or irritability. Can take 2-3 weeks before optimal benefits realized.

(Continued)

BRAND NAME	GENERIC NAME	Hours Effective	PREPARATIONS	COMMENTS
Wellbutrin	bupropion	6	75-100mg Tablet	Almost as effective as stimulants for all symptoms of ADHD without exacerbating co-morbid behaviors (irritability, mood suppression, anxiety tics). Needs 2-3 doses a day of regular and SR. One dose of XL can last all day, but very difficult to titrate dose in children with only 150-300mg dosages. Very rare lowering of seizure threshold. Short-acting Wellbutrin Brand Name not available. Three days or longer to see optimal benefit.
Wellbutrin SR	bupropion	8	100-150-200mg	
Wellbutrin XL	bupropion	12-16	150-300mg Tablet	
Qelbree	viloxazine	8	100-150-200mg Capsule	Works in similar manner to Strattera (atomoxetine). Approved by the FDA for the treatment of ADHD in April 2021. Minimal clinical experience with this medication yet. May be a good option for children with co-morbid behaviors, especially mood.

Karniski, Updated 2022.

NOTES

CHAPTER 1

1. K. W. Lange, S. Reichl, K. M. Lange, L. Tucha, and O. Tucha, "The History of Attention Deficit Hyperactivity Disorder," *Attention Deficit Hyperactivity Disorder* 2, no. 4 (2010): 241–55, doi:10.1007/s12402-010-0045-8.

2. American Psychiatric Association, *Diagnostic and Statistical Manual of Mental Disorders*, 5th ed., 2013, https://doi.org/10.1176/appi.books.9780890425596.

3. American Psychiatric Association, *Diagnostic and Statistical Manual of Mental Disorders*, 5th ed.

4. Council on Scientific Affairs, American Medical Association, L. Goldman et al., "Diagnosis and Treatment of Attention Deficit Hyperactivity Disorder in Children and Adolescents," *Journal of the American Medical Association*, 279 (1998): 1100.

CHAPTER 2

1. E. W. Skogli, M. H. Teicher, P. N. Andersen, K. T. Hovik, and M. Øie, "ADHD in Girls and Boys—Gender Differences in Co-existing Symptoms and Executive Function Measures," *BioMed Central Psychiatry*, 13 (2013): 298, doi:10.1186/1471-244X-13-298.

CHAPTER 3

1. M. R. Lee, "The History of Ephedra (ma-huang)," *Journal of the Royal College of Physicians Edinburgh* 41, no. 1 (March 2011): 78–84, doi:10.4997/JRCPE.2011.116. PMID: 21365072.

2. Harry G. Preuss, *Obesity: Epidemiology, Pathophysiology, and Prevention*, 2nd ed. (Boca Raton, FL: CRC Press, 2012), https://books.google.com/books?id=6oHRBQAAQBAJ&pg=PA692#v=onepage&q&f=false.

3. https://en.wikipedia.org/wiki/Nagai_Nagayoshi.

4. https://en.wikipedia.org/wiki/Charles_Bradley_(doctor).

5. C. Bradley, "Behaviour of Children Receiving Benzedrine," *American Journal of Psychiatry*, 94 (1937): 577–85, https://ajp.psychiatryonline.org/doi/abs/10.1176/ajp.94.3.577.

6. C. Bradley and M. Bowen, "Amphetamine (Benzedrine) Therapy of Children's Behavior Disorders," *American Journal of Orthopsychiatry*, 11 (1940): 92–103.

7. Bradley and Bowen, "Amphetamine (Benzedrine) Therapy of Children's Behavior Disorders."

8. Bradley, "Behaviour of Children Receiving Benzedrine."

9. Bradley, "Behaviour of Children Receiving Benzedrine."

10. Bradley and Bowen, "Amphetamine (Benzedrine) Therapy of Children's Behavior Disorders."

11. https://en.wikipedia.org/wiki/Charles_Bradley_(doctor).

12. https://en.wikipedia.org/wiki/Obetrol.

13. T. E. Wilens, S. V. Faraone, J. Biederman, and S. Gunawardene, "Does Stimulant Therapy of Attention-Deficit/Hyperactivity Disorder Beget Later Substance Abuse? A Meta-Analytic Review of the Literature," *Pediatrics* 1, no. 111 (2003): 179–85, doi:10.1542/peds.111.1.179.

14. *U.S. Pharmacist*, 2002, http://www.cesar.umd.edu/cesar/drugs/ritalin.asp.

15. Hearings before the Subcommittee to Investigate Juvenile Delinquency of the Committee on the Judiciary United States Senate, 92nd Cong., 1st sess., Legislative Hearings on S. 674, "To Amend the Controlled Substances Act to Move Amphetamines and Certain other Stimulant Substances from Schedule III of Such Act to Schedule II, and for Other Purposes" July 15 and 16, 1971. Printed for the use of the Committee on the Judiciary, U.S. Government Printing Office, Washington, DC, 1972.

16. https://timesmachine.nytimes.com/timesmachine/1970/06/30/78152146.html?pageNumber=17.

17. R. Mayes and A. Rafalovich, "Suffer the Restless Children: The Evolution of ADHD and Paediatric Stimulant Use, 1900–80," *History of Psychiatry* 18, no.

72 pt. 4 (December 2007): 435–57, doi:10.1177/0957154X06075782. PMID: 18590022.

18. Edward T. Ladd, "Pills for Classroom Peace?," *Saturday Review*, November 21, 1970, 53, 66–68+.

19. J. E. Jackson, "The Coerced Use of Ritalin for Behavior Control in Public Schools: Legal Challenges," *Clearinghouse Review* 10, no. 3 (July 1976): 181–93. PMID: 11664661.

CHAPTER 4

1. R. Thomas, S. Sanders, J. Doust, E. Beller, and P. Glasziou, "Prevalence of Attention-Deficit/Hyperactivity Disorder: A Systematic Review and Meta-Analysis," *Pediatrics*, 4 (2015): 135, www.pediatrics.org/cgi/content/full/135/4/e994.

2. Rae Thomas, Sharon Sanders, Jenny Doust, Elaine Beller, and Paul Glasziou, "Prevalence of Attention-Deficit/Hyperactivity Disorder: A Systematic Review and Meta-analysis," *Pediatrics* 135, no. 4 (April 2015): e994–e1001, doi:10.1542/peds.2014-3482.

3. Melissa L. Danielson, Rebecca H. Bitsko, Reem M. Ghandour, Joseph R. Holbrook, Michael D. Kogan, and Stephen J. Blumberg, "Prevalence of Parent-Reported ADHD Diagnosis and Associated Treatment among U.S. Children and Adolescents, 2016," *Journal of Clinical Child and Adolescent Psychology* 47, no. 2 (2018): 199–212, doi:10.1080/15374416.2017.1417860.

4. S. V. Faraone, J. Sergeant, C. Gillberg, and J. Biederman, "The Worldwide Prevalence of ADHD: Is It an American Condition?," *World Psychiatry* 2, no. 2 (June 2003): 104–13. PMID: 16946911; PMCID: PMC1525089.

5. https://www.childstats.gov/americaschildren/tables/pop1.asp.

6. Alan Zametkin, Elizabeth Schroth, and Dara Faden, "The Role of Brain Imaging in the Diagnosis and Management of ADHD," *ADHD Report: Special Issue—Focus on Assessment*, 13, no. 5 (2005): 11–14.

7. S. V. Faraone, T. Banaschewski, D. Coghill, Y. Zheng, J. Biederman, and M. A. Bellgrove, et al., "The World Federation of ADHD International Consensus Statement: 208 Evidence-Based Conclusions about the Disorder," *Neuroscience and Biobehavioral Reviews*, 128 (September 2021): 789–818, doi:10.1016/j.neubiorev.2021.01.022. Epub 2021 Feb 4. PMID: 33549739; PMCID: PMC8328933.

8. Steven Pliszka, MD, "Practice Parameter for the Assessment and Treatment of Children and Adolescents with Attention-Deficit/Hyperactivity Disorder," doi:https://doi.org/10.1097/chi.0b013e318054e724.

9. J. A. Grahn, J. A. Parkinson, and A. M. Owen, "The Role of the Basal Ganglia in Learning and Memory: Neuropsychological Studies," *Behavioural Brain Research* 199, no. 1 (April 12, 2009): 53–60, doi:10.1016/j.bbr.2008.11.020. Epub 2008 Nov 18. PMID: 19059285.

10. J. A. Grahn, J. A. Parkinson, and A. M. Owen, "The Cognitive Functions of the Caudate Nucleus," *Progress in Neurobiology* 86, no. 3 (November 2008): 141–55, doi:10.1016/j.pneurobio.2008.09.004. Epub 2008 Sep 7. PMID: 18824075.

11. N. Makris, J. Biederman, E. M. Valera, et al., "Cortical Thinning of the Attention and Executive Function Networks in Adults with Attention-Deficit/Hyperactivity Disorder," *Cerebral Cortex* 17, no. 6 (2007): 1364–75, doi:10.1093/cercor/bhl047; L. J. Seidman, E. M. Valera, N. Makris, et al., "Dorsolateral Prefrontal and Anterior Cingulate Cortex Volumetric Abnormalities in Adults with Attention-Deficit/Hyperactivity Disorder Identified by Magnetic Resonance Imaging," *Biological Psychiatry* 60, no. 10 (2006): 1071–80, doi:10.1016/j.biopsych.2006.04.031; S. D. S. Noordermeer, M. Luman, C. U. Greven, et al., "Structural Brain Abnormalities of Attention-Deficit/Hyperactivity Disorder with Oppositional Defiant Disorder," *Biological Psychiatry* 82, no. 9 (2017): 642–50, doi:10.1016/j.biopsych.2017.07.008; S. Carmona, O. Vilarroya, A. Bielsa, et al., "Global and Regional Gray Matter Reductions in ADHD: A Voxel-Based Morphometric Study," *Neuroscience Letters* 389, no. 2 (2005): 88–93, doi:10.1016/j.neulet.2005.07.020; X. R. Yang, N. Carrey, D. Bernier, and F. P. MacMaster, "Cortical Thickness in Young Treatment-Naive Children with ADHD," *Journal of Attention Disorders* 19, no. 11 (2015): 925–30, doi:10.1177/1087054712455501; P. Shaw, J. Lerch, D. Greenstein, et al., "Longitudinal Mapping of Cortical Thickness and Clinical Outcome in Children and Adolescents with Attention-Deficit/Hyperactivity Disorder," *Archives of General Psychiatry* 63, no. 5 (2006): 540–49, doi:10.1001/archpsyc.63.5.540; S. H. Mostofsky, K. L. Cooper, W. R. Kates, M. B. Denckla, and W. E. Kaufmann, "Smaller Prefrontal and Premotor Volumes in Boys with Attention-Deficit/Hyperactivity Disorder," *Biological Psychiatry* 52, no. 8 (2002): 785–94, doi:10.1016/s0006-3223(02)01412-9.

12. L. J. Seidman, J. Biederman , L. Liang, et al., "Gray Matter Alterations in Adults with Attention-Deficit/Hyperactivity Disorder Identified by Voxel Based Morphometry, *Biological Psychiatry* 69, no. 9 (2011): 857–66, doi:10.1016/j.biopsych.2010.09.053; L. J. Norman, C. Carlisi, S. Lukito, et al., "Structural and Functional Brain Abnormalities in Attention-Deficit/Hyperactivity Disorder and Obsessive-Compulsive Disorder: A Comparative Meta-Analysis," *JAMA Psychiatry* 73, no. 8 (2016): 815–25, doi:10.1001/jamapsychiatry.2016.0700 (published correction appears in *JAMA Psychiatry* 74, no. 10 [October 1,

2017]: 1079, and *JAMA Psychiatry* 75, no. 3 [March 1, 2018]: 303); Carmona, Vilarroya, Bielsa, et al., "Global and Regional Gray Matter Reductions in ADHD: A Voxel-Based Morphometric Study."

13. Seidman, Biederman, Liang, et al., "Gray Matter Alterations in Adults with Attention-Deficit/Hyperactivity Disorder Identified by Voxel Based Morphometry"; Y. Luo, J. M. Halperin, and X. Li, "Anatomical Substrates of Symptom Remission and Persistence in Young Adults with Childhood Attention Deficit/Hyperactivity Disorder," *European Neuropsychopharmacology*, 33 (2020): 117–25, doi:10.1016/j.euroneuro.2020.01.014.

14. C. A. Marshall, Z. D. Brodnik, O. V. Mortensen, et al., "Selective Activation of Dopamine D3 Receptors and Norepinephrine Transporter Blockade Enhances Sustained Attention," *Neuropharmacology*, 148 (2019): 178–88, doi:10.1016/j.neuropharm.2019.01.003.

CHAPTER 5

1. L. S. Goldman, M. Genel, R. J. Bezman, and P. J. Slanetz, "Diagnosis and Treatment of Attention-Deficit/Hyperactivity Disorder in Children and Adolescents," *Council on Scientific Affairs, American Medical Association, JAMA* 279, no. 14 (April 8, 1998): 1100–07, doi:10.1001/jama.279.14.1100. PMID: 9546570.

2. This chart was constructed with data obtained from the U.S. National Library of Medicine (PubMed Central ncbi.nlm.nih.gov/pmc/). The number of research articles published was determined by searching for all papers published with each of the specific medications named that co-occurred with "ADHD." Thus, the search terms were "methylphenidate ADHD," "amphetamine ADHD," and so on. It should be noted that many papers were excluded if they concerned methylphenidate but not ADHD. In addition, some research papers referenced ADHD and two or more medications. Those papers would then be counted more than once. But for practical purposes, these numbers are a close approximation to the numbers of research papers published each year.

3. S. Cortese, N. Adamo, C. Del Giovane, et al., "Comparative Efficacy and Tolerability of Medications for Attention-Deficit Hyperactivity Disorder in Children, Adolescents, and Adults: A Systematic Review and Network Meta-Analysis," *Lancet Psychiatry* 5, no. 9 (2018): 727–38.

4. S. V. Faraone and J. Biederman J, "What Is the Prevalence of Adult ADHD? Results of a Population Screen of 966 Adults," *Journal of Attention Disorders* 9, no. 2 (November 2011): 384–91, doi:10.1177/1087054705281478. PMID: 16371661.

5. T. W. Frazier, E. A. Youngstrom, Jeffrey Glutting, and M. W. Watkins, "ADHD and Achievement: Meta-Analysis of the Child, Adolescent, and Adult Literatures and a Concomitant Study with College Students," *Journal of Learning Disabilities* 40, no. 1 (2007): 49–65; C. Galera, M. Melchior, J. F. Chastang, M. P. Bouvard, and E. Fombonne, "Childhood and Adolescent Hyperactivity-Inattention Symptoms and Academic Achievement 8 Years Later: The GAZEL Youth Study," *Psychological Medicine* 39, no. 11 (2009): 1895–906; K. Murphy and R. A. Barkley, "Attention Deficit Hyperactivity Disorder Adults: Comorbidities and Adaptive Impairments," *Comprehensive Psychiatry*, 37 (1996): 393–401; S. Mannuzza and R. G. Klein, "Long-Term Prognosis in Attention-Deficit/Hyperactivity Disorder," *Child and Adolescent Psychiatric Clinics of North America* 9, no. 3 (2000): 711–26; I. M. Loe and H. M. Feldman, "Academic and Educational Outcomes of Children with ADHD," *Ambulatory Pediatrics* 7, 1 suppl (January–February 2007): 82–90, doi:10.1016/j.ambp.2006.05.005, PMID: 17261487.

6. Barkley, Murphy, and Fischman, *ADHD in Adults: What the Science Says*; Galera, Melchior, Chastang, Bouvard, and Fombonne, "Childhood and Adolescent Hyperactivity-Inattention Symptoms and Academic Achievement 8 Years Later"; Loe and Feldman, "Academic and Educational Outcomes of Children with ADHD."

7. R. A. Barkley, M. Fischer, C. S. Edelbrock, and L. Smallish, "The Adolescent Outcome of Hyperactive Children Diagnosed by Research Criteria: I. An 8-Year Prospective Follow-Up Study"; B. S. G. Molina, S. P. Hinshaw, J. M. Swanson, L. E. Arnold, B. Vitiello, P. S. Jensen, et al., "The MTA at 8 Years: Prospective Follow-Up of Children Treated for Combined Type ADHD in a Multisite Study," *Journal of the American Academy of Child and Adolescent Psychiatry* (2009), https://www.ncbi.nlm.nih.gov/pmc/articles/PMC3068222/.

8. Murphy and Barkley, "Attention Deficit Hyperactivity Disorder Adults: Comorbidities and Adaptive Impairments."

9. J. Biederman, S. V. Faraone, T. J. Spencer, et al., "Functional Impairment in Adults with Self-Reports of Diagnosed ADHD: A Controlled Study of 1001 Adults in the Community," *Journal of Clinical Psychiatry* 67, no. 4 (2006): 524–40; Galera, Melchior, Chastang, Bouvard, and Fombonne, "Childhood and Adolescent Hyperactivity-Inattention Symptoms and Academic Achievement 8 Years Later"; R. G. Klein, S. Mannuzza, M. A. Olazagasti, E. Roizen, J. A. Hutchison, E. C. Lashua, and F. X. Castellanos, "Clinical and Functional Outcome of Childhood Attention-Deficit/Hyperactivity Disorder 33 Years Later," *Archives of General Psychiatry* (2012): 1–9; S. Mannuzza, R. G. Klein, A. Bessler, P. Malloy, and M. LaPadula, "Adult Outcome of Hyperactive Boys. Educational Achievement, Occupational Rank, and Psychiatric Status," *Archives of General Psychiatry* 50, no. 7 (1993): 565–76.

10. J. Biederman, M. C. Monuteaux, T. Spencer, T. E. Wilens, and S. V. Faraone, "Do Stimulants Protect against Psychiatric Disorders in Youth with ADHD? A 10-Year Follow-Up Study," *Pediatrics* 124, no. 1 (2009): 71–78, https://doi.org/10.1542/peds.2008-3347.

11. Biederman, Faraone, Spencer, et al., "Functional Impairment in Adults with Self-Reports of Diagnosed ADHD"; R. A. Barkley, M. Fischer, L. Smallish, and K. Fletcher, "Young Adult Outcome of Hyperactive Children: Adaptive Functioning in Major Life Activities," *Journal of the American Academy of Child and Adolescent Psychiatry* 45, no. 2 (2006): 192–202.

12. Biederman, Faraone, Spencer, et al., "Functional Impairment in Adults with Self-Reports of Diagnosed ADHD"; Murphy and Barkley, "Attention Deficit Hyperactivity Disorder Adults: Comorbidities and Adaptive Impairments."

13. Murphy and Barkley, "Attention Deficit Hyperactivity Disorder Adults: Comorbidities and Adaptive Impairments."

14. J. Biederman and S. V. Faraone, "The Effects of Attention-Deficit/ Hyperactivity Disorder on Employment and Household Income," *Medscape General Medicine* 8, no. 3 (2006): 12.

15. Barkley, Fischer, Smallish, and Fletcher, "Young Adult Outcome of Hyperactive Children: Adaptive Functioning in Major Life Activities"; P. A. Graziano, A. Reid, J. Slavec, A. Paneto, J. P. McNamara, and G. R. Geffken, "ADHD Symptomatology and Risky Health, Driving, and Financial Behaviors in College: The Mediating Role of Sensation Seeking and Effortful Control," *Journal of Attention Disorders* 19, no. 3 (March 2015): 179–90; A. R. Altszuler, T. F. Page, E. M. Gnagy, S. Coxe, A. Arrieta, B. S. G. Molina, and W. E. Pelham Jr., "Financial Dependence of Young Adults with Childhood ADHD," *Journal of Abnormal Child Psychology*, 44 (2016): 1217–29; T. P. Beauchaine, I. Ben-David, and A. Sela, "ADHD, Delay Discounting, and Risky Financial Behaviors: A Preliminary Analysis of Self-Report Data," *PLOS One* 12, e0176933 (2017).

16. A. Fernández-Jaén, D. Martín Fernández-Mayoralas, and S. López-Arribas, et al., "Social and Leadership Abilities in Attention Deficit/Hyperactivity Disorder: Relation with Cognitive-Attentional Capacities," *Actas Espanolas de Psiquiatria* 40, no. 3 (2012): 136–46; S. P. Becker, K. McBurnett, S. P. Hinshaw, and L. J. Pfiffner, "Negative Social Preference in Relation to Internalizing Symptoms among Children with ADHD Predominantly Inattentive Type: Girls Fare Worse Than Boys," *Journal of Clinical Child and Adolescent Psychology* 42, no. 6 (2013): 784–95, doi:10.1080/15374416.2013.828298; J. Biederman, S. V. Faraone, T. J. Spencer, E. Mick, M. C. Monuteaux, and M. Aleardi, "Functional Impairments in Adults with Self-Reports of Diagnosed ADHD:

A Controlled Study of 1001 Adults in the Community," *Journal of Clinical Psychiatry* 67, no. 4 (2006): 524–40, doi:10.4088/jcp.v67n0403.

17. Biederman, Faraone, Spencer, et al., "Functional Impairments in Adults with Self-Reports of Diagnosed ADHD."

18. S. Mannuzza and R. G. Klein, "Long-Term Prognosis in Attention-Deficit/Hyperactivity Disorder," *Child and Adolescent Psychiatric Clinics of North America* 9, no. 3 (2000): 711–26.

19. Biederman, Faraone, Spencer, et al., "Functional Impairments in Adults with Self-Reports of Diagnosed ADHD."

20. Barkley, Fischer, Smallish, and Fletcher, "Young Adult Outcome of Hyperactive Children."

21. Barkley, Fischer, Smallish, and Fletcher, "Young Adult Outcome of Hyperactive Children."

22. Biederman, Faraone, Spencer, et al., "Functional Impairments in Adults with Self-Reports of Diagnosed ADHD"; Klein, Mannuzza, Olazagasti, Roizen, Hutchison, Lashua, and Castellanos, "Clinical and Functional Outcome of Childhood Attention-Deficit/Hyperactivity Disorder 33 Years Later."

23. Murphy and Barkley, "Attention Deficit Hyperactivity Disorder Adults: Comorbidities and Adaptive Impairments."

24. R. L. Aguirre Castaneda, S. Kumar, R. G. Voigt, C. L. Leibson, W. J. Barbaresi, A. L. Weaver, J. M. Killian, and S. K. Katusic, "Childhood Attention-Deficit/Hyperactivity Disorder, Sex, and Obesity: A Longitudinal Population-Based Study," *Mayo Clinic Proceedings* 91, no. 3 (March 2016): 352–61, doi:10.1016/j.mayocp.2015.09.017. Epub 2016 Feb 4. PMID: 26853710; PMCID: PMC5264451.

25. C. A. Martin, N. Papadopoulos, T. Chellew, N. J. Rinehart, and E. Sciberras, "Associations between Parenting Stress, Parent Mental Health and Child Sleep Problems for Children with ADHD and ASD: Systematic Review," *Research in Developmental Disabilities*, 93 (2019): 103463, doi:10.1016/j.ridd.2019.103463.

26. S. Dalsgaard, S. C. Ostergaard, J. F. Leckman, P. B. Mortensen, and M. G. Pedersen, "Mortality in Children, Adolescents, and Adults with Attention Deficit Hyperactivity Disorder: A Nationwide Cohort Study," *Lancet* 385, no. 9983 (2015): 2190–6; B. Franke, G. Michelini, P. Asherson, et al., "Live Fast, Die Young? A Review on the Developmental Trajectories of ADHD across the Lifespan," *European Neuropsychopharmacology* 28, no. 10 (2018):1059–88, doi:10.1016/j.euroneuro.2018.08.001.

27. G. Shoval, E. Visoki, T. M. Moore, G. E. DiDomenico, S. T. Argabright, N. J. Huffnagle, A. F. Alexander-Bloch, R. Waller, L. Keele, T. D. Benton, R. E. Gur, and R. Barzilay, "Evaluation of Attention-Deficit/

Hyperactivity Disorder Medications, Externalizing Symptoms, and Suicidality in Children," *JAMA network open* 4, no. 6 (2021): e2111342, https://doi.org/10.1001/jamanetworkopen.2021.11342.

28. M. Weiss, L. T. Hechtman, and G. Weiss, *ADHD in Adulthood: A Guide to Current Theory, Diagnosis, and Treatment* (Baltimore: Johns Hopkins University Press, 1999).

29. Weiss, Hechtman, and Weiss, *ADHD in Adulthood: A Guide to Current Theory, Diagnosis, and Treatment*; Barkley, Fischer, Smallish, and Fletcher, "Young Adult Outcome of Hyperactive Children"; M. H. Chen, J. W. Hsu, K. L. Huang, Y. M. Bai, N. Y. Ko, T. P. Su, C. T. Li, W. C. Lin, S. J. Tsai, T. L. Pan, W. H. Chang, and T. J. Chen, "Sexually Transmitted Infection among Adolescents and Young Adults with Attention-Deficit/Hyperactivity Disorder: A Nationwide Longitudinal Study," *Journal of the American Academy of Child and Adolescent Psychiatry* 57, no. 1 (January 2018): 48–53, doi:10.1016/j.jaac.2017.09.438. Epub 2017 Nov 10. PMID: 29301669; Barkley, Fischer, Smallish, and Fletcher, "Young Adult Outcome of Hyperactive Children."

30. Murphy and Barkley, "Attention Deficit Hyperactivity Disorder Adults: Comorbidities and Adaptive Impairments."

31. Z. Chang, P. Lichtenstein., B. M. D'Onofrio, A. Sjolander, and H. Larsson, "Serious Transport Accidents in Adults with Attention-Deficit/Hyperactivity Disorder and the Effect of Medication: A Population-Based Study," *JAMA Psychiatry* 71, no. 3 (2014): 319–25; Murphy and Barkley, "Attention Deficit Hyperactivity Disorder Adults: Comorbidities and Adaptive Impairments"; R. A. Barkley, D. C. Guevremont, A. D. Anastopoulos, G. J. DuPaul, and T. L. Shelton, "Driving-Related Risks and Outcomes of Attention Deficit Hyperactivity Disorder in Adolescents and Young Adults: A 3- to 5-Year Follow-Up Survey," *Pediatrics* 92, no. 2 (1993): 212–18; R. A. Barkley, K. R. Murphy, G. I. DuPaul, and T. Bush, "Driving in Young Adults with Attention Deficit Hyperactivity Disorder: Knowledge, Performance, Adverse Outcomes and the Role of Executive Functioning," *Journal of the International Neuropsychological Society* 8, no. 5 (2002): 655–72; R. Fried, C. Petty, C. Surman, et al., "Characterizing Impaired Driving in Adults with Attention-Deficit/Hyperactivity Disorder: A Controlled Study," *Journal of Clinical Psychiatry*, 67 (2006): 567–74; R. Barkley, "Driving Impairments in Teens and Adults with Attention-Deficit/Hyperactivity Disorder," *Psychiatric Clinics of North America*, 27 (2004): 233–60; A. Swensen, H. G. Birnbaum, R. Ben Hamadi, P. Greenberg, P. Y. Cremieux, and K. Secnik, "Incidence and Costs of Accidents among Attention-Deficit/Hyperactivity Disorder Patients," *Journal of Adolescent Health* 35, no. 4 (2004): 346, e1-346.e3469; Roy Arunima, Annie A. Garner, Jeffrey N. Epstein, Betsy Hoza, J. Quyen Nichols, Brooke S.

G. Molina, James M. Swanson, L. Eugene Arnold, and Lily Hechtman, "Effects of Childhood and Adult Persistent Attention-Deficit/Hyperactivity Disorder on Risk of Motor Vehicle Crashes: Results From the Multimodal Treatment Study of Children with Attention-Deficit/Hyperactivity Disorder," *Journal of the American Academy of Child and Adolescent Psychiatry* 59, no. 8 (2020): 952, doi:10.1016/j.jaac.2019.08.007.

32. Swensen, Birnbaum, Hamadi, Greenberg, Cremieux, and Secnik, "Incidence and Costs of Accidents among Attention-Deficit/Hyperactivity Disorder Patients."

33. Z. Chang, P. D. Quinn, K. Hur, et al., "Association between Medication Use for Attention-Deficit/Hyperactivity Disorder and Risk of Motor Vehicle Crashes," *JAMA Psychiatry* 74, no. 6 (2017): 597–603, doi:10.1001/jamapsychiatry.2017.0659; Chang, Lichtenstein, D'Onofrio, Sjolander, and Larsson, "Serious Transport Accidents in Adults with Attention-Deficit/Hyperactivity Disorder and the Effect of Medication."

34. Biederman, Faraone, Spencer, et al., "Functional Impairments in Adults with Self-Reports of Diagnosed ADHD."

35. R. Mannuzza, R. G. Klein, and J. L. Moulton, "Lifetime Criminality among Boys with Attention Deficit Hyperactivity Disorder: A Prospective Follow-Up Study into Adulthood Using Official Arrest Records," *Psychiatry Research* 160, no. 3 (2008): 237–46.

36. S. Dalsgaard, P. B. Mortensen, M. Frydenberg, and P. H. Thomsen, "Long-Term Criminal Outcome of Children with Attention Deficit Hyperactivity Disorder," *Criminal Behaviour and Mental Health* 23, no. 2 (2013): 86–98; Mannuzza, Klein, and Moulton, "Lifetime Criminality among Boys with Attention Deficit Hyperactivity Disorder"; P. Lichtenstein, L. Halldner, J. Zetterqvist, A. Sjolander, E. Serlachius, S. Fazel, N. Langstrom, and H. Larsson, "Medication for Attention Deficit-Hyperactivity Disorder and Criminality," *New England Journal of Medicine* 367, no. 21 (2012): 2006–14.

37. H. P. Upadhyaya and M. J. Carpenter, "Is Attention Deficit Hyperactivity Disorder (ADHD) Symptom Severity Associated with Tobacco Use?," *American Journal of Addiction* 17, no. 3 (2008): 295–98; E. E. Van Voorhees, J. T. Mitchell, F. J. McClernon, J. C. Beckham, and S. H. Kollins, "Sex, ADHD Symptoms, and Smoking Outcomes: An Integrative Model," *Medical Hypotheses* 78, no. 5 (2012): 585–93, doi:10.1016/j.mehy.2012.01.034.

38. R. C. Kessler, L. Adler, R. Barkley, J. Biederman, C. K. Conners, O. Delmer, . . . A. M. Zaslavsky, "The Prevalence and Correlates of Adult ADHD in the United States: Results from the National Comorbidity Survey

Replication," *American Journal of Psychiatry*, 163 (2006): 716–23; J. Biederman, T. E. Wilens, and E. Mick, "Pyschoactive Substance Use Disorders in Adults with Attention Deficit Hyperactivity Disorder (ADHD): Effects of ADHD and Psychiatric Comorbidity," *American Journal of Psychiatry*, 152 (1995): 1642–58; Murphy and Barkley, "Attention Deficit Hyperactivity Disorder Adults: Comorbidities and Adaptive Impairments."

39. T. E. Wilens, S. V. Faraone, J. Biederman, and S. Gunawardene, "Does Stimulant Therapy of Attention-Deficit/Hyperactivity Disorder Beget Later Substance Abuse? A Meta-Analytic Review of the Literature," *Pediatrics* 111, no. 1 (2003): 179–85, doi:10.1542/peds.111.1.179.

40. H. G. Birnbaum, R. C. Kessler, S. W. Lowe, et al., "Costs of Attention Deficit-Hyperactivity Disorder (ADHD) in the US: Excess Costs of Persons with ADHD and Their Family Members in 2000," *Current Medical Research and Opinion*, 21 (2005): 195–206.

41. T. J. Spencer, A. Brown, L. J. Seidman, et al., "Effect of Psychostimulants on Brain Structure and Function in ADHD: A Qualitative Literature Review of Magnetic Resonance Imaging-Based Neuroimaging Studies," *Journal of Clinical Psychiatry* 74, no. 9 (2013): 902–17, doi:10.4088/JCP.12r08287; T. Frodl and N. Skokauskas, "Meta-Analysis of Structural MRI Studies in Children and Adults with Attention Deficit Hyperactivity Disorder Indicates Treatment Effects," *Acta Psychiatrica Scandinavica* 125, no. 2 (2012): 114–26, doi:10.1111/j.1600-0447.2011.01786.x; Lizanne J. S. Schweren, Patrick de Zeeuw, and Sarah Durston, "MR Imaging of the Effects of Methylphenidate on Brain Structure and Function in Attention-Deficit/Hyperactivity Disorder, *European Neuropsychopharmacology* 23, no. 10 (2013): 1151–64, ISSN 0924-977X; L. J. Schweren, P. de Zeeuw, and S. Durston, "MR Imaging of the Effects of Methylphenidate on Brain Structure and Function in Attention-Deficit/Hyperactivity Disorder," *European Neuropsychopharmacology* 23, no. 10 (October 2013): 1151–64, doi:10.1016/j.euroneuro.2012.10.014. Epub 2012 Nov 17. PMID: 23165220; C. Pretus, J. A. Ramos-Quiroga, V. Richarte, et al., "Time and Psychostimulants: Opposing Long-Term Structural Effects in the Adult ADHD Brain. A Longitudinal MR Study," *European Neuropsychopharmacology* 27, no. 12 (2017): 1238–47, doi:10.1016/j.euroneuro.2017.10.035; Avis R. Brennan and Amy F. T. Arnsten, "Neuronal Mechanisms Underlying Attention Deficit Hyperactivity Disorder: The Influence of Arousal on Prefrontal Cortical Function," *Annals of the New York Academy of Sciences*, 1129 (2008): 236–45, doi:10.1196/annals.1417.007; A. Moreno-Alcázar, J. A. Ramos-Quiroga, J. Radua, et al., "Brain Abnormalities in Adults with Attention Deficit Hyperactivity Disorder Revealed by Voxel-Based Morphometry,"

Psychiatry Research: Neuroimaging, 254 (2016): 41–47, doi:10.1016/j.pscychresns.2016.06.002; S. Maier, E. Perlov, E. Graf, et al., "Discrete Global But No Focal Gray Matter Volume Reductions in Unmedicated Adult Patients with Attention-Deficit/Hyperactivity Disorder," *Biological Psychiatry* 80, no. 12 (2016): 905–15, doi:10.1016/j.biopsych.2015.05.012; H. Hart, J. Radua, T. Nakao, D. Mataix-Cols, and K. Rubia, "Meta-Analysis of Functional Magnetic Resonance Imaging Studies of Inhibition and Attention in Attention-Deficit/Hyperactivity Disorder: Exploring Task-Specific, Stimulant Medication, and Age Effects," *JAMA Psychiatry* 70, no. 2 (2013): 185–98, doi:10.1001/jamapsychiatry.2013.277; A. M. Onnink, M. P. Zwiers, M. Hoogman, et al., "Brain Alterations in Adult ADHD: Effects of Gender, Treatment and Comorbid Depression," *European Neuropsychopharmacology* 24, no. 3 (2014): 397–409, doi:10.1016/j.euroneuro.2013.11.011; L. J. Schweren, C. A. Hartman, M. P. Zwiers, et al., "Stimulant Treatment History Predicts Frontal-Striatal Structural Connectivity in Adolescents with Attention-Deficit/Hyperactivity Disorder," *European Neuropsychopharmacology* 26, no. 4 (2016): 674–83, doi:10.1016/j.euroneuro.2016.02.007; T. Nakao, J. Radua, K. Rubia, and D. Mataix-Cols, "Gray Matter Volume Abnormalities in ADHD: Voxel-Based Meta-Analysis Exploring the Effects of Age and Stimulant Medication," *American Journal of Psychiatry* 168, no. 11 (2011): 1154–63, doi:10.1176/appi.ajp.2011.11020281; M. Hoogman, J. Bralten, D. P. Hibar, M. Mennes, M. P. Zwiers, L. Schweren, K. van Hulzen, S. E. Medland, E. Shumskaya, N. Jahanshad, P. Zeeuw, E. Szekely, G. Sudre, T. Wolfers, A. Onnink, J. T. Dammers, J. C. Mostert, Y. Vives-Gilabert, G. Kohls, E. Oberwelland, . . . B. Franke, "Subcortical Brain Volume Differences in Participants with Attention Deficit Hyperactivity Disorder in Children and Adults: A Cross-Sectional Mega-Analysis," *Lancet Psychiatry* 4, no. 4 (2017): 310–19, https://doi.org/10.1016/S2215-0366(17)30049-4.

42. M. L. Wolraich, J. F. Hagan Jr., C. Allan, E. Chan, D. Davison, M. Earls, et al.; Subcommittee on Children and Adolescents with Attention-Deficit/Hyperactive Disorder. "Clinical Practice Guideline for the Diagnosis, Evaluation, and Treatment of Attention-Deficit/Hyperactivity Disorder in Children and Adolescents," *Pediatrics* 144, no. 4 (October 2019): e20192528, doi:10.1542/peds.2019-2528. Erratum in *Pediatrics* 145, no. 3 (March 2020), PMID: 31570648; PMCID: PMC7067282.

43. S. Pliszka; AACAP Work Group on Quality Issues, "Practice Parameter for the Assessment and Treatment of Children and Adolescents with Attention-Deficit/Hyperactivity Disorder," *Journal of the American Academy of Child and Adolescent Psychiatry* 46, no. 7 (July 2007): 894–921, doi:10.1097/chi.0b013e318054e724. PMID: 17581453.

CHAPTER 6

1. M. Berkovitch, E. Pope, J. Phillips, and G. Koren, "Pemoline-Associated Fulminant Liver Failure: Testing the Evidence for Causation," *Clinical Pharmacology Therapy* 57, no. 6 (1995): 696–98, doi:10.1016/0009-9236(95)90233-3; P. J. Marotta and E. A. Roberts, "Pemoline Hepatotoxicity in Children," *Journal of Pediatrics* 132, no. 5 (1998): 894–97, doi:10.1016/s0022-3476(98)70329-4.

2. https://www.fda.gov/about-fda/what-we-do.

3. https://www.fda.gov/about-fda/fda-basics/fact-sheet-fda-glance.

4. https://www.forbes.com/sites/matthewherper/2017/10/16/the-cost-of-developing-drugs-is-insane-a-paper-that-argued-otherwise-was-insanely-bad/?sh=31404b322d45.

5. R. Feldman, "May Your Drug Price Be Evergreen," *Journal of Law and the Biosciences*, 5, no. 3 (2018): 590–647, doi:10.1093/jlb/lsy022, 601.

6. Feldman, "May Your Drug Price Be Evergreen," 618.

7. S. Dickson, "Effect of Evergreened Reformulations on Medicaid Expenditures and Patient Access from 2008 to 2016," *Journal of Managed Care & Specialty Pharmacy* 25, no. 7 (2019): 780–92, doi:10.18553/jmcp.2019.18366.

8. Feldman, "May Your Drug Price Be Evergreen," 618.

9. https://www.forbes.com/sites/matthewherper/2017/10/16/the-cost-of-developing-drugs-is-insane-a-paper-that-argued-otherwise-was-insanely-bad/?sh=31404b322d45.

10. S. C. Chow, "Bioavailability and Bioequivalence in Drug Development," *Wiley Interdisciplinary Reviews: Computational Statistics* 6, no. 4 (2014): 304–12, doi:10.1002/wics.1310.

11. https://www.fda.gov/drugs/development-approval-process-drugs/orange-book-preface#_ftn5 Orange Book 21 CFR 314.3(b).

12. Katherine Eban, *Bottle of Lies* (New York: HarperCollins, 2019).

13. Eban, *Bottle of Lies*, 131.

14. Eban, *Bottle of Lies*, 365.

15. Feldman, "May Your Drug Price Be Evergreen," 601.

16. Eban, *Bottle of Lies*, 116.

17. Eban, *Bottle of Lies*, 348.

18. Eban, *Bottle of Lies*.

19. Eban, *Bottle of Lies*, 342.

20. Eban, *Bottle of Lies*, 369.

21. https://www.statista.com/statistics/238702/us-total-medical-prescriptions-issued/.

CHAPTER 7

1. J. S. Markowitz and K. S. Patrick, "The Clinical Pharmacokinetics of Amphetamines Utilized in the Treatment of Attention-Deficit/Hyperactivity Disorder," *Journal of Child and Adolescent Psychopharmacology* 27, no. 8 (2017): 678–89, doi:10.1089/cap.2017.0071.

2. D. J. Heal and D. M. Pierce, "Methylphenidate and Its Isomers: Their Role in the Treatment of Attention-Deficit Hyperactivity Disorder Using a Transdermal Delivery System," *CNS Drugs* 20, no. 9 (2006): 713–38, doi:10.2165/00023210-200620090-00002, PMID: 16953648; D. Quinn, "Does Chirality Matter? Pharmacodynamics of Enantiomers of Methylphenidate in Patients with Attention-Deficit/Hyperactivity Disorder," *Journal of Clinical Psychopharmacology* 28, no. 3, suppl 2 (2008): S62–66, doi:10.1097/JCP.0b013e3181744aa6; N. R. Srinivas, J. W. Hubbard, D. Quinn, and K. K. Midha, "Enantioselective Pharmacokinetics and Pharmacodynamics of Dl-Threo-Methylphenidate in Children with Attention Deficit Hyperactivity Disorder," *Clinical Pharmacology & Therapeutics* 52, no. 5 (1992): 561–68, doi:10.1038/clpt.1992.185.

3. G. A. Alles, "Comparative Physiological Actions of the Optically Isomeric Phenisopropylamines," *University of California Publications in Pharmacology*, 1 (1939): 129–50.

4. S. Berman, R. Kuczenski, J. McCracken, et al., "Potential Adverse Effects of Amphetamine Treatment on Brain and Behavior: A Review," *Molecular Psychiatry*, 14 (2009): 123–42, https://doi.org/10.1038/mp.2008.90; T. B. Fay and M. A. Alpert, "Cardiovascular Effects of Drugs Used to Treat Attention-Deficit/Hyperactivity Disorder, Part 2: Impact on Cardiovascular Events and Recommendations for Evaluation and Monitoring," *Cardiology in Review* 27, no. 4 (2019): 173–78, doi:10.1097/CRD.0000000000000234; M. D. St. Amour, D. D. O'Leary, J. Cairney, and T. J. Wade, "What Is the Effect of ADHD Stimulant Medication on Heart Rate and Blood Pressure in a Community Sample of Children?," *Canadian Journal of Public Health* 109, no. 3 (2018): 395–400, doi:10.17269/s41997-018-0067-0.

5. K. S. Patrick and J. S. Markowitz, "Pharmacology of Methylphenidate, Amphetamine Enantiomers and Pemoline in Attention-Deficit Hyperactivity Disorder," *Human Psychopharmacology: Clinical and Experimental* 12, no. 6 (1997): 527–46, https://doi.org/10.1002/(SICI)1099-1077(199711/12)12:6 <527::AID-HUP932>3.0.CO;2-U.

6. S. Cortese, N. Adamo, C. Del Giovane, C. Mohr-Jensen, A. J. Hayes, S. Carucci, L. Z. Atkinson, L. Tessari, T. Banaschewski, D. Coghill, C. Hollis, E. Simonoff, A. Zuddas, C. Barbui, M. Purgato, H. C. Steinhausen, F. Shokraneh, J. Xia, and A. Cipriani, "Comparative Efficacy and Tolerability of Medications

for Attention-Deficit Hyperactivity Disorder in Children, Adolescents, and Adults: A Systematic Review and Network Meta-Analysis," *Lancet Psychiatry* 5, no. 9 (2018): 727–38, doi:10.1016/S2215-0366(18)30269-4, Epub 2018 August 7, PMID: 30097390, PMCID: PMC6109107.

7. Cortese, Adamo, Del Giovane, et al., "Comparative Efficacy and Tolerability of Medications for Attention-Deficit Hyperactivity Disorder in Children, Adolescents, and Adults."

8. "Attention Deficit Hyperactivity Disorder: Diagnosis and Management," NICE guideline (NG87), March 14, 2018. Last updated September 13, 2019, https://www.nice.org.uk/guidance/ng87/chapter/Recommendations #medication.

9. https://www.additudemag.com/adhd-medication-for-adults-and -children/.

10. https://www.healthline.com/health/adhd/celebrities#8.-Simone-Biles.

11. https://www.gracepointwellness.org/3-adhd/article/60778-famous -people-with-adhd.

CHAPTER 8

1. O. J. Storebø, E. Ramstad, H. B. Krogh, et al., "Methylphenidate for Children and Adolescents with Attention Deficit Hyperactivity Disorder (ADHD)," *Cochrane Database of Systematic Reviews*, 11 (2015): CD009885, doi:10.1002/14651858.CD009885.pub2.

2. O. J. Storebø, N. Pedersen, E. Ramstad, et al., "Methylphenidate for Attention Deficit Hyperactivity Disorder (ADHD) in Children and Adolescents—Assessment of Adverse Events in Non-Randomised Studies," *Cochrane Database of Systematic Reviews* 5, no. 5 (2018): CD012069; A. J. Cerrillo-Urbina, A. García-Hermoso, M. J. Pardo-Guijarro, M. Sánchez-López, J. S. Santos-Gómez, and V. Martínez-Vizcaíno, "The Effects of Long-Acting Stimulant and Nonstimulant Medications in Children and Adolescents with Attention-Deficit/Hyperactivity Disorder: A Meta-Analysis of Randomized Controlled Trials," *Journal of Child and Adolescent Psychopharmacology* 28, no. 8 (2018): 494–507, doi:10.1089/cap.2017.0151.

3. D. Chierrito de Oliveira, P. Guerrero de Sousa, C. Borges Dos Reis, et al., "Safety of Treatments for ADHD in Adults: Pairwise and Network Meta-Analyses," *Journal of Attention Disorders* 23, no. 2 (2019): 111–20, doi:10.1177/1087054717696773.

4. Storebø, Ramstad, Krogh, et al., "Methylphenidate for Children and Adolescents with Attention Deficit Hyperactivity Disorder (ADHD)."

5. S. Punja, L. Shamseer, L. Hartling, L. Urichuk, B. Vandermeer, J. Nikles, and S. Vohra, "Amphetamines for Attention Deficit Hyperactivity Disorder (ADHD) in Children and Adolescents," *Cochrane Database of Systematic Reviews* 4, no. 2 (2016): CD009996, doi:10.1002/14651858.CD009996.pub2, PMID: 26844979.

6. S. V. Faraone, J. Biederman, C. P. Morley, and T. J. Spencer, "Effect of Stimulants on Height and Weight: A Review of the Literature," *Journal of the American Academy of Child and Adolescent Psychiatry* 47, no. 9 (2008): 994–1009, doi:10.1097/CHI.ObO13e31817eOea7.

7. V. Sung, H. Hiscock, E. Sciberras, and D. Efron, "Sleep Problems in Children with Attention-Deficit/Hyperactivity Disorder: Prevalence and the Effect on the Child and Family," *Archives of Pediatrics and Adolescent Medicine*, 162 (2008): 336–42, doi:10.1001/archpedi.162.4.336; P. Corkum, R. Tannock, and H. Moldofsky, "Sleep Disturbances in Children with Attention-Deficit/Hyperactivity Disorder," *Journal of the American Academy of Child and Adolescent Psychiatry*, 37 (1998): 637–46, doi:10.1097/00004583-199806000-00014; S. Cortese, S. V. Faraone, E. Konofal, and M. Lecendreux, "Sleep in Children with Attention-Deficit/Hyperactivity Disorder: Meta-Analysis of Subjective and Objective Studies," *Journal of the American Academy of Child and Adolescent Psychiatry* 48, no. 9 (2009): 894–908, doi:10.1097/CHI.0b013e3181ac09c9; M. A. Stein, "Unravelling Sleep Problems in Treated und Untreated Children with ADHD," *Journal of Child and Adolescent Psychopharmacology* 9, no. 3 (1999): 157–68, https://doi.org/10.1089/cap.1999.9.157.

8. M. Cohen-Zion and S. Ancoli-Israel, "Sleep in Children with Attention-Deficit Hyperactivity Disorder (ADHD): A Review of Naturalistic and Stimulant Intervention Studies," *Sleep Medicine Reviews* 8, no. 5 (2004): 379–402, doi:10.1016/j.smrv.2004.06.002.

9. S. C. O. S. Padilha, S. Virtuoso, F. S. Tonin, H. H. L. Borba, and R. Pontarolo, "Efficacy and Safety of Drugs for Attention Deficit Hyperactivity Disorder in Children and Adolescents: A Network Meta-Analysis," *European Child and Adolescent Psychiatry* 27, no. 10 (2018): 1335–45, doi:10.1007/s00787-018-1125-0.

10. M. A. Stein, C. S. Sarampote, I. D. Waldman, A. S. Robb, C. Conlon, P. L. Pearl, D. O. Black, K. E. Seymour, and J. H. Newcorn, "A Dose-Response Study of OROS Methylphenidate in Children with Attention-Deficit/Hyperactivity Disorder," *Pediatrics* 112, no. 5 (2003): e404, https://doi.org/10.1542/peds.112.5.e404.

11. I. M. Verweij, N. Romeijn, D. J. Smit, et al., "Sleep Deprivation Leads to a Loss of Functional Connectivity in Frontal Brain Regions," *BMC Neuroscience* 15, no. 88 (2014), https://doi.org/10.1186/1471-2202-15-88; A. Lundahl, K. M. Kidwell, T. R. Van Dyk, and T. D. Nelson, "A Meta-Analysis

of the Effect of Experimental Sleep Restriction on Youth's Attention and Hyperactivity," *Developmental Neuropsychology* 40, no. 3 (2015): 104–21, doi:10.1080/87565641.2014.939183.

12. I. Janjua and R. D. Goldman, "Sleep-Related Melatonin Use in Healthy Children," *Canadian Family Physician* 62, no. 4 (2016): 315–17.

13. K. M. Kidwell, T. R. Van Dyk, A. Lundahl, and T. D. Nelson, "Stimulant Medications and Sleep for Youth with ADHD: A Meta-Analysis," *Pediatrics* 136, no. 6 (2015): 1144–53, doi:10.1542/peds.2015-1708.

14. E. Efron, K. Lycett, and E. Sciberras, "Use of Sleep Medication in Children with ADHD," *Journal of Clinical Sleep Medicine* 15, no. 4 (2014): 472–75, doi:10.1016/j.sleep.2013.10.018.

15. L. M. Bendz and A. C. Scates, "Melatonin Treatment for Insomnia in Pediatric Patients with Attention-Deficit/Hyperactivity Disorder," *Annals of Pharmacotherapy* 44, no. 1 (2010): 185–91, doi:10.1345/aph.1M365.

16. J. A. Owens and S. Moturi, "Pharmacologic Treatment of Pediatric Insomnia," *Child and Adolescent Psychiatry Clinics of North America* 18, no. 4 (2009): 1001–16, doi:10.1016/j.chc.2009.04.009.

17. C. Cummings, Canadian Paediatric Society, Community Paediatrics Committee, "Melatonin for the Management of Sleep Disorders in Children and Adolescents," *Paediatrics & Child Health* 17, no. 6 (2012): 331–36.

18. Efron, Lycett, and Sciberras, "Use of Sleep Medication in Children with ADHD."

19. R. B. Sangal, J. Owens, A. J. Allen, V. Sutton, K. Schuh, and D. Kelsey, "Effects of Atomoxetine and Methylphenidate on Sleep in Children with ADHD," *Sleep* 29, no. 12 (2006): 1573–85, https://doi.org/10.1093/sleep/29.12.1573.

20. Gina Pera, The Tragic Truth of Prescription Adderall, or "Madderall" https://adhdrollercoaster.org/?s=madderall.

21. Kamath Tallur and Robert A. Minns, "Tourette's Syndrome," *Paediatrics and Child Health* 20, no. 2 (2010): 88–93.

22. T. Knight, T. Steeves, L. Day, M. Lowerison, N. Jette, and T. Pringsheim, "Prevalence of Tic Disorders: A Systematic Review and Meta-Analysis," *Pediatric Neurology*, 47 (2012): 77–90.

23. J. Biederman, F. A. Lopez, S. W. Boellner, and M. C. Chandler, "A Randomized, Double-Blind, Placebo-Controlled, Parallel-Group Study of SLI381 Adderall XR in Children with attention-Deficit/Hyperactivity Disorder," *Pediatrics*, 110 (2002): 258–66; M. L. Wolraich, L. L. Greenhill, and W. Pelham, et al., "Randomized, Controlled Trial of OROS Methylphenidate Once a Day in Children with Attention-Deficit/Hyperactivity Disorder," *Pediatrics*, 108 (2001): 883–92; V. Roessner, M. Robatzek, G. Knapp, T. Banaschewski, and A. Rothenberger, "First-Onset Tics in Patients with

Attention-Deficit-Hyperactivity Disorder: Impact of Stimulants," *Developmental Medicine & Child Neurology* 48, no. 7 (2006): 616–21, doi:10.1017/S0012162206001290; S. F. Law and R. J. Schachar, "Do Typical Clinical Doses of Methylphenidate Cause Tics in Children Treated for Attention-Deficit Hyperactivity Disorder?," *Journal of the American Academy of Child and Adolescent Psychiatry* 38, no. 8 (1999): 944–51, doi:10.1097/00004583-199908000-00009; M. H. Bloch, K. E. Panza, A. Landeros-Weisenberger, and J. F. Leckman, "Meta-Analysis: Treatment of Attention-Deficit/Hyperactivity Disorder in Children with Comorbid Tic Disorders," *Journal of the American Academy of Child and Adolescent Psychiatry* 48, no. 9 (2009): 884–93, doi:10.1097/CHI.0b013e3181b26e9f.

24. C. K. Varley, J. Vincent, P. Varley, and R. Calderon, "Emergence of Tics in Children with Attention Deficit Hyperactivity Disorder Treated with Stimulant Medications," *Comprehensive Psychiatry* 42, no. 3 (2001): 228–33, doi:10.1053/comp.2001.23145.

25. S. C. Cohen, J. M. Mulqueen, E. Ferracioli-Oda, et al., "Meta-Analysis: Risk of Tics Associated with Psychostimulant Use in Randomized, Placebo-Controlled Trials," *Journal of the American Academy of Child and Adolescent Psychiatry* 54, no. 9 (2015): 728–36, doi:10.1016/j.jaac.2015.06.011.

26. K. D. Gadow, J. Sverd, J. Sprafkin, E. E. Nolan, and S. Grossman, "Long-Term Methylphenidate Therapy in Children with Comorbid Attention-Deficit Hyperactivity Disorder and Chronic Multiple Tic Disorder," *Archives of General Psychiatry*, 56 (1999): 330–36; K. D. Gadow and J. Sverd, "Stimulants for ADHD in Child Patients with Tourette's Syndrome: The Issue of Relative Risk," *Journal of Developmental & Behavioral Pediatrics*, 11 (1990): 269–71; https://jaacap.org/article/S0890-8567(09)62182-1/fulltext.

27. C. Yang, X. Cheng, Q. Zhang, D. Yu, J. Li, and L. Zhang, "Interventions for Tic Disorders: An Updated Overview of Systematic Reviews and Meta Analyses," *Psychiatry Research*, 287 (May 2020): 112905, doi:10.1016/j.psychres.2020.112905, Epub 2020 Mar 1, PMID: 32163785.

28. Steven Pliszka; The AACAP Work Group on Quality Issues, "Practice Parameter for the Assessment and Treatment of Children and Adolescents with Attention-Deficit/Hyperactivity Disorder," *AACAP Official Action* 46, no. 7 (July 1, 2007): 894–921, https://doi.org/10.1097/chi.0b013e318054e724.

29. T. Sichilima and M. J. Rieder, "Adderall and Cardiovascular Risk: A Therapeutic Dilemma," *Paediatrics & Child Health* 14, no. 3 (2009): 193–95, doi:10.1093/pch/14.3.193.

30. K. Couper, O. Putt, R. Field, K. Poole, W. Bradlow, A. Clarke, G. C. Perkins, P. Royle, J. Yeung, and S. Taylor-Phillips, "Incidence of Sudden Cardiac Death in the Young: A Systematic Review," *British Medical Journal Open* 10, no. 10 (October 7, 2020): e040815, doi:10.1136/bmjopen-2020-040815.

PMID: 33033034; PMCID: PMC7542928; H. Liu, W. Feng, and D. Zhang, "Association of ADHD Medications with the Risk of Cardiovascular Diseases: A Meta-Analysis," *European Child and Adolescent Psychiatry* 28, no. 10 (October 2019): 1283–93, doi:10.1007/s00787-018-1217-x. Epub 2018 Aug 24. PMID: 30143889.

31. https://doi.org/10.1097/chi.0b013e318054e724; R. R. Liberthson, "Sudden Death from Cardiac Causes in Children and Young Adults," *New England Journal of Medicine*, 334 (1996): 1039–44; Villalaba, "Follow-Up Review of AERS Search."

32. K. K. Man, E. W. Chan, D. Coghill, I. Douglas, P. Ip, L. P. Leung, M. S. Tsui, W. H. Wong, and I. C. Wong, "Methylphenidate and the Risk of Trauma," *Pediatrics* 135, no. 1 (2015): 40–48, doi:10.1542/peds.2014-1738, Epub 2014 Dec 15, PMID: 25511122; K. K. C. Man, P. Ip, E. W. Chan, et al., "Effectiveness of Pharmacological Treatment for Attention-Deficit/Hyperactivity Disorder on Physical Injuries: A Systematic Review and Meta-Analysis of Observational Studies," *CNS Drugs* 31, no. 12 (2017): 1043–55, doi:10.1007/s40263-017-0485-1.

33. H. Liu, W. Feng, and D. Zhang, "Association of ADHD Medications with the Risk of Cardiovascular Diseases: A Meta-Analysis," *European Child and Adolescent Psychiatry* 28, no. 10 (2019): 1283–93, doi:10.1007/s00787-018-1217-x.

34. L. Hennissen, M. J. Bakker, T. Banaschewski, et al., "Cardiovascular Effects of Stimulant and Non-Stimulant Medication for Children and Adolescents with ADHD: A Systematic Review and Meta-Analysis of Trials of Methylphenidate, Amphetamines and Atomoxetine," *CNS Drugs* 31, no. 3 (2017): 199–215, doi:10.1007/s40263-017-0410-7.

35. T. B. Fay and M. A. Alpert, "Cardiovascular Effects of Drugs Used to Treat Attention-Deficit/Hyperactivity Disorder, Part 2: Impact on Cardiovascular Events and Recommendations for Evaluation and Monitoring," *Cardiology in Review* 27, no. 4 (2019): 173–78, doi:10.1097/CRD.0000000000000234; M. D. St. Amour, D. D. O'Leary, J. Cairney, and T. J. Wade, "What Is the Effect of ADHD Stimulant Medication on Heart Rate and Blood Pressure in a Community Sample of Children?," *Canadian Journal of Public Health* 109, no. 3 (2018): 395–400, doi:10.17269/s41997-018-0067-0; S. Berman, R. Kuczenski, J. McCracken, et al., "Potential Adverse Effects of Amphetamine Treatment on Brain and Behavior: A Review," *Molecular Psychiatry*, 14 (2009): 123–42, https://doi.org/10.1038/mp.2008.90.

36. J. Biederman, T. J. Spencer, T. E. Wilens, J. B. Prince, and S. V. Faraone, "Commentary: Treatment of ADHD with Stimulant Medications: Response to Nissen Perspective in the New England Journal of Medicine," *Journal of the American Academy of Child and Adolescent Psychiatry* 45 (2006): 1147–50.

CHAPTER 9

1. L. Reale, B. Bartoli, M. Cartabia, et al., "Comorbidity Prevalence and Treatment Outcome in Children and Adolescents with ADHD," *European Child and Adolescent Psychiatry* 26, no. 12 (2017): 1443–57, doi:10.1007/s00787-017-1005-z; P. S. Jensen, S. P. Hinshaw, H. C. Kraemer, et al., "ADHD Comorbidity Findings from the MTA Study: Comparing Comorbid Subgroups," *Journal of the American Academy of Child and Adolescent Psychiatry* 40, no. 2 (2001): 147–58, doi:10.1097/00004583-200102000-00009; S. Brem, E. Grünblatt, R. Drechsler, P. Riederer, and S. Walitza, "The Neurobiological Link between OCD and ADHD," *Attention Deficit Hyperactivity Disorder* 6, no. 3 (2014): 175–202, doi:10.1007/s12402-014-0146-x.

2. S. Brem, E. Grünblatt, R. Drechsler, P. Riederer, and S. Walitza, "The Neurobiological Link between OCD and ADHD," Attention Deficit Hyperactivity Disorder 6, no. 3 (2014): 175–202, doi:10.1007/s12402-014-0146-x.

3. Jensen, Hinshaw, Kraemer, et al., "ADHD Comorbidity Findings from the MTA Study."

4. Reale, Bartoli, Cartabia, et al., "Comorbidity Prevalence and Treatment Outcome in Children and Adolescents with ADHD."

5. R. A. Barkley, "Emotional Dysregulation Is a Core Component of ADHD," in R. A. Barkley, ed., *Attention-Deficit Hyperactivity Disorder: A Handbook for Diagnosis and Treatment* (New York: Guilford, 2015), 81–115.

6. T. M. Achenbach, "The Child Behavior Profile: I. Boys Aged 6–11," *Journal of Consulting and Clinical Psychology* 46, no. 3 (1978): 478–88, doi:10.1037//0022-006x.46.3.478.

7. L. Borza, "Cognitive-Behavioral Therapy for Generalized Anxiety," *Dialogues in Clinical Neuroscience* 19, no. 2 (2017): 203–8, doi:10.31887/DCNS.2017.19.2/lborza.

8. C. G. Coughlin, S. C. Cohen, J. M. Mulqueen, E. Ferracioli-Oda, Z. D. Stuckelman, and M. H. Bloch, "Meta-Analysis: Reduced Risk of Anxiety with Psychostimulant Treatment in Children with Attention-Deficit/Hyperactivity Disorder," *Journal of Child and Adolescent Psychopharmacology* 25, no. 8 (2015): 611–17.

9. A. M. Wehry, K. Beesdo-Baum, M. M. Hennelly, S. D. Connolly, and J. R. Strawn, "Assessment and Treatment of Anxiety Disorders in Children and Adolescents," *Current Psychiatry Reports* 17, no. 7 (2015): 52, doi:10.1007/s11920-015-0591-z.

10. Z. D. Stuckelman, J. M. Mulqueen, E. Ferracioli-Oda, et al., "Risk of Irritability with Psychostimulant Treatment in Children with ADHD: A Meta-Analysis," *Journal of Clinical Psychiatry* 78, no. 6 (2017): e648–55, doi:10.4088/JCP.15r10601.

CHAPTER 10

1. Novartis, Ritalin LA package insert.
2. F. A. Bokhari and G. M. Fournier, "Entry in the ADHD Drugs Market: Welfare Impact of Generics and Me-Too's," *Journal of Industrial Economics* 61, no. 2 (2013): 339–92, doi:10.1111/joie.12017.
3. Bokhari and Fournier, "Entry in the ADHD Drugs Market: Welfare Impact of Generics and Me-Too's."
4. https://adhdrollercoaster.org/adhd-medications/authorized-generic -concerta-update-6-1-19/.
5. https://www.fda.gov/drugs/drug-safety-and-availability/questions-and -answers-regarding-methylphenidate-hydrochloride-extended-release-tablets -generic; https://www.fda.gov/drugs/drug-safety-and-availability/methylphenidate -hydrochloride-extended-release-tablets-generic-concerta-made-mallinckrodt-and -kudco; http://www.ncbop.org/PDF/CONCERTA_METHYLPHENIDATE _FAQ.pdf; http://www.fda.gov/drugs/drugsafety/ucm422569.htm.
6. https://www.drugs.com/availability/generic-metadate-cd.html.
7. T. E. Wilens, S. W. Boellner, F. A. López, J. M. Turnbow, S. B. Wigal, A. C. Childress, H. B. Abikoff, and M. J. Manos, "Varying the Wear Time of the Methylphenidate Transdermal System in Children with Attention-Deficit/ Hyperactivity Disorder," *Journal of the American Academy of Child and Adolescent Psychiatry* 47, no. 6 (2008): 700–708, doi:10.1097/CHI.0b013e31816bffdf, PMID: 18434918.
8. Wilens, Boellner, López, Turnbow, Wigal, Childress, Abikoff, and Manos, "Varying the Wear Time of the Methylphenidate Transdermal System in Children with Attention-Deficit/Hyperactivity Disorder."
9. E. M. Warshaw, L. Squires, Y. Li, R. Civil, and A. S. Paller, "Methylphenidate Transdermal System: A Multisite, Open-Label Study of Dermal Reactions in Pediatric Patients Diagnosed with ADHD," *Primary Care Companion to the Journal of Clinical Psychiatry* 12, no. 6 (2010): PCC.10m00996, doi:10.4088/PCC.10m00996pur.
10. R. L. Findling, S. B. Wigal, O. G. Bukstein, et al., "Long-Term Tolerability of the Methylphenidate Transdermal System in Pediatric Attention-Deficit/

Hyperactivity Disorder: A Multicenter, Prospective, 12-Month, Open-Label, Uncontrolled, Phase III Extension of Four Clinical Trials," *Clinical Therapeutics* 31, no. 8 (2009): 1844–55, doi:10.1016/j.clinthera.2009.08.002; Warshaw, Squires, Li, Civil, and Paller, "Methylphenidate Transdermal System: A Multisite, Open-Label Study of Dermal Reactions in Pediatric Patients Diagnosed with ADHD."

11. http://www.corepsych.com/daytrana-tips-the-add-patch-system-works/.

12. https://www.ismp.org/resources/requirement-1-patch-should-stick-patient.

13. E. M. Warshaw, A. S. Paller, J. F. Fowler, M. J. Zirwas, "Practical Management of Cutaneous Reactions to the Methylphenidate Transdermal System: Recommendations from a Dermatology Expert Panel Consensus Meeting," *Clinical Therapeutics* 30, no. 2 (2008): 326–37, doi:10.1016/j.clinthera.2008.01.022.

14. FDA Drug Safety Communication: "FDA Reporting Permanent Skin Color Changes Associated with Use of Daytrana Patch (Methylphenidate Transdermal System) for Treating ADHD," https://www.fda.gov/drugs/drug-safety-and-availability/fda-drug-safety-communication-fda-reporting-perma-nent-skin-color-changes-associated-use-daytrana.

15. https://www.ismp.org/resources/requirement-1-patch-should-stick-patient.

16. M. D. Moen and S. J. Keam, "Dexmethylphenidate Extended Release: A Review of Its Use in the Treatment of Attention-Deficit Hyperactivity Disorder," *CNS Drugs* 23, no. 12 (2009): 1057–83, doi:10.2165/11201140-000000000-00000.

17. https://www.medscape.com/viewarticle/911569; A. Childress, S. Mehrotra, J. Gobburu, et al., "Single-Dose Pharmacokinetics of HLD20, a Delayed-Release and Extended-Release Methylphenidate Formulation in Healthy Adults and in Adolescents and Children with Attention-Deficit/ Hyperactivity Disorder," *Journal of Child and Adolescent Psychopharmacology*, 28 (2017): 10–18; F. R. Sallee, "Early Morning Functioning in Stimulant-Treated Children and Adolescents with Attention-Deficit/Hyperactivity Disorder and Its Impact on Caregivers," *Journal of Child and Adolescent Psychopharmacology*, 25 (2015): 558–65; S. R. Pliszka, T. E. Wilens, S. Bostrom, et al., "Efficacy and Safety of KLD200, Delayed-Release and Extended-Release Methylphenidate, in Children with Attention-Deficit/Hyperactivity Disorder," *Journal of Child and Adolescent Psychopharmacology*, 27 (2017): 474–82.

18. https://kempharm.com/kempharm-completes-kp415-pre-nda-meet-ing-with-fda/; https://www.globenewswire.com/news-release/2020/07/28/2068550/0/en/KemPharm-Announces-Issuance-of-Two-Additional-U-S-Patents-Governing-KP415-and-KP484.html; https://investors.kempharm.com/news-releases/news-release-details/kempharm-announces-fda-approval-azstarystm-serdexmethylphenidate/.

CHAPTER 11

1. L. E. Arnold, P. H. Wender, K. McCloskey, and S. H. Snyder, "Levoamphetamine and Dextroamphetamine: Comparative Efficacy in the Hyperkinetic Syndrome: Assessment by Target Symptoms," *Archives of General Psychiatry* 27, no. 6 (1972): 816–22, doi:10.1001/archpsyc.1972.01750300078015.

2. Arnold, Wender, McCloskey, and Snyder, "Levoamphetamine and Dextroamphetamine: Comparative Efficacy in the Hyperkinetic Syndrome."

3. D. J. Heal, S. L. Smith, J. Gosden, and D. J. Nutt, "Amphetamine, Past and Present—A Pharmacological and Clinical Perspective," *Journal of Psychopharmacology* 27, no. 6 (2013): 479–96, doi:10.1177/0269881113482532.

4. J. S. Markowitz and K. S. Patrick, "The Clinical Pharmacokinetics of Amphetamines Utilized in the Treatment of Attention-Deficit/Hyperactivity Disorder," *Journal of Child and Adolescent Psychopharmacology* 27, no. 8 (2017): 678–89, doi:10.1089/cap.2017.0071.

5. https://adhdrollercoaster.org/?s=madderall.

6. https://www.ncbi.nlm.nih.gov/pmc/articles/PMC4090185/.

7. S. P. Kane, "The Top 300 of 2019," ClinCalc DrugStats Database, Version 2019.10. ClinCalc, https://clincalc.com/DrugStats/Top300Drugs.aspx (retrieved March 12, 2019).

8. https://www.mydayis-pro.com/adverse-reactions.

9. Markowitz and Patrick, "The Clinical Pharmacokinetics of Amphetamines Utilized in the Treatment of Attention-Deficit/Hyperactivity Disorder."

CHAPTER 12

1. L. Scahill, "Alpha-2 Adrenergic Agonists in Children with Inattention, Hyperactivity and Impulsiveness," *CNS Drugs*, 23, suppl 1 (2009): 43–49, https://doi.org/10.2165/00023210-200923000-00006.

2. J. T. Coull, C. Büchel, K. J. Friston, and C. D. Frith, "Noradrenergically Mediated Plasticity in a Human Attentional Neuronal Network," *NeuroImage* 10, no. 6 (1999): 705–15, https://doi.org/10.1006/nimg.1999.0513.

3. R. D. Hunt, R. B. Minderaa, and D. J. Cohen, "Clonidine Benefits Children with Attention Deficit Disorder and Hyperactivity: Report of a Double-Blind Placebo-Crossover Therapeutic Trial," *Journal of the American Academy of Child Psychiatry* 24, no. 5 (1985): 617–29, doi:10.1016/s0002-7138(09)60065-0.

4. E. Harstad, J. Shults, W. Barbaresi, et al., "α2-Adrenergic Agonists or Stimulants for Preschool-Age Children with Attention-Deficit/Hyperactivity Disorder" (published online ahead of print, May 4, 2021), *JAMA*, e216118. doi:10.1001/jama.2021.6118.

5. Harstad, Shults, Barbaresi, et al., "α2-Adrenergic Agonists or Stimulants for Preschool-Age Children with Attention-Deficit/Hyperactivity Disorder."

6. J. Kerbeshian and L. Burd, "A Clinical Pharmacological Approach to Treating Tourette Syndrome in Children and Adolescents," *Neuroscience and Biobehavioral Reviews* 12, nos. 3–4 (1988): 241–45, https://doi.org/10.1016/s0149-7634(88)80051-4.

7. T. Pringsheim, L. Hirsch, D. Gardner, and D. A. Gorman, "The Pharmacological Management of Oppositional Behaviour, Conduct Problems, and Aggression in Children and Adolescents with Attention-Deficit Hyperactivity Disorder, Oppositional Defiant Disorder, and Conduct Disorder: A Systematic Review and Meta-Analysis. Part 1: Psychostimulants, Alpha-2 Agonists, and Atomoxetine," *Canadian Journal of Psychiatry. Revue Canadienne de Psychiatrie* 60, no. 2 (2015): 42–51, https://doi.org/10.1177/070674371506000202.

8. Philip L. Hazell et al., "A Randomized Controlled Trial of Clonidine Added to Psychostimulant Medication for Hyperactive and Aggressive Children," *Journal of the American Academy of Child and Adolescent Psychiatry* 42, no. 8 (2011): 886–94, doi:10.1097/01.CHI.0000046908.27264.00; Harstad, Shults, Barbaresi, et al., "α2-Adrenergic Agonists or Stimulants for Preschool-Age Children with Attention-Deficit/Hyperactivity Disorder."

9. D. Kolar, A. Keller, M. Golfinopoulos, L. Cumyn, C. Syer, and L. Hechtman, "Treatment of Adults with Attention-Deficit/Hyperactivity Disorder," *Neuropsychiatric Disease and Treatment* 4, no. 2 (2008): 389–403, https://doi.org/10.2147/NDT.S6985.

10. B. C. Strange, "Once-Daily treatment of ADHD with Guanfacine: Patient Implications. *Neuropsychiatric Disease and Treatment* 4, no. 3 (2008): 499–506, https://doi.org/10.2147/ndt.s1711; S. V. Faraone, K. McBurnett, F. R. Sallee, J. Steeber, and F. A. López, "Guanfacine Extended Release: A Novel Treatment for Attention-Deficit/Hyperactivity Disorder in Children and Adolescents," *Clinical Therapeutics* 35, no. 11 (2013): 1778–93, https://doi.org/10.1016/j.clinthera.2013.09.005; R. M. Bilder, S. K. Loo, J. J. McGough, F. Whelan, G. Hellemann, C. Sugar, M. Del'Homme, A. Sturm, J. Cowen, G. Hanada, and J. T. McCracken, "Cognitive Effects of Stimulant, Guanfacine, and Combined Treatment in Child and Adolescent Attention-Deficit/Hyperactivity Disorder," *Journal of the American Academy of Child and Adolescent Psychiatry* 55, no. 8 (2016): 667–73, https://doi.org/10.1016/j.jaac.2016.05.016.

11. J. M. Halperin, J. H. Newcorn, K. E. McKay, L. J. Siever, and V. Sharma, "Growth Hormone Response to Guanfacine in Boys with Attention Deficit Hyperactivity Disorder: A Preliminary Study," *Journal of Child and Adolescent Psychopharmacology* 13, no. 3 (2003): 283–94, https://doi.org/10.1089/104454603322572615.

12. Strange, "Once-Daily Treatment of ADHD with Guanfacine: Patient Implications."

13. Strange, "Once-Daily Treatment of ADHD with Guanfacine: Patient Implications."

14. Strange, "Once-Daily Treatment of ADHD with Guanfacine: Patient Implications."

15. Pringsheim, Hirsch, Gardner, and Gorman, "The Pharmacological Management of Oppositional Behaviour, Conduct Problems, and Aggression in Children and Adolescents with Attention-Deficit Hyperactivity Disorder, Oppositional Defiant Disorder, and Conduct Disorder: A Systematic Review and Meta-Analysis. Part 1."

16. J. T. McCracken, J. J. McGough, S. K. Loo, et al., "Combined Stimulant and Guanfacine Administration in Attention-Deficit/Hyperactivity Disorder: A Controlled, Comparative Study," *Journal of the American Academy of Child and Adolescent Psychiatry*, 55 (2016): 657–66.

17. J. L. Gayleard and M. P. Mychailyszyn, "Atomoxetine Treatment for Children and Adolescents with Attention-Deficit/Hyperactivity Disorder (ADHD): A Comprehensive Meta-Analysis of Outcomes on Parent-Rated Core Symptomatology," *Attention Deficicit Hyperactivity Disorder* 9, no. 3 (2017): 149–60.

18. G. Rezaei, S. A. Hosseini, A. Akbari Sari, et al., "Comparative Efficacy of Methylphenidate and Atomoxetine in the Treatment of Attention Deficit Hyperactivity Disorder in Children and Adolescents: A Systematic Review and Meta-Analysis," *Medical Journal of the Islamic Republic of Iran*, 30 (2016): 325; K. P. Garnock-Jones and G. M. Keating, "Atomoxetine: A Review of Its Use in Attention-Deficit Hyperactivity Disorder in Children and Adolescents," *Paediatric Drugs* 11, no. 3 (2009): 203–26, doi:10.2165/00148581-200911030-00005.

19. J. Biederman, S. B. Wigal, T. J. Spencer, J. J. McGough, and D. A. Mays, "A Post Hoc Subgroup Analysis of an 18-Day Randomized Controlled Trial Comparing the Tolerability and Efficacy of Mixed Amphetamine Salts Extended Release and Atomoxetine in School-Age Girls with Attention-Deficit/Hyperactivity Disorder," *Clinical Therapeutics* 28, no. 2 (2006): 280–93, doi:10.1016/j.clinthera.2006.02.008.

20. J. Y. Cheng, R. Y. Chen, J. S. Ko, and E. M. Ng, "Efficacy and Safety of Atomoxetine for Attention-Deficit/Hyperactivity Disorder in Children and Adolescents-Meta-Analysis and Meta-Regression Analysis," *Psychopharmacology (Berl)* 194, no. 2 (2007): 197–209, doi:10.1007/s00213-007-0840-x.

21. W. Verbeeck, S. Tuinier, and G. E. Bekkering, "Antidepressants in the Treatment of Adult Attention-Deficit Hyperactivity Disorder: A Systematic Review," *Advances in Therapy* 26, no. 2 (2009): 170–84, doi:10.1007/

s12325-009-0008-7; T. E. Wilens, B. R. Haight, J. P. Horrigan, et al., "Bupropion XL in Adults with Attention-Deficit/Hyperactivity Disorder: A Randomized, Placebo-Controlled Study," *Biological Psychiatry* 57, no. 7 (2005): 793–801, doi:10.1016/j.biopsych.2005.01.027; Biederman, "Attention-Deficit/Hyperactivity Disorder: A Life-Span Perspective," *Journal of Clinical Psychiatry*, 59, suppl 7 (1998): 4–16; Q. X. Ng, "A Systematic Review of the Use of Bupropion for Attention-Deficit/Hyperactivity Disorder in Children and Adolescents," *Journal of Child and Adolescent Psychopharmacology* 27, no. 2 (2017): 112–16, doi:10.1089/cap.2016.0124.

22. Wilens, Haight, Horrigan, et al., "Bupropion XL in Adults with Attention Deficit/Hyperactivity Disorder."

23. S. Pliszka S; AACAP Work Group on Quality Issues, "Practice Parameter for the Assessment and Treatment of Children and Adolescents with Attention-Deficit/Hyperactivity Disorder," *Journal of the American Academy of Child and Adolescent Psychiatry* 46, no. 7 (July 2007): 894–921, doi:10.1097/chi.0b013e318054e724. PMID: 17581453.

24. A. W. Peck, W. C. Stern, and C. Watkinson, "Incidence of Seizures during Treatment with Tricyclic Antidepressant Drugs and Bupropion," *Journal of Clinical Psychiatry* 44, no. 5, pt. 2 (1983): 197–201; Pliszka; AACAP Work Group on Quality Issues, "Practice Parameter for the Assessment and Treatment of Children and Adolescents with Attention-Deficit/Hyperactivity Disorder."

INDEX

Actavis Pharmaceuticals, 199–200

Adderall, 53, 55, 77, 93, 106–108, 118, 131–132, 140, 141, 148, 153, 160, 171, 175–176, 191, 228, 230, 235–237, 239, 244, 247, 262, 276, 277, 278

Adhansia XR, 106–108,113, 203–204, 215, 272

ADD vs. ADHD, 7

ADHD affects
learning, 6, 10, 23, 34, 58, 59, 65–72, 77–79, 86, 93, 179, 180, 181, 182, 183, 187, 189, 191, 253
self-esteem, 23, 47, 59, 67, 71, 170, 195
social behavior, 8–10, 52, 66, 68–69, 72, 94, 96, 99, 143, 181–183, 185, 189, 191

ADHD caused by neurological differences in the brain, 72–77
prefrontal cortex, 75–76, 79, 98, 150, 252
fronto-striato-cerebellar projections, 75–76, 79, 98

caudate nucleus, 75–76, 79, 98

ADHD core behaviors, 101
blurts out, 9
distractibility, 6, 8, 10, 14, 21, 26, 30, 41, 47, 64, 65, 68–70, 72, 76, 78, 79, 85, 86, 96, 97, 101, 103–104, 142–143, 147, 152, 168, 176, 177, 230, 252–254, 261, 263, 268
fidgety, 9
focusing, difficulty, 8, 13, 14, 15, 17, 21–22, 25–27, 30, 31, 35, 36–37, 42, 43, 55, 57, 64–66, 71, 72, 76–77, 81–83, 85–87, 94, 97, 101, 103, 116, 136–137, 164, 177–178, 183, 190, 252, 253–256, 260
follow-through, 8
hyperactivity, 6–9, 9, 22–23, 43, 58, 67, 72, 78, 85–89, 92, 93–94, 97, 101, 148, 156, 177, 191, 236, 252–256, 259–260, 261, 263
impulsivity, 6–9, 22–25, 30, 34, 66–70, 78, 85–86, 93–97, 101,

104, 158, 163, 168–170, 177, 191, 192, 195, 230, 252–256, 259–260, 261
inattention, 7, 8, 11, 23, 25–26, 34, 35–38, 59, 72, 76, 77, 79, 92, 101, 261, 263
interrupts, 9, 168, 169
listening, not, 8
memory, 8, 77, 79, 147
normal, all ADHD behaviors can be, 9, 63–66
organization, 8, 64, 67, 75, 77, 79, 93, 101, 177
productive behaviors, 66, 69
planning, 75, 79
tasks, avoids, 8
playing quietly, difficulty, 9
seated, cannot stay, 9
talks frequently, 9
ADHD evolved, 67–71
ADHD Diagnosis, 7–14, 42–43
American Medical Association Consensus Statement, 1998, 11
boy:girl ratio, 23
diagnostic test unavailable, 63–64
denial, 22–23
over diagnosed, 61–67
subjectivity, 10–11, 14, 65
symptoms are normal behaviors, 65–68
ADHD non-medication treatments
applied kinesiology (realigning bones in the skull), 99
candida yeast infection treatment, 99
EEG biofeedback (training to increase brain-wave activity), 99
megavitamins and mineral supplements, 99

motion-sickness medication (to treat the inner ear), 99
optometric vision training, 99
sugar, reduced in diet, 99
ADHD not caused by
cell phones, 71–72
lack of sleep, 71–72
poor parental discipline, 71–72
poor teachers, 71–72
sugar, 71–72
TV, 71–72
video games, 71–72
ADHD outcomes, long-term
cost to society, 97
driving, 95, 101
education, 94, 101
employment, 94, 101
family life, 94, 101
finances, 94, 101
health, 94–95, 101
illegal activities, 95, 101
medication effect, 96
persists into adulthood, 93–97
sexual activity, 95, 101
social life, 94, 101
substance abuse, 95, 101, 244
Adverse Event Reporting System (FAERS) database, 212
Adzenys ER Liquid, 106–108, 114, 228, 231, 233, 234, 238–240, 278, 279
Adzenys XR ODT, 106–108, 114, 228, 232, 234, 238–239, 277, 280
aggression, 24–25, 68, 184, 190, 195, 260
Alles, Gordon, 50
American Academy of Child and Adolescent Psychiatry, 72
American Medical Association, 11, 89

American Medical Association
Scientific Counsel, 89–91
American Psychiatric Association, 6,
8, 9
Amphetamine Transdermal System,
106–108, 248–249, 279
flexible duration, 248–249
flexible dosing, 248–249
crash-resistant, 248–249
compliance, 248–249
anger, 8, 24, 190, 260
antihistamines, 154–155
anxiety, 8, 100, 156, 179, 180, 184–
186, 189, 190, 191, 264, 266,
281, 282
appetite and growth, 53–54, 84–85,
116, 127, 140–146, 172, 198,
209, 211, 230–231, 256–257,
260
amphetamines impact appetite
more than methylphenidate,
135, 141, 232, 235, 236
child, what to say to your child, 145
diets, 144
dose-related, 139, 140–141, 217
growth, 141–142
growth hormone, 257, 259
Jornay PM, 222–223
levo-amphetamine, 131
non-stimulants, minimal effect on
appetite, 141, 146, 252, 254,
257, 259
management of appetite problems,
142–145
methylphenidate less likely to
cause, 134, 135, 141
Mydayis, 241–242
Obetrol, designed to reduce
appetite, 53
prevention, 142–143

stopping medication, 146
Strattera, 262
supplements, 144–145
time-related, 140, 141, 220
vacations from medication,
143–144
applied kinesiology (realigning bones
in the skull), 99
Aptensio XR, 106–108, 113, 203–
204, 215, 271
Ativan, 190
Atomoxetine, 91–93, 106–108,
134, 141, 146, 156–157, 166,
170–171, 176, 192, 251–252,
261–263, 281, 290
attention, 8, 77, 79, 101, 252–254
*Attention Deficit Disorder: A Different
Perspective* (Hartmann), 67
ADHD subtypes
Attention Deficit Disorder with
Hyperactivity, 6
Attention Deficit Disorder
without Hyperactivity, 6
Attention Deficit Hyperactivity
Disorder, Primarily
Hyperactive/Impulsive Type,
7–8
Attention Deficit Hyperactivity
Disorder, Primarily
Hyperactive/Impulsive Type,
7–8
Attention Deficit Hyperactivity
Disorder, Primarily Inattentive
Type, 7–8
Azstarys, 106–108, 214, 222–224, 228,
273

bed-wetting, 143, 144
behavior management training,
99–100

Benzedrine, 50–53, 56, 227, 230
Biles, Simone, 138
bioequivalence, 118–119, 121–124, 239
blurts out, 9
Bottle of Lies (Eban), 120
Bradley, Charles, 51–53, 56, 227, 228, 230, 245
Bradley, Emma, 50
Bradshaw, Terry, 138
brain areas affected by ADHD
    prefrontal cortex, 75–76, 79, 98, 150, 252
    fronto-striato-cerebellar projections, 75–76, 79, 98
    caudate nucleus, 75–76, 79, 98
bupropion, 92, 93, 106–108, 141, 170, 251–252, 264, 265–266, 282

caffeine, 148
California Institute of Technology, 50
candida yeast infection treatment, 99
Cardiac
    atomoxetine, 176
    blood pressure, 176
    evaluations, 176
    increased heart rate, 176
    non-stimulants, 176
    Strattera, 176
    sudden death, 175–176
Catapres, 93, 106–108, 134, 174–175, 192, 207, 251–259, 281
Catapres-TTS, 174, 192, 207, 248, 251, 254, 258, 281
caudate nucleus, 75–76, 79, 98
celebrities with ADHD
    Phelps, Michael, 138
    Biles, Simone, 138
    Timberlake, Justin, 138
    Levine, Adam, 138

Watson, Emma, 138
Kelly, Scott, 138
Bradshaw, Terry, 138
Jordan, Michael, 138
Van Gogh, Vincent, 138
Lincoln, Abraham, 138
Edison, Thomas, 138
Einstein, Albert, 138
Celexa, 190
Center for Pediatric Psychopathology, 62
Centre for Research in Evidence-Based Practice, 62
Children's Memorial Hospital, Boston, 4
CIBA, 55–56
clonidine, 91–93, 106–108, 134, 141, 146, 156, 166, 170–171, 174–175, 192, 248, 251–262, 281
co-morbidity
    anxiety, 8, 100, 156, 179, 180, 184–186, 189, 190, 191, 264, 266, 281, 282
    Ativan, 190
    benzodiazepine, 190
    Celexa, 190
    compulsions, 156, 173, 179, 186–192, 255, 264, 277, 281
    irritability, 46, 116, 126, 135, 157–167, 170–172, 183, 191, 194, 206, 210, 211, 215, 221, 237, 251–253, 254, 256, 261–264, 277, 281, 282
    irritability, time-related, 140, 156, 157–167, 216, 221, 235, 248, 257, 259, 270, 272, 273, 275, 276, 277, 278, 280, 281
    Mood Disorder, 25, 179
    mood suppression, 54, 100, 116, 123, 163, 167–170, 182–184,

189–190, 192, 210, 251–252, 262

mood variability, 126, 164–165, 170, 253, 255–257, 264

Lexapro, 190

Librium, 190

Oppositional Defiant Disorder, 25, 179–184, 189, 192, 255

Paxil, 190

Prozac, 190

selective serotonin reuptake inhibitor (SSRI), 190

treatment, 189–192

Valium, 190

Xanax, 190

Zoloft, 190

compliance, 195, 206, 211, 248, 275

compulsions, 156, 173, 186–192, 255, 264, 277, 281

Frequency, 179

Concerta, 47, 77, 93, 104, 106–108, 113, 117, 118, 126, 128, 129, 141, 148, 153, 178, 197–201, 202, 204, 208, 209, 215–216, 223, 225, 242, 247, 262, 272

Congress, US, 57

Cotempla XR-ODT, 106–108, 113, 114, 219–220, 273, 274

Counseling, 52, 62, 99, 100, 186, 189, 191

crash-resistant, 46, 126, 206, 207, 210, 248

Crichton, Sir Alexander, 5

Cylert, 106

Dayatrana, 77, 106–108, 113, 114, 118, 126, 129, 132, 147, 206–214, 215, 217, 242, 247, 248, 249, 258, 272, 273, 275, 278, 280

application of skin patch, 213

compliance, 206, 211

crash-resistant, 206, 210

flexible dosing, 206, 209–210

flexible duration, 206, 208–209

side effects, calamine, 212

side effects, Calmoseptine, 211

side effects, contact dermatitis 211

side effects, leukoderma 212

side effects, olive oil, 212

side effects, steroid cream, 212

side effects, zinc oxide, 212

denial, 30

developmental pediatrician, definition, 4

Dexedrine, 52, 53, 56, 57, 77, 93, 106–108, 118, 131, 132, 160, 228, 229–232, 234, 235, 236, 237, 238, 247, 255, 276

Dexedrine liquid, 228, 229, 231, 277, 279

Dexedrine Spansule, 106–108, 114, 228, 234, 238, 242, 245, 247, 255–256, 277, 278, 280

Destrostat, 106–108, 131, 160, 230, 232, 235, 245, 276

Diagnostic and Statistical Manual of Mental Disorders, 6–7, 11, 14, 65

distractibility, 6, 8, 10, 14, 21, 26, 30, 41, 47, 64, 65, 68–70, 72, 76, 78, 79, 85, 86, 96, 97, 101, 103–104, 142–143, 147, 152, 168, 176, 177, 230, 252–254, 261, 263, 268

Diversion, 54, 243–247

Doctors without Borders, 122

dopamine, 76–78, 131, 251–252, 262, 263

double-blind trials, 59

driving, 95, 96, 144, 195
Drug Spending Research Institute of
    the Pew Charitable Trust, 114
Dynavel XR Liquid, 106–108, 114,
    132, 228, 231, 233, 234, 239,
    240, 278, 279

Edeleano, Lazar, 49
Edison, Thomas, 138
education, 94, 101
EEG biofeedback (training to increase
    brain-wave activity), 99
effect size, 91–92, 262, 266
Einstein, Albert, 138
Emma Pendleton Bradley Home, 50
emotional hypersensitivity, 170–171,
    183
emotional lability, 126, 157–167, 170–
    171, 181, 195, 196, 198, 207, 210,
    215, 234, 241, 252–254, 270, 271
    treatment with non-stimulant,
    165–167
Emovit, 263
employment, 94, 101
ephedra plant, 49, 109
ephedrine, 49
European Network for Hyperkinetic
    Disorders, 134
Evekeo, 106–108, 160, 232, 245, 276
Evekeo ODT, 106–108, 114, 228,
    232, 277, 280
evergreening, 10–115, 118, 204, 225
exclusivity, 112–115, 118, 199, 243, 245
executive function training, 71

family life, effect of ADHD on, 94,
    101
Federal Food, Drug, and Cosmetic
    Act, 53
Fidgety Phil, 5

fidgety, 9
Finances, effect of ADHD on, 94, 101
flexible dosing, 206, 207, 208–209,
    211, 248–249, 258, 273, 275
flexible duration, 206, 207, 208–209,
    211, 248–249, 275
Focalin, 106–108, 118, 130, 160, 214–
    215, 223, 224, 228, 242, 270
Focalin XR, 106–108, 113, 214–216,
    228, 237, 270, 271
focusing, difficulty, 8, 13, 14, 15,
    17, 21–22, 25–27, 30, 31, 35,
    36–37, 42, 43, 55, 57, 64–66,
    71, 72, 76–77, 81–83, 85–87,
    94, 97, 101, 103, 116, 136–137,
    164, 177–178, 183, 190, 252,
    253–256, 260
food and amphetamines, 249
Food and Drug Administration, 53,
    55, 106, 107, 110–115, 119–
    124, 131, 159, 175, 190, 200,
    203, 204, 207, 208, 212, 214,
    223, 230, 235–237, 242, 245–
    246, 248, 249, 255, 261, 263,
    265, 266, 273, 278, 280, 282
    inspections, 110–111, 119–122
Freud, Sigmund, 52
fronto-striato-cerebellar projections,
    75–76, 79
frustration, 16, 25–26, 36, 40, 57, 178,
    182, 183, 189, 267

Gallagher, Cornelious, 57
generic medications, 111–124, 132–
    133, 154, 196, 197, 199–201,
    202, 203, 204, 205, 206, 214,
    217, 231, 233, 234, 240, 243,
    247, 252, 258
    China, 120, 122
    India, 120, 122

GoodRx, 132–134, 194, 197, 214, 234, 240
growth chart, 142
growth hormone, 257, 259
guanfacine, 91, 92, 93, 106–108, 134, 141, 146, 156, 166, 170–171, 174–175, 192, 251–260, 262, 281
guilt, parent's and child's, 1–2, 4, 25–29, 33, 35–36,38, 105, 168

Hartmann, Thom, 67
headaches, 51, 64, 116, 171–172
health, effect of ADHD on, 94–95, 101
history of ADHD medication, 49–59
Hoffman, Heinrich, 5
hyperactivity, 6–9, 9, 22–23, 43, 58, 67, 72, 78, 85–89, 92, 93–94, 97, 101, 148, 156, 177, 191, 236, 252–256, 259–260, 261, 263
hyperkinetic reaction of childhood, 6

illegal activities, effect of ADHD on, 95, 101
impulsivity, 6–9, 22–25, 30, 34, 66–70, 78, 85–86, 93–97, 101, 104, 158, 163, 168–170, 177, 191, 192, 195, 230, 252–256, 259–260, 261
impulsivity vs. spontaneity, 163, 168–170, 184
inattention, 7, 8, 11, 23, 25–26, 34, 35–38, 59, 72, 76, 77, 79, 92, 101, 261, 263
Inquiry into the Nature and Origin of Mental Derangement (Crichton 1763), 5
insomnia, 116, 146–157, 251–252, 254, 259, 261, 262, 263

intelligence, 7, 25, 31, 34, 36–37, 70, 71, 170, 177, 181, 267, 268
interrupts, 9, 168, 169
Intuniv, 93, 106–108, 174, 192, 251–260, 281
irritability, 46, 116, 126, 135, 157–167, 170–172, 183, 191, 194, 206, 210, 211, 215, 221, 237, 251–253, 254, 256, 261–264, 277, 281, 282
    time-related, 140, 156, 157–167, 216, 221, 235, 248, 257, 259, 270, 272, 273, 275, 276, 277, 278, 280, 281
    Adderall, 237, 239

Janssen Pharmaceuticals, 197–200
Jordan, Michael, 138
Jornay PM, 106–108, 113, 197, 220–223, 272, 273

Kapvay, 93, 106–108, 174–175, 192, 251–258, 281
Kefauver-Harris amendment to the Federal Food, Drug, and Cosmetic Act, 53
Kelly, Scott, 138

Lannett Pharmaceuticals, 202
learning disability, 10, 58–59
leukemia compared to ADHD, 63–64
Levine, Adam, 138
Lexapro, 190, 265
Librium, 190
Lincoln, Abraham, 138
LiquiXR technology, 217, 240
lis-dex-amphetamine, 93, 106–108, 243–244, 247, 278, 280
lysine, 244–247

Madderall, 171, 237
Markowitz, John S., 237
Massachusetts General Hospital, 62
Maynard, Robert, *Omaha Pupils Given "Behavior Drugs,"* 57
Medicaid, 114
medication vacations, 143–144, 152–153
megavitamins, 99
melatonin, 155–156
memory, 8, 77, 79, 147
mental state, 164
Metadate CD, 77, 93, 106–108, 113, 114, 118, 126, 153, 201–204, 208, 215, 217, 220, 221, 223, 234, 237, 241, 271
Metadate ER, 201, 271
methamphetamine, 49–50, 53–54, 235
Methylin, 114, 160, 205–206, 270, 272
Methylin chewable, 106–108, 114, 205–206, 218, 270, 274
Methylin ER, 205–206, 271
Methylin liquid, 114, 205–206, 207, 217, 270, 274
mineral supplements, 99
mirror-image molecules, 125, 129–132, 214, 223–225, 228, 229, 235–237
mirror-image molecules, dextro-amphetamine vs. levo-amphetamine, 131, 228, 235–236
mirror-image molecules, dextro-methylphenidate vs. levo-methylphenidate, 130, 224, 228
mixed amphetamine salts, 235–238, 241, 247
mood
    Mood Disorder, 25, 179
    mood suppression, 54, 100, 116, 123, 163, 167–170, 182–184,
        189–190, 192, 210, 251–252, 262
    mood variability, 126, 164–165, 170, 253, 255–257, 264
parents, mother / father perceptions, 38, 46–47, 65, 128
motion-sickness medication (to treat the inner ear), 99
MRI scans of areas of brain affected by ADHD, 64, 76
Multimodal Treatment of Attention Deficit Hyperactivity Disorder (MTA) study, 99–100
Mydayis, 106–108, 114, 241–242, 278

Nagai, Nagayoshi, 49–50
National Drug Code (NDC), 200–202
National Institute for Health and Care Excellence, 134
National Survey of Children's Health, 62
neuron, 73–78
    defined, 73–75
    picture, 74
neurotransmitters, 73–79, 251, 252, 262, 263
    dopamine, 76–78, 131, 251–252, 262, 263
    norepinephrine, 76–78, 251–252, 261, 262, 263
    serotonin, 190, 263–264
nightmares, 147–148
non-stimulant medications for the treatment of ADHD, 92, 251–266
norepinephrine, 76–78, 251–252, 261, 262, 263
Noven Pharmaceuticals, 207, 213, 214, 248

obesity, 53, 55, 131, 140, 230, 235, 236

Obetrol, 54, 235–236
    precursor to Adderall, 53–55, 131, 140, 235, 236
    treatment of obesity, 53–54, 235–237
Oppositional Defiant Disorder, 25, 179–184, 189, 192, 255
optometric vision training, 99
Orally Dissolving Tablet, 128, 129, 132, 193, 219–220, 227, 228
    Adzenys XR-ODT, 106–108, 114, 228, 232, 234, 238–239, 277, 280
    Cotempla XR-ODT, 106–108, 113, 114, 219–220, 273, 274
    Evekeo ODT, 106–108, 114, 228, 232, 277, 280
organization, 8, 64, 67, 75, 77, 79, 93, 101, 177
Osmotic-Controlled Release Oral Delivery System (OROS), 198–200

Panizzon, Leandro, 55
patent for medications, 112
Patriot Pharmaceuticals, 197, 200–201, 272
Paxil, 190
pharmaceutically equivalent, 118–119
Phelps, Michael, 137–138
Phenylisopropylamine, 49
prefrontal cortex, 75–76, 79, 98, 150, 252
prescriptions, number written per year (4.5 billion), 123
prevalence of ADHD, 62, 67, 109
Procentra Liquid, 106–108, 114, 131, 228, 233, 239, 240, 245, 277, 279
pro-drug
    Azstarys, 223–225, 273

Vyvanse, 243–245, 278
Prozac, 190, 261
pseudoephedrine, 49

Qelbree, 106–108, 251–252, 263–264, 282
QuilliChew ER, 106–108, 114, 206, 218, 272, 274
Quillivant XR liquid, 105, 106–108, 114, 206, 207, 216–219, 240, 270, 272, 274

rapid eye movements (REM), 147
research studies published since 1970, 90–91
restless leg syndrome, 147
Rexar Pharmaceuticals, 54–55
risk-taking, 34, 68, 184
Ritalin, 55–58, 77, 93, 103–108, 116–118, 126, 129, 132, 141, 148, 158–166, 194–197, 201, 205–206, 208, 215, 222, 230, 270
Ritalin LA, 77, 106–108, 113, 126, 167, 194–198, 201–204, 208–209, 215, 217, 220–221, 234, 237, 241, 255–256, 270, 271, 272
Ritalin SR, 106–108, 194–197, 206, 270, 271

salts, mixed amphetamine, 54–55, 235–237, 238–239, 241–242, 247
sedation, 156, 254, 257, 259–260, 262, 266
seizures, 264, 266, 282
sexual activity, 95
Shakespeare, 147
Shire Pharmaceuticals, 55, 230, 235–237, 243–246
side effects, 3 main types
    dose-related, 139, 140, 148, 149, 153, 170,

time-related, 140, 141, 143, 148–
151, 153, 157, 171–172
idiosyncratic, 139, 140, 170
appetite and growth, 53–54, 84–85,
116, 127, 140–146, 172, 198,
209, 211, 230–231, 256–257, 260
amphetamines impact appetite
more than methylphenidate,
135, 141, 232, 235, 236
child, what to say to your child,
145
diets, 144
dose-related, 139, 140–141, 217
growth, 141–142
growth hormone, 257, 259
Jornay PM, 222–223
levo-amphetamine, 131
non-stimulants, minimal effect on
appetite, 141, 146, 252, 254,
257, 259
management of appetite problems,
142–145
methylphenidate less likely to
cause, 134, 135, 141
Mydayis, 241–242
Obetrol, designed to reduce
appetite, 53
preventioin, 142–143
stopping medication, 146
Strattera, 262
supplements, 144–145
time-related, 140, 141, 220
vacations from medication,
143–144
side effects, cardiac, 175–176
sudden death, 175–176
blood pressure, 176
heart rate increased, 176
non-stimulants, 176
atomoxetine, 176
Strattera, 176, 262

side effects, emotional lability, 116,
157–167
management, 165–167, 170–171,
210
management with non-stimulant,
166
time-related, 126, 157–167,
170–171
idiosyncratic, 170–171
non-stimulants, 170–171, 252,
262
methylphenidate vs. amphetamine,
171
side effects, headaches, 116, 171–172
time-related, 171–172
side effects, mood suppression, 167–
170, 282
zombie effect, 116, 117, 167–170
dose related, 167–170
side effects, sleep difficulties, 72, 116,
146–157
antihistamines, 154–155
benefit to sleep, through stimulant
medication, 147–148
management of sleep difficulties,
146–157
management, non-stimulants,
156–157
management, clonidine, 156
management, guanfacine, 156
management, atomoxetine,
156–157
melatonin, 155–156
stimulant medication affects sleep,
147–149
stimulant medication, dose-related,
149, 153
stimulant medication, time-
related, 127, 148–150, 153
vacation from medication, 152–
153

side effects, stomachaches, 116,
171–173
time-related, 171–173
side effects, tics, 172–175
definition, 172–173
frequency, 173
stimulant medication, 173–174
non-stimulant medications,
174–175
clonidine, 174–175
Catapres, 174–175
Catapres TTS, 174–175
Kapvay, 174–175
Guanfacine, 174–175
Singh, Dr. G. N., 122
sleep difficulties, 72, 116, 146–157
antihistamines, 154–155
benefit to sleep, through stimulant
medication, 147–148
management of sleep difficulties,
146–157
management, non-stimulants,
156–157
management, clonidine, 156
management, guanfacine, 156
management, atomoxetine,
156–157
melatonin, 155–156
stimulant medication affects sleep,
147–149
stimulant medication, dose-related,
149, 153
stimulant medication, time-
related, 127, 148–150, 153
vacation from medication, 152
153
sleep study, 157
Smith, Klein & French, 50, 52, 227,
230
SODAS, 196, 215
speed (methamphetamine), 54, 235

spheroidal oral drug absorption systen
(SODAS), 196, 215
spontaneity vs. impulsivity, 163, 168–
170, 184
stereo-isomers, 125, 129–132, 214,
223–225, 228, 229, 235–237
stereo-isomers, dextro-amphetamine
vs. levo-amphetamine, 131, 228,
235–236
stereo-isomers, dextro-
methylphenidate vs. levo-
methylphenidate, 130, 224, 228
side effects, stomachaches, 116, 171–
173, 262
time-related, 171–173
stories (Danny, child)
aggression, 24
frustration, early, 22
frustration, deepening, 25
frustration, 31
guilt, blames his brain, 26
guilt, blames himself, 33
optimistic on first day of school,
17
variability, 30
stories (Liz, mother)
aggression, 24
diagnosis of ADHD by
pediatrician, 12–13
frustration and guilt, 35–36
generic medications, 115–116
guilt, 25
guilt about medication, 1–2
inattention, 31–32
irritability, 157 159
medication response, 43–46
medication response, 81–83
multiple medications available to
treat ADHD, 103–105
optimistic on first day of school, 17
parent perceptions, 38

task, staying on, 22
variability, 30
variability, 33
what to say to your child before
    starting medication, 135–137
Strattera, 93, 106–108, 134, 146,
    156–157, 176, 192, 251–252,
    261–262, 263, 281, 282
stroke symptoms compared to ADHD
    symptoms, 64–65
substance abuse, 95, 101, 224, 244,
    246
    diversion, 54, 243–247
    reduced by taking stimulant
        medication, 54
sudden-death, 175–176
sugar reduced in diet, 71, 99, 145
synapse, 73–76, 78–79, 86

Takeda, 243
talks frequently, 9
Tampa Day School, vi, 70
temper-tantrums, 178
Tenex, 93, 106–108, 134, 174, 192,
    251, 259, 260, 281
Thalidomide, 53
therapeutic range, 162–165
tics, 156, 172–175, 253
    Catapres, 174–175
    Catapres TTS, 174–175
    clonidine, 174–175
    compulsions, 173
    definition, 172–173
    Guanfacine, 174–175
    frequency, 173
    Kapvay, 174–175
    stimulant medication, 173–174
Timberlake, Justin, 138
Tourette's syndrome, 173, 255

transporter protein, 74–79
Tris Pharma, 240
tutoring, 4, 9, 71

UCB Pharmaceuticals, 202
UNICEF, 122
University in Queensland, Australia,
    62
University of South Florida, 4, 309

Valium, 190
Van Gogh, Vincent, 138
variability, 30, 65, 126, 205, 209, 210,
    258
viloxazine, 91, 106–108, 251–252,
    263–264, 282
Vivalan, 263
vomiting, 172, 262
Vyvanse, 47, 53, 77, 93, 106–108, 114,
    118, 127, 128, 131, 141, 148,
    149, 153, 191, 209, 230, 234,
    242, 243–247, 265, 278
Vyvanse chewable, 106–108, 228, 243,
    278, 280

Watson, Emma, 138
Wellbutrin, 93, 106–108, 251, 252,
    264–266, 282
Wellbutrin SR, 106–108, 251–252,
    264, 282
Wellbutrin XL, 106–108, 251, 264,
    282

Xanax, 190

Zenzedi, 106–108, 131, 229–231,
    232, 235, 239, 240, 245, 276
Zoloft, 190
Zyban, 265

ABOUT THE AUTHOR

Walt Karniski is a developmental pediatrician. He trained at Boston Children's Hospital, affiliated with Harvard Medical Center. He was director of the Division of Developmental Pediatrics at the University of South Florida in Tampa, Florida, for fifteen years. He then opened a private practice and for twenty years, evaluated and treated children with ADHD, autism, anxiety, learning disabilities, and other developmental difficulties. During that time, he developed and operated three private schools for children with ADHD, anxiety, and learning disabilities. Over the forty years he has been practicing, he has evaluated and treated close to ten thousand children. He has been director of a child abuse program and a program for enhancing development in children born prematurely. He has also conducted numerous studies of brain activity in children. He has approached each child as a unique individual, with distinctive strengths and weaknesses, where the diagnosis does not matter as much as understanding the specific needs of that child.

CPSIA information can be obtained
at www.ICGtesting.com
Printed in the USA
BVHW040852020522
634488BV00014B/2